In Vitro Toxicity Testing

In Vitro Toxicity Testing

Applications to Safety Evaluation

edited by
John M. Frazier
The Johns Hopkins University
School of Hygiene and
Public Health
Baltimore, Maryland

Marcel Dekker, Inc.   New York • Basel • Hong Kong

ISBN: 0-8247-8614-9

This book is printed on acid-free paper.

MARCEL DEKKER, INC.
270 Madison Avenue, New York, New York 10016

Current printing (last digit):
10 9 8 7 6 5 4 3 2 1

PRINTED IN THE UNITED STATES OF AMERICA

Preface

The use of in vitro model systems as a component of the chemical safety hazard evaluation process is not a new phenomenon. In vitro studies of drug metabolism and mechanisms of toxic action have historically supported toxicological considerations and in many cases clarified questions that arose in whole-animal testing. What is new is the emphasis on in vitro testing systems as a major component of the initial phases of the evaluation process even before any in vivo testing is conducted. The concepts of both intrinsic cellular toxicity, which defines (it is hoped at a mechanistic level) the adverse cellular response to chemicals and formulations, and tier testing, where in vitro testing systems can screen for potent toxicants, provide the basis for new strategies for toxicological evaluations.

The purpose of this book is to review the status of in vitro toxicity testing methods in the context of chemical safety evaluation. Other books have focused specifically on testing protocols (1) or the use of in vitro models in mechanistic studies (2). This is not the objective of this book. The focus here is to place in vitro toxicity testing in perspective with respect to how the results of such testing can be used to make toxicological decisions. Authors of the chapters on target-organ toxicity were asked three questions:

1. What are the potential in vivo toxicological responses that must be evaluated?

2. What are the current in vitro testing systems available to make such evaluations?
3. What are the limitations of the available technology and, thus, what are the research/developmental needs to attain the ultimate goal of predicting in vivo toxicity?

In addition to the discussion of target organ toxicity, several chapters evaluate generic issues, such as validation, testing strategies, and regulatory acceptance. These issues are not confined to questions of target organ toxicity, but address more universal concerns relating to the ultimate utilization of available methods in chemical safety/hazard considerations.

The field of in vitro toxicity testing is a rapidly evolving scientific endeavor. Initially, the scientific approaches to toxicity testing were focused mainly on applying existing technologies from other fields of biomedical research to the problem at hand. In more recent years we have seen a shifting of emphasis to second-generation methods that are designed to address the in vitro toxicity testing problem from a more mechanistic approach. In coming years the new approaches will move through the cycle of research, development, validation, and ultimately acceptance by both the scientific and regulatory communities. In the past (for example, with the Ames Assay) this cycle has taken 10-15 years to come full term. It is hoped that with a better understanding of what this cycle involves and the establishment of formal mechanisms to attain these goals, the cycle can be shortened and thus the fruits of technological progress can be utilized to their fullest in our quest to protect the health and safety of the general public, workers, and our natural biological resources.

John M. Frazier

REFERENCES

1. Williams, G. M., Dunkel, V. C., Ray, V. A. (1983). *Cellular Systems for Toxicity Testing*, In: *Annals of the New York Academy of Sciences*, Vol. 407, The New York Academy of Sciences, New York.
2. Rauckman, E. J., Padilla, G. M. (1987). *The Isolated Hepatocyte: Use in Toxicology and Xenobiotic Biotransformations*, Academic Press, Inc., New York.

Contents

Contributors

Daniel Acosta The University of Texas at Austin, Austin, Texas

June A. Bradlaw Center for Food and Applied Nutrition, Food and Drug Administration, Washington, D.C.

Leon H. Bruner Miami Valley Laboratories, Human and Environmental Safety Division, The Proctor & Gamble Company, Cincinnati, Ohio

David J. Brusick Hazleton Washington, Inc., Vienna, Virginia

Vincent A. DeLeo College of Physicians and Surgeons, Columbia University, New York, New York

John M. Frazier Center for Alternatives to Animal Testing, The Johns Hopkins University School of Hygiene and Public Health, Baltimore, Maryland

Shayne Cox Gad Becton Dickson and Company, Research Triangle Park, North Carolina

Sidney Green Center for Food Safety and Applied Nutrition, Food and Drug Administration, Washington, D.C.

André Guillouzo Hôpital de Pontchaillou, Unité de Recherche Hepatologique U49, Institut National de la Santé et de la Recherche Médicale, Rennes, France

Barbara F. Hales McGill University, Montreal, Quebec, Canada

Alan L. Harvey Department of Physiology and Pharmacology, University of Strathclyde, Glasgow, Scotland

Kenneth Ramos Texas A&M University, College Station, Texas

Glenn F. Rush Eli Lilly and Company, Greenfield, Indiana

Neill H. Stacey Occupational Health Division, National Institute of Occupational Health and Safety, and the University of Sydney, Sydney, Australia

Charles A. Tyson SRI International, Menlo Park, California

Patricia D. Williams Investigative Toxicology, Medical Research Division, American Cyanamid Company, Pearl River, New York

1

General Perspectives on In Vitro Toxicity Testing

John M. Frazier

The Johns Hopkins University School of Hygiene and Public Health
Baltimore, Maryland

INTRODUCTION

The objective of toxicity testing is to develop an adequate database to make reasonable and reliable judgments concerning the safe use of chemicals for societal needs. Historically, this objective has been attained by relying mainly on in vivo experimental animal models to provide the data which is subsequently utilized to make decisions concerning the impact of chemicals, products, and formulations on human health and welfare. In vitro models have played an important role in this process, particularly in mechanistic investigations; however, in the overall perspective in vivo studies far outweigh in vitro contributions. The current approach to safety evaluations has evolved over the last 60 years; when it began in the 1920s and 1930s, in vivo models were the only practical approach to the problem. Considering such an approach, which has worked extremely well in the context of public health and safety, the question arises as to why many feel it is necessary to undertake changes.

There are four factors which contribute to the argument for change. The first is logistical. Thousands of new chemicals and commercial products are introduced into the human environment each year. In addition, tens of thousands of existing chemicals have never been adequately evaluated for their toxicological properties. It is singularly impossible to develop a complete toxicological database on all of these chemicals using the classic whole animal toxicity testing procedures. New toxicological approaches must be established to provide minimum acceptable databases for these materials. Second, existing toxicity testing methodology using whole animals is expensive both in terms of dollars and time. New testing methods, which are faster and cheaper, can significantly reduce the economic burden to industry of bringing a new product to market. Third, society demands that new commercial products not present an undue risk to the consumer, yet significant concern about the use of animals in toxicological considerations has been voiced. Some segments of society feel it is inappropriate to use sentient organisms in toxicological testing, while others are concerned about the humane treatment of test animals which is felt to be in conflict with testing guidelines. The development of alternative testing methods which encompass the three Rs (refinement, reduction, and replacement) and their incorporation into accepted testing practices are viewed as improvements over the current testing situation. Finally, but certainly not least, there is a scientific imperative for changing the current testing situation. Dramatic advances in biotechnology both in the area of cell, tissue, and organ culture as well as in bioanalytical techniques provide new tools for toxicity testing and research. The application of these technological advances to toxicity testing must be implemented to provide the strongest scientific basis for the toxicological evaluation process. Taken together these four factors make a strong argument for the continued evolution of toxicity testing to include alternative toxicity testing methods as an integral component of the chemical safety evaluation process.

OBJECTIVES OF TOXICITY TESTING

The purpose of toxicity testing is to provide an adequate database to make decisions concerning the toxicological properties of chemicals and commercial products. In some situations, the purpose is to decide whether a material will be safe under the conditions of expected use. This process is referred to as safety evaluation and would apply, for example, to the development of new drugs. In these cases, the expected exposure is defined by the proposed uses of the product. In other situations, the objective is to establish the safe limits of exposure to a new material to define the appropriate conditions of use. This process is called hazard evaluation and would contribute to the introduction of new industrial chemicals or household products. Both of these processes—safety and hazard evaluations—utilize similar experimental tools to accomplish their goals.

Decisions which require toxicological information are diverse in nature and range from selecting which newly discovered chemical entities should be further developed for commercial purposes to establishing a legally binding safe level of exposure for a food additive. Toxicological information which is used in the decision-making process can be derived from various sources: (1) historical databases, (2) structure-activity relationships, (3) in vivo toxicological testing data from whole animal testing, (4) in vivo toxicological testing data from clinical trials, human volunteer studies, and/or epidemiological studies, and (5) in vitro toxicological testing data. Historical databases provide toxicological data about related chemicals and formulations. Often a new product may be a variation in the formulation of a previously existing product. Therefore, the available toxicological database on the existing product may be useful in toxicological decisions concerning the new product. When totally new materials are developed there may be no historical database on chemicals of similar structure. By decomposing the new chemical structurally into toxicologically relevant fragments and applying existing structure-activity relationships, it is possible to obtain a theoretical prediction of the potential toxicological reactivities of the new product (1). A third source of information is obtained from in vivo animal toxicity testing. This source of information has evolved to be the main basis for most toxicological decisions. The various types of in vivo animal testing are listed in Table 1. Human in vivo toxicological data are obtained in chemical trials of drugs, in human volunteer studies (particularly skin testing for irritation and hypersensitivity reactions), and from epidemiological studies once the product is out on the market (this would include accidental exposures, consumer complaints, and suicide attempts). Finally, toxicological data are obtained from in vitro toxicity testing and mechanistic studies. All of these sources of information contribute to our ability to make rational toxicological decisions.

This wealth of toxicological information sources must be viewed with caution. Much of the toxicological information is obtained from model systems;

Table 1 The main categories of in vivo animal toxicity testing

Acute toxicity testing[a]
Subchronic toxicity testing[a]
Chronic toxicity testing[a]
Reproductive toxicity testing
Teratogenicity testing
Ocular irritation testing
Dermal irritation testing
Hypersensitivity testing
Phototoxicity testing
Toxicokinetic studies[a]
Behavioral testing[a]

[a]Routes of exposure (oral, dermal, inhalation, i.v.) may vary depending on expected use of the product and its physical/chemical properties

i.e., biological systems other than the organism of primary concern, human beings. Many products, such as industrial chemicals or household commercial products, cannot be tested in humans on ethical grounds. Therefore, until the product is actually in use little in vivo human toxicological data are available. Even when there is extensive in vivo animal data as well as human data from clinical trials, it is not possible to *prove* that a product is completely safe under expected conditions of use. The best that the toxicologist can do is to conclude that the weight of evidence infers that the probability of adverse responses in the exposed population will be acceptably small. It should be recognized that the term "acceptable" will depend on the benefits accrued by the population at risk. Thus, the acceptable probability of adverse responses will be much higher for an antineoplastic drug than for a food additive.

The focus of this book is on the contribution that in vitro toxicity testing can make in the toxicological decision-making process (2). For this reason, it is important to classify in vitro toxicity tests into various categories depending on the types of roles they play in a testing strategy and the level of toxicological information they provide. With respect to the type of testing, in vitro toxicity tests can be classified into three categories: (1) screening tests, (2) adjunct tests, and (3) replacement tests. Screening tests provide preliminary data for decision-making purposes, and, as the name implies, more definitive testing, whether in vivo or in vitro, will follow. Adjunct tests provide useful data for ultimate decision-making purposes, whether by corporations or regulatory agencies, but in and of themselves are not sufficient. Thus, adjunct toxicity tests provide information which is directly taken into consideration in marketing or regulatory decisions. Finally, replacement tests are those which provide sufficient information to make decisions which had previously been made on the basis of another existing test. These three categories are based on the role the test plays in decision-making processes.

A second scheme to categorize tests is based on the level of toxicological information provided: (1) toxicity potential (hazard identification), (2) toxicity potency, and (3) hazard. Tests which evaluate toxicity potential are designed to give a qualitative evaluation (often a yes/no response) of whether a particular toxicological response is possible and should be investigated further. The next higher level of tests are those which can directly measure relative potency of test materials and thus rank materials as to their relative toxicity. Since the scale for evaluating responses is dependent on the test system employed, the data provided indicate relative toxicities and are not intended to be interpreted as absolute measures of toxicity. Finally, tests which predict hazard, i.e., the probability of a given toxicological response in an organism as a function of exposure, provide the highest level of toxicological information and the data provided by such methods can be incorporated into the risk assessment process.

The importance in classifying in vitro toxicity tests using this two component scheme is that the criteria for validation and acceptance of new methods will vary from one category to another. Thus, proper classification of a test will maximize the chances that the test will be implemented in the safety/hazard evaluation process.

IN VITRO TOXICITY TESTING

The various roles that in vitro toxicity testing can play in toxicological evaluations relate to the fundamental concept that toxicological effects are a consequence of the interaction of the toxicant and/or a reactive metabolite with a molecular target on or within a sensitive cell type. Thus, the response of cellular systems in culture to test chemicals can be related to the central events in the toxicological process (Fig. 1). For this reason, in vitro toxicity testing systems can be effectively utilized in various aspects of safety/hazard evaluations, including but not limited to: (1) ranking chemicals for their potency, (2) identifying mechanisms of toxic action, and (3) identifying potential target organ toxicity.

The ranking of chemicals for their toxicity to cells in vitro provides useful toxicological information. It is clear from the toxicological process described in Figure 1 that many factors in addition to the specific cellular response to chemicals determine the overall dose-response relationships in vivo. However, the central component of the process is the interaction of the toxicant and/or its metabolites with molecular targets located on or within the cell. Thus, an evaluation of the relative potency of a new chemical in cellular systems, in comparison with known benchmark chemicals, will provide an indication of the potential hazard of a new chemical at a fundamental level. There are limitations to the interpretation of this data in the context of in vivo toxicological responses. These limitations are mainly due to the complex modulation of the in vitro response by kinetic, interactive and repair processes in vivo. However, a new chemical which elicits severe toxic responses in cells at extremely low concentrations (submicromolar concentrations) will in all likelihood have limited commercial applications due to in vivo toxicity.

The concept of potency based on a single in vitro measurement can be expanded to include a spectrum of endpoint measurements which together can be used in a diagnostic sense to elucidate the mechanisms of action of a toxicant. Mechanistic studies using in vitro systems are not new and have been a component of the safety/hazard evaluation process for many years. However, in the past these studies were usually conducted late in the development process, often to resolve mechanistic questions which arose in animal studies. The concept proposed here is to utilize multiple endpoint measurements in a decision tree design to rapidly evaluate the intrinsic cellular toxicity of a chemical as an initial step in the toxicological evaluation process. Having

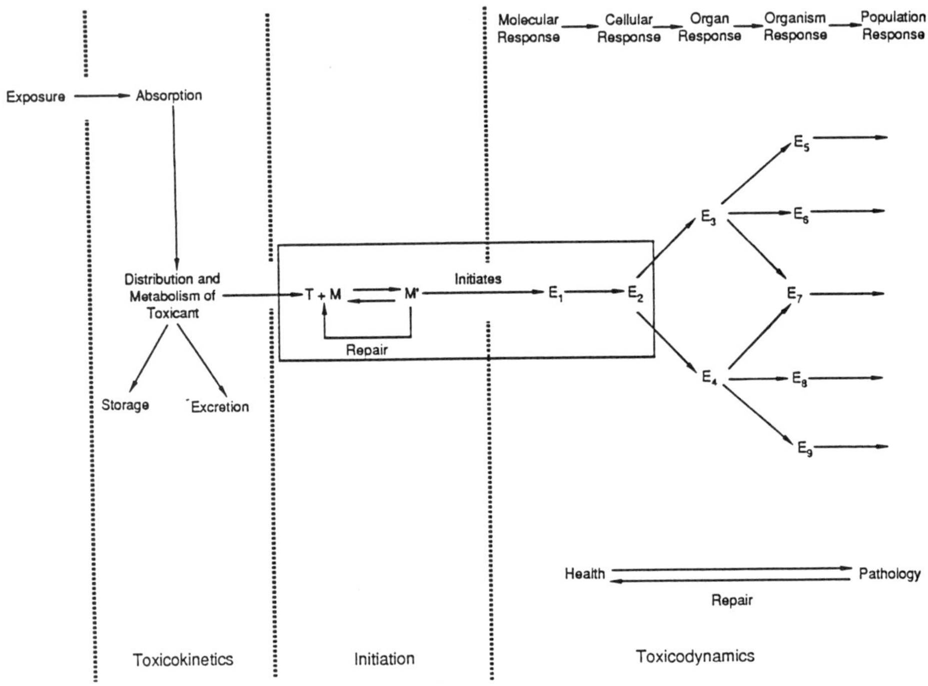

Figure 1 Diagram of the toxicological process. Expression of toxicity in any biological system is the culmination of many interacting processes including toxicokinetics, initiation, and toxicodynamics. Toxicokinetic processes control the delivery of the active form of the toxicant, T, to the site of interaction with molecular targets, M. The molecular interaction between the active form of the toxicant and the molecular target results in alterations in cellular macromolecules, M′, which initiates the cascade of biological events referred to as toxicodynamics. These events begin at the molecular and cellular level and ultimately propagate to higher levels of biological organization. In vitro toxicity testing systems can evaluate the toxicological events at the molecular and cellular levels (indicated by the central box in the figure) which are at the core of the toxicological process. (Reprinted from Frazier, J. M. (1990) by permission of Mary Ann Liebert, Inc. Publishers.)

this information up front will allow for better design of animal studies which may follow or, better yet, the information developed may be adequate to undertake the toxicological decision making at hand without resorting to in vivo studies.

A third use for in vitro toxicity testing systems is in the area of target organ toxicity identification. By using a spectrum of cell types representative of various potential target organs (hepatocytes, proximal tubular cells, neurons, cardiac myocytes, etc.) it would be possible to determine if any particular cell type is significantly more sensitive to an unknown toxicant. If metabolic activation is a question of concern, the representative cell types could be cultured in the presence and absence of a metabolizing system, either a cell-free extract (S9) or cocultured with isolated hepatocytes. Identification of sensitive cell types could improve in vivo toxicity testing by suggesting specific clinical measurements which should be included in the in vivo experimental design to improve chances of detecting adverse effects.

These three examples—potency testing, mechanisms identification, and target organ identification—are indicative of the role in vitro toxicity testing systems can play in the safety/hazard evaluation process. Some of the advantages of using in vitro toxicity testing systems are outlined in Table 2. Two points of particular interest are the rapidity of in vitro tests and the feasibility of using human cells. The first point, rapid turnaround of test results, reduces the time required for developing toxicological information on a potentially new product. This ultimately translates into a shortening of the time between new product discovery and introduction of product on the market. It also allows for a more rapid identification of nonviable products, thus reducing the investment of resources into products which will never make it to market. The other point to note from Table 2 is that the in vitro approach allows for the use of human cells and tissues which open numerous

Table 2 Advantages of In Vitro Toxicity Testing Systems

Allow for control of environmental conditions
Eliminate interactive systemic effects
Utilize large number of test organisms (cells) per dose level
Reduce variability between experiments
Allow for simultaneous and/or repeated sampling over time
Make feasible complex interactive toxicity experiments
Are often quicker and cheaper
Require smaller quantities of test chemicals
Produce smaller quantities of toxic waste
Utilize human cells
Reduce intact animal usage

possibilities for toxicological studies in the target organism of concern—human beings—which are prohibited in vivo owing to ethical considerations. Use of human cells eliminates one of the more difficult extrapolation processes—interspecies extrapolation. Thus, in vitro studies can be conducted using human hepatocytes, proximal tubular cells, etc., which are directly applicable to human toxicological considerations.

Utilization of in vitro toxicity testing systems is not without significant limitations at the present time. The major barrier which must be faced is the in vitro - in vivo extrapolation problem. The issues involved are illustrated in the diagram of the toxicological process in Figure 1. In vitro toxicity testing systems are focused on the initiation process and the subsequent molecular and cellular responses. The problem of how to relate in vitro concentrations which produce cellular toxicity to equivalent in vivo dosages is outstanding at this point in time. This issue must be resolved by the development of better tools for predictive toxicokinetics. A key component in the solution to this problem is the development of physiologically based toxicokinetic modeling (3). On the other side of the toxicological process are the factors which modulate the toxicological response, in particular cellular and tissue repair processes, and the interactive influence between different cell types (e.g., immunological responses). If our knowledge of basic mechanisms of toxicological processes was more fully developed, it might be possible to identify biological markers for these interactions (e.g., release of cytokines) which would signal activation of these interactive process. Unfortunately, at this stage in the development of toxicology as a science there are many critical areas of knowledge which are lacking. Another important limitation to the in vitro approach relates to prediction of chronic toxicities. Again, the mechanistic basis of many of these pathological processes is poorly understood and thus in vitro approaches cannot be developed on a rational basis. In the light of these uncertainties in mechanistic toxicology, many current in vitro approaches are of a more empirical nature than would be desired.

ROLE OF IN VITRO TOXICITY TESTING IN SAFETY/HAZARD EVALUATION

In the short run, in vitro toxicity testing will play an increasing role in screening testing and as adjuncts employed in both tier testing strategies and mechanistic studies. In these roles in vitro toxicity testing is already making significant contributions. For example, in the cosmetic industry, where many new products are variations in formulations of previously marketed products, a tier testing strategy has evolved which begins with an evaluation of the historical database. If there are no apparent toxicological concerns, the new product is tested by a small battery of in vitro toxicity tests. If the results of these studies are consistent with results for previously documented formulations which are known to be safe, the product is tested by human volunteers. If all goes well at each stage of the evaluation the product can be taken to market. This tier testing strategy eliminates redundant animal testing of similar products yet provides a rational basis for decision making.

Obviously, this particular tier testing strategy is limited in its application to the special case where the new formulation is a variation on existing products. In industries where exotic chemical entities are synthesized on a regular basis, such as pharmaceutical and agrochemical industries, this approach will not work today. The ability of in vitro toxicity testing systems to replace totally in vivo animal studies in testing strategies is still limited to special cases. However, as discussed above, the use of in vitro toxicity testing systems early in the toxicological evaluation process will allow for better and more efficient designs of animal studies.

As mentioned previously, the major limitation to the replacement of in vivo animal testing with in vitro toxicity testing approaches is the issue of in vitro-in vivo extrapolation. The critical question is how to utilize the in vitro toxicity testing database to make intelligent predictions of in vivo toxicity. This problem has not been thoroughly explored and the extrapolation techniques must be developed; a successful resolution of this problem will require a significant research effort. In vitro toxicity testing provides a concentration-response relationship for some relevant marker of toxicity in some particular cell types. The goal is to predict what the dose-response relationships will be in vivo. Assuming human cells are employed in the testing system so that species extrapolations are not a concern, then two components must be incorporated into the in vitro-in vivo extrapolation: the toxicokinetic component, which would predict the exposure dose of the chemical that results in extracellular concentrations at the target tissue equivalent to the concentrations in vitro, and the toxicodynamic component, which would modulate the in vitro cellular response by various factors, such as tissue repair processes or induction of inflammatory reactions. Experimental and theoretical techniques to predict the appropriate correction factors must be investigated and incorporated into an in vitro-in vivo extrapolation algorithm.

Finally, when both testing and extrapolation techniques have been established, it may be possible to conduct a significant portion of the safety/hazard evaluations on the basis of these newer technologies. A possible scheme for toxicological evaluations in the future would include in vitro toxicity testing, structure-activity methodologies (which would draw heavily on historical databases), physiologically based toxicokinetic modeling and in vitro

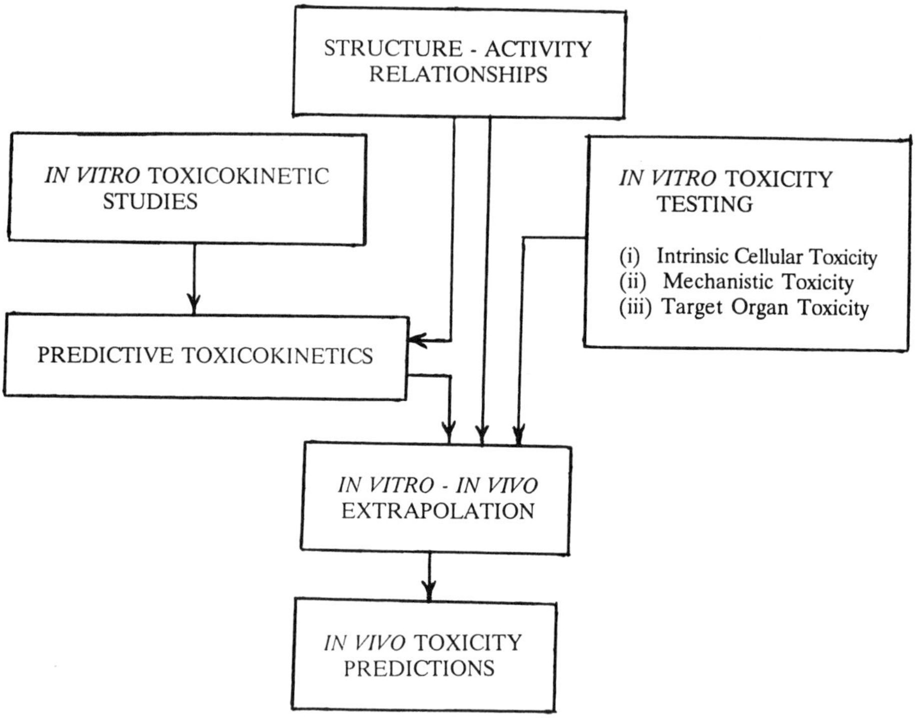

Figure 2 A proposed scheme for toxicological evaluations based on in vitro and computer technologies.

toxicokinetic studies, and finally the in vitro-in vivo extrapolation process to integrate the data provided by the various techniques to make predictions of in vivo toxicity (Fig. 2). Focused research will be needed to implement fully this global approach; however, in the meantime piecewise implementation of various components of the process will continue to improve the safety/hazard evaluation process.

REFERENCES

1. Rosenkranz, H. S. (1991). An expert system approach to the prediction and elucidation of the structural basis of toxicological activities. In *Alternative Methods in Toxicology—In Vitro Toxicology: Mechanisms and New Technologies*. vol. 8. A. M. Goldberg (Ed.). Mary Ann Liebert, New York. In press.
2. Goldberg, A. M., and Frazier, J. M. (1989). Alternatives to animals in toxicity testing. *Sci. Amer.* **261**: 24-30.

3. Anderson, M. E. (1991). The role of physiollogical modelling in reducing animal use in toxicology research. In *Alternative Methods in Toxicology—In Vitro Toxicology: Mechanisms and New Technologies*. Vol. 8. A.M. Goldberg (Ed.). Mary Ann Liebert, New York. In press.
4. Frazier, J. M. 1990. Multiple endpoint measurements to evaluate the intrinsic cellular toxicity of chemicals. *In Vitro Toxicol.* **3**: 349-357.

2

In Vitro Technology, Trends, and Issues

Charles A. Tyson

SRI International
Menlo Park, California

Neill H. Stacey

National Institute of Occupational Health and Safety, and
University of Sydney
Sydney, Australia

INTRODUCTION

The partial or total substitution of in vitro methods for whole animal assays is already established in fact and therefore in principle. Some examples illustrating this point are given in Table 1. Many other examples come to mind that are more difficult to document in terms of specific numbers of animals conserved. Short-term assays for genotoxicity fit into that category. They continue to be used widely even though their shortcomings individually or in combination have been cited (1,2), and they must certainly be considered "substitutes" at the preliminary testing stage. Some companies have gone so far as to discontinue whole animal testing altogether, replacing it with in vitro or other alternative approaches (3).

Many new developments have occurred in the testing field over the last 5 years, during which time there has been a dramatic surge in interest in alternative approaches to whole animal testing. The result is a large increase in number, quality, and sophistication of in vitro systems and in the instrumentation and bioanalytical techniques used in toxicological investigations and screening. Although progress has been made on a broad front, developments in three areas that have spurred considerable activity are (1) new substrata and techniques for growth or differentiation, (2) more powerful and versatile analytical techniques for mechanistic investigations, and (3) semi-

Table 1 Examples of Animal Replacement and Reduction by In Vitro Methods

In vitro assay	Whole animal test replaced	Reduction in animal usage	Reference
Pregnancy test	Rabbits	Total	4
Limulus amebocyte lysate (LAL) test for bacterial endotoxins	Pyrogen test in rabbits	Total	4
Insulin	Quantal mouse convulsion method	630 to 1[a]	5
Vitamins and hormones	Chicks and rats	Total	4
Neurotoxic esterase assay for delayed neurotoxicity	Hens	Substantial	6
Isolated perfused rabbit eye for corrosive agents	Rabbit	Substantial	7
Human tumor cell line screens for anti-cancer activity	Mice	Total	8

[a]Prospects for total elimination of animal usage possible with improved high pressure liquid chromatography (HPLC) columns.

automated and automated procedures to improve assay reproducibility and the economics of in vitro testing.

This chapter begins with a brief general overview of in vitro systems and techniques available for in vitro toxicology. Recent advances illustrating progress in culture methodology, analytical techniques, instrumentation, and automation equipment will be discussed next. Finally, areas are identified in which further technical and conceptual advances are needed for the full exploitation of these approaches to toxicity testing.

SYSTEMS AVAILABLE

Structure-Activity Relationships

The development and application of structure-activity relationships (SARs) to the understanding and prediction of the toxic potentials for chemicals have become more important and more often used in recent years (9). Among many examples are the prediction of carcinogenic potential of aromatic amines and the delayed neurotoxicity of organophosphate compounds (6,10,

11). When the relationship is determined principally by either the physicochemical or electronic properties of the chemicals, mathematical expressions can be formulated that allow reasonable predictions of toxic potential without testing in biological systems. Examples are the dependence of toxic potency on octanol/water partition coefficients (12) and estimation of the inherent hepatotoxic potential of dinitrotoluenes using the lowest unoccupied molecular orbital (LUMO) theory (13).

The applications are by no means always straightforward. For example, relatively minor changes in the chemical structure of receptor agonists and antagonists can result in very different pharmacological or toxicological effects. An interesting example illustrating the intricacies of SARs is the peripheral neuropathy that results from exposure to *n*-hexane (14). From SAR considerations alone it might be predicted, albeit simplistically, that pentane or heptane would produce a similar toxicity, perhaps differing only in magnitude, the dose required, or time for emergence of the lesion. This turns out not to be so; neither chemical has been associated with peripheral neuropathy. More concerted investigations have shown that biotransformation of *n*-hexane produces a metabolite with a γ-diketone moeity that is a critical requirement for neuropathy to develop. Thus, purely structural considerations of the parent chemicals alone would be misleading for estimating toxic potential.

Uncovering this kind of mechanistic information requires an initial commitment to basic research and the use of a considerable number of animals. That may seem contrary to the aim of reducing animal experimentation, but by enhancing our understanding of chemical-mediated toxicity in this way, we can develop techniques for improved risk assessment, and the use of fewer animals over the long run can be the result. With *n*-hexane as an example, it should now be possible to screen all aliphatics with the potential to form γ-diketone metabolites by SARs or in established in vitro metabolic systems such as microsomes or freshly isolated hepatocytes without the need for conducting whole animal studies. Furthermore, these in vitro tissues are available from humans, which in fact somewhat reduces the uncertainty associated with animal-to-human extrapolation.

Molecular and Receptor Interactions

Interactions at the molecular and receptor levels will be considered together here because there is often an overlap between them. In vitro binding studies on chemicals having or suspected of having carcinogenic potential have yielded valuable information on structures likely to interact directly with the genetic material deoxyribonucleic acid (DNA) (14). This approach has not been routinely used because of ambiguities in interpreting results. However, when the results are clearly negative (no significant binding is found above the level of detection for the methods used), they can be interpreted in conjunction with other data to mitigate concerns that such chemicals might be genotoxic.

Use of receptors in drug development is now well established, and there is every reason to anticipate similar applications in toxicological screening. Interaction of organophosphates with neurotoxic esterase, which is the key to the delayed neurotoxicity of some of these compounds, has been described in cultured cells (15), but the effects of organophosphate on cholinesterase are also important and provide an example of how receptor interactions could well be used for screening (16).

Such molecular and receptor interactions will be areas of greater development in future in vitro toxicology. For example, it is possible that screening techniques now using animals to detect the purity of commercial therapeutic preparations could well employ suitable in vitro assays using receptors if analytical techniques are unavailable.

Subcellular Preparations

Currently, subcellular fractions are not often used for toxicological investigations primarily designed for risk assessment except as metabolic activation systems in genotoxicity assays. Their main use apart from this is for studies at the molecular level, such as investigations of toxic metabolite formation in microsomal fractions in vitro and covalent binding to macromolecules for a better understanding of the toxic sites of chemical action. Probably as many subcellular systems as there are organelles can be used for such investigations, including mitochondria (17), lysosomal and membrane preparations, endoplasmic reticulum fragments, and nuclear capsules among others. Because they are separated from their native environment in the intact cell, they often provide only qualitative information on the potential for a specific effect. The absence of the cellular milieu can significantly distort interpretations quantitatively and sometimes qualitatively as well. An excellent example comes from the studies of Mandel and colleagues (18), who found the dependence of Na^+/K^+-ATPase activity on cellular ATP content in intact renal proximal tubules to be very different from that in isolated membranes.

Microorganisms

Microorganisms have found limited but important applications in toxicology. The Ames test is unquestionably the best known and most extensively employed among mutagenesis assays to identify suspect carcinogens. A recent publication presented data to indicate that nonmutagenic carcinogens induce intrachromosomal recombination in yeast (19) that might ultimately increase the predictive value of microorganisms for this application. Other possible uses for microorganisms in toxicology include fungi to evaluate the phototoxic potential of chemicals (20) and ciliated protozoa or luminescent bacteria as an alternative indicator of ocular irritancy (21,22).

Cells

Isolated cells are by far the most extensively and intensively used in vitro systems for toxicological studies. These systems include freshly isolated cells in suspension, primary cell cultures, cell lines, cell strains, and cocultures. Grisham and Smith (23) have compared the strengths and weaknesses of various cell preparations. Primary cultures seem most often the system of choice, mainly because they retain their original capabilities and properties to a greater extent in isolation and therefore mimic in vivo responses most closely. Cocultures may be even better in this regard (24); however, their complexity requires more effort to optimize conditions that will accurately replicate in vivo responses.

The advantages and disadvantages of in vitro toxicological studies and screening have been reviewed in many reports, including those of Stammati et al. (25), Grisham and Smith (23), Rowan and Goldberg (26), Atterwill and Steele (27), Flint (28), Enger (29), and Atterwill and Walum (30), among others. Table 2 essentially represents a composite.

Many different cell types have been proposed and employed in toxicological tests to date. This can be best appreciated simply by scanning the contents of this monograph. In Table 3, we list some examples of the general cell types used. Many of these groups include cells derived from human sources. A list of specific cell types used for toxicological investigations has been provided by Stammati et al. (25) from the literature. Examples of applications are presented in Table 4.

As can be appreciated from the wide variety of cells used and the research to which they have been applied, a great deal of experimental work has been conducted with cells in vitro. It is surprising, therefore, that until recently, except for genotoxicity testing, little effort had gone into validating these systems. Accumulating data to identify the most promising systems for extensive validation, modifying them to correct or minimize the number of "false negatives" or "positives" they produce, and particularly obtaining the funding and resources to conduct these investigations expeditiously are formidable problems. But progress, although slow for both scientists and those interested in animal use reduction, is being made.

Table 2 Advantages and Disadvantages of In Vitro Systems in Toxicity Assessment with Emphasis on Cells

Advantages
Improved efficiency, reduced cost
Reduction in use of experimental animals
Smaller amounts of chemical required
Greater control over nature of cell population
Direct control over extracellular medium, chemical concentration, duration of exposure
Freedom from potential confounding factors such as hormones, nervous system, or immunity
Replicates available from same stock
Disadvantages
Loss of in vivo organ morphology
Selected loss of in vivo organ-specific functions
Loss of possible mitigating influences such as hormones, nervous system, or immunity
Generally a static system resulting in progressive loss of nutrients and accumulation of metabolic end products
Generally short-term and at present of limited, if any, value in estimating subchronic or chronic toxicity

Table 3 Examples of Cells In Vitro That Have Been Used in Toxicological Studies

Fibroblasts from various species
Lymphoblastoid
Ascites sarcoma
Lymphocytes
Keratinocytes
Liver cells, mainly hepatocytes
Hepatoma
Kidney, medullary and cortical cells
Lung, various types
Brain-derived cell types
Dorsal root ganglia cell cultures
Testicular cell cultures
Sertoli cells
Bladder cells
Heart cells
Cells from cerebral microvessels
Adipocytes

Table 4 Examples of Applications of Cells In Vitro in Toxicology

General cytotoxicity, mainly related to acute toxicity, including lethality, skin and eye damage
Organ-specific toxicity
Mechanisms of toxicity
Biotransformation to toxic metabolites
Genotoxicity, (e.g., unscheduled DNA synthesis)
Reproductive toxicity
Mixture toxicity
Comparative toxicity
Photosensitivity

Multicellular Tissue Pieces

Various preparations obtained initially from fresh tissues are available for toxicological investigations, including slices, cubes, aggregates, and explants. They generally share a common disadvantage of poor retention of viability; the pieces are often too thick to allow enough oxygen penetration, resulting in limited lifetime in isolation. Furthermore, the ability of added chemicals to penetrate the tissue fully may be compromised. Although tissue pieces were used extensively before the improvement of methods for cell isolation and culture, they have been employed less frequently in recent years. Nevertheless, because of their retention of three-dimensional structure, as pointed out by Kotin (31) and others, they do allow investigation of the interactions among adjacent cell types on exposure to toxic stimuli.

Improvements in the technology associated with the supply of such tissue pieces and their maintenance in vitro offer promise of their expanded use in the future. Tissue lifespans have been increased sixfold or more, compared with the previous lifetime for slices from these tissues. For example, liver slices, used rarely over the last 20 years in toxicological studies, may now be available with a suitable viability profile (32). This allows histological examination of a toxic response for direct comparison with in vivo response. Brendel, Gandolfi, and colleagues have successfully applied the technique to the isolation of kidney cortical slices and slices from other organs as well (33). Another recent development that may prove useful in thyroid toxicity is a miniorgan culture of thyroid tissue (34). With adherence to particular experimental conditions, viable tissue was maintained for several weeks. This system is apparently superior to cellular aggregates, which have also been suggested for toxicological studies (35). The latter, even though they are derived from normal tissue, may have limited scope because they rapidly develop fetal tissue properties in culture suspension.

Other tissue pieces to find use in toxicological investigations include esophageal, tracheal, and pancreatic ductal fragments for study of cell injury (36); ciliated trachea for cytotoxicity studies of compounds derived from cigarette smoke (37); epidermal slices for detection of skin corrosives (38); ventricular strips for cardiotoxicity (39); and fetal explants of mouse sensory and neuromuscular tissues for examination of neurotoxic chemicals (40). While this list is by no means all inclusive, the use of these tissue pieces has been limited, especially in comparison with that of cell cultures.

Isolated Organs

Isolated intact organs have historically had a place in toxicology studies. However, their limitations, such as a relatively short period of viability, and the advent of cell culture have restricted their use. Furthermore, not much advantage is gained in time and resources as with cell cultures, for example, and virtually none in terms of conserving animal usage. Some toxic effects, such as interference with bile formation, still require the intact organ for comprehensive examination, but even that may be measurable in cell culture in the near future with the use of hepatocyte doublets (41).

In general, isolated organ techniques will continue to have a relatively limited impact on in vitro toxicology, particularly for testing purposes.

OTHER TEST SYSTEMS

Some systems used for toxicological in vitro tests do not fit neatly into the above categories. The reason is probably related to the toxic effect under study; the procedures are essentially for detecting teratogenic effects, and target organ tissue specificity in that case is secondary to mimicking the developing organism. Such systems include chick embryo culture (42), postimplantation rat embryo culture (43) and the chorioallantoic membrane (44, 45). While there is some debate over whether these should truly be classified as in vitro systems, it seems well accepted that they do not constitute what is normally meant by in vivo in this context.

TESTING CONSIDERATIONS

Table 5 provides a qualitative comparison of the properties of the various in vitro systems available. Immediately obvious is the fact that none perfectly matches the properties of the intact system. The aim of in vitro methods development is to optimize the in vitro response to chemicals, versus the in vivo response, to the maximum extent possible, balanced against the time and resources that must be committed to the project (i.e., the cost-benefit ratio).

Table 5 Properties of In Vitro Systems

Preparation and consequences	Level of tissue organization	Reproducibility	Expression similar to in vivo	Genetic alteration by mutation and/or selection	Environmental control
Intact system (no consequence)	+ + + +	+ + + +	+ + + +	+	+
Organ culture (remove influences of whole organism)	+ + + +	+ + + +	+ to + + +	+	+ +
Tissue culture (remove influences of whole organ isms)	+ + +	+ + +	+ to + + +	+	+ + +
Primary cell cultures (disrupt intercellular relationships)	0	+ +	+ to + + +	+	+ + + +
Cell lines (intercellular relationships are reduced; cell proliferation is enhanced, at times with little control)	0	+ + + +	+ to + + +	+ to + + + +	+ + + +

Key: + + + + = high degree; + + + = Moderate degree; + + = Modest degree; + = some degree; 0 = None.

Source: Excerpted from Ref. 46. Adapted from R. M. Nardone and L. A. Ouellette, *Scope of "Alternatives:" Overview of the State of the Art,* contract report prepared for the Office of Technology Assessment, U.S. Congress, July 1984.

In optimizing in vitro response, there are several factors to be considered when dealing with such systems in general for toxicological studies and screening. Many of these factors assume much greater if not critical importance when the data are used for risk assessment. These aspects will be discussed in a later section on standardization and validation in the general sense, while this section will detail, with examples, those factors that must be considered when providing data that should be readily interpretable to a broad audience. Because cells are the most widely used in vitro system, most comments and examples will be related directly to them but presumably should be more or less applicable to other systems as well. The review by Stark et al. (47) on this topic and the report on technical problems associated with in vitro toxicity testing systems (48) should also be consulted.

System

The system must be carefully chosen and the rationale clearly stated. With cells, for example, the source should be clearly defined; if primary cultures are being used, the characteristics of the donor animal should be detailed to allow conformity and reproducibility across laboratories. In an interlaboratory comparison of a cell transformation assay, the source of cells was a major factor affecting comparability (49). Use of a cloned cell or cells from a single source would have clear advantages in this regard. If differentiated cells are used, assays are needed to document retention of functional capabilities under the culture conditions. Reference chemicals and one or two simple, reproducible, and appropriate assays to assess the functional status of the cells are routinely included in the protocols. The method of preparing and handling cells should be documented because, for example, some enzymes used in cell isolation procedures can affect such functions as uptake of certain substrates. This can also result from increasing time in culture as recently documented (50).

The cell density at which experimental procedures are conducted is also important. Increasing cell density with a constant aqueous concentration of added liposoluble chemical could result in decreased individual cell concentration, thereby affecting the toxic response either individually or relative to other cells in a test set.

Media

The choice of media also requires careful consideration and documentation. For example, Medium 199, a physiological-like medium in composition, has been reported to be much superior to a simple Tris buffered balanced salt solution for hepatocyte incubations (51). The optimal medium composition will differ depending on the cell type. These media are supplemented with various additives that can complicate the comparison and interpretation of results from different laboratories.

A recent example that stirred considerable controversy in the literature is the role of intracellular and extracellular calcium as a common mediator in chemical-induced cell death. Reports from different groups led essentially to opposite conclusions with seemingly no explanation for the differences. The critical factor was eventually ascribed to use by one group of an incubation medium containing vitamin E, whereas the media used in other studies had none (52). The importance of varying calcium concentrations in the media under the particular conditions of the study and in the presence of particular toxicants can also be appreciated.

The sulfhydryl-containing tripeptide, reduced glutathione (GSH), is generally accepted as playing a major role in protecting cells against various toxicants. Thus, media with different amounts of GSH or precursor amino acids may well lead to different toxicities on exposure to chemicals.

It is common practice to use incubation media with fetal calf serum (FCS) or some other source of protein such as bovine serum albumin (BSA). Problems may arise with changes in the FCS over time; many of the constituents remain undefined, and the source of serum can be a major factor influencing variability among studies (49). There are now several commercially available protein-free synthetic media that are apparently able to support cells to the same extent as FCS. FCS or BSA in the medium can influence chemical-mediated cytotoxicity significantly (47,53). Chemicals that form complexes with proteins can have their free concentrations reduced by orders of magnitude in the presence of protein, and the protein/chemical ratio in the medium has a significant impact on the quantitative toxic potential.

Gaseous Atmosphere

The gaseous atmosphere of the incubation vessel is another important variable. Maier (54) recently reminded us of the varying oxygen tensions down the liver lobule and the need to give this factor appropriate consideration when performing in vitro hepatocellular experiments. Use of inappropriately high oxygen concentrations has led to results in vitro that seemed different from the known in vivo response. For example, some early attempts to demonstrate lipid peroxidation induced by carbon tetrachloride in hepatocytes in vitro were unsuccessful, at variance with the known in vivo response to the chemical. It was subsequently determined that this anomalous result was related to the use of an atmosphere containing 95% oxygen; at 20% or lower O_2 concentrations, lipid peroxidation was readily demonstrable (55).

Test Chemical

Factors related to the chemical being tested must also be considered. The choice of concentrations, the timing of exposure and sampling, chemical solubility and stability, and changes in osmolarity and pH all are important determinants of the toxic response. Chemicals that are volatile at 37 °C will have lower than nominal dissolved concentration as the chemical redistributes between airspace and the incubation medium. If the flasks or culture dishes are unsealed, some material will inevitably escape over time, further reducing the concentration.

Interactions among chemicals may also affect the toxic response, sometimes in unexpected ways. For example, piperonyl butoxide, a commonly used inhibitor of cytochrome P-450, potentiated $CHCl_3$ in its toxicity to rat renal proximal tubules in vitro (56); a similar observation was made earlier on rodents treated with both under appropriate conditions (57). Other possibilities include interactions with antimicrobial agents or interference by test chemicals with the determination of toxic parameters (e.g., inhibition of alanine aminotransferase by cadmium).

Cocultures

Cocultures are increasingly being examined for their potential as test systems when more than one cell type is needed to produce a particular effect. Coculturing differentiated target cells like hepatocytes with another cell type is also being done to a limited extent to stabilize the culture system (54,58). When cocultures are used, factors such as differential accumulation by the different cell types and possible differential metabolism may have an influence on the results. If reactive metabolites are involved in the toxicity, the ability to traverse relatively long distances from one cell to another may be a further limiting factor.

SAMPLE STORAGE

Once samples have been taken they may need to be stored until time permits their assay. Stability should be ascertained before reliance can be placed on such values, as is done in whole animal studies. A point to remember is that frozen storage of incubation media for later enzyme assay such as alanine aminotransferase can cause differentially lower values compared with those anticipated after frozen storage of plasma (59).

STATISTICAL ANALYSIS

The statistical analysis of data for appropriate interpretation of the results is standardized for some types of tests. In newly evolving tests, standardization of both the mode of presentation and data analysis is an area that needs attention to facilitate rapid and meaningful comparison of results from different laboratories. The importance of data handling and analysis in assessing the toxicity of the joint action of two (or more) chemicals has been discussed by Pounds and Kodell (60). In general, it is appropriate to obtain expert advice on the statistical analysis of data, especially for tests that are destined to be used regularly.

TECHNICAL ADVANCES

Advances In Culture Methodology and Systems Availability

One of the most challenging problems for cell biologists has been the development of culture techniques that promote the growth or retention of differentiation. It is now well documented that the composition of the attachment matrix can greatly influence success in this effort. For example, changes in the differentiated state of the cells during longer-term cultures of rat and, to a lesser extent, human hepatocytes on single-layer, collagen-coated dishes are reduced appreciably by employing collagen sandwiches, rat liver epithelial cells, basement membrane matrix (e.g., Matrigel), or extracellular liver matrix material, as attachment substratum (58,61,62).

More recently, newer materials such as cellulosic fibers apparently have eliminated the need even for extracellular matrix components in some cases. PC12 cells that are anchored and grown on cellulosic fibers exhibit nerve growth factor-induced differentiated characteristics, in contrast to cells grown on traditional culture dishes (63). Other cell types that were not possible a short time ago can now be grown because of such advances. Cocultures can be prepared even in small multiwell plates by permitting one cell type to attach to the bottom of the well and adding the second attached to commercially available inserts. Several laboratories attach or grow epithelial cells on collagen-coated membranes, beads, or nylon mesh to allow metabolite exchange through the membrane and to more faithfully simulate spatial relationships and response characteristics in vivo (4,64). Test skins from a mixture of cells (keratinocytes), collagen, and other dermal components are under development for a number of applications (65). Jumblatt and colleagues used multilayer rabbit corneal epithelial cells in a wound-healing assay they developed for eye irritants (66,67).

Cell or tissue preparations for use in testing with these versatile systems are also commercially available. They include normal human epithelial keratinocytes that are prepackaged and grown in the user's laboratory with supplied culture medium, human umbilical vein endothelial cells for vascular pathology and wound-healing research, melanocytes, dermal fibroblasts, mammary epithelial cells, human corneal epithelial cells, and smooth muscle cells. The National Testing Corporation (now named Ropak Laboratories Irvine, California) offers a cellular system composed of matrix protein as a screen for eye irritation (68). Some of these systems have undergone fairly extensive validation testing and further refinements to identify the applications and test chemical classes for which they have the most value.

Advances in Analytical Techniques and Instrumentation

The technical advances in culturing techniques are being matched by those in analytical techniques and instrumentation. The classic array of biochemical indicators used traditionally for monitoring cell characteristics and chemical-induced changes is constantly being expanded and even displaced by fluorescent, electrophysiological, structural, and other techniques. A number of these are listed in Table 6.

Table 6 Special Bioanalytical Techniques and Instrumentation for In Vitro Toxicology

Fluorescent indicators
Flow cytometers
Anchored-dependent cell techniques
Confocal microscopy
Multiparameter-digitized data recording
Patch clamping
Nuclear magnetic resonance (NMR) spectroscopy
Electron spin resonance (ESR)
Multidish cultures
Microplate readers

Fluorescent Indicators

Advances in instrumentation together with a burgeoning collection of constituent-specific fluorescent probes and other indicators are now being applied aggressively and imaginatively to the study of toxicity mechanisms. The onset of cell death may be assessed by monitoring changes in cell constituents resulting from a rapid increase in nonspecific permeability of the plasma membrane. Subcellular and organelle-specific changes can also be monitored by fluorimetric techniques. Table 7 lists many currently available fluroescent probes and their applications.

Flow Cytometry

Flow cytometric techniques now make possible the on-line measurement of these subcellular effects as well as structural changes like blebbing that often precede them, in cell suspension systems (70). Monitoring intracellular Ca^{2+} levels has received a great deal of attention in recent years because of its vital role as a messenger in regulation and control of cellular functions, such as glycogenolysis and gluconeogenesis, transport and secretion of fluids and electrolytes, growth and division of cells, and neurological activity, among others (71). The toxicological consequences of deregulation through an increase in cystosolic Ca^{2+} can be varied and profound (72).

Anchored-Dependent Cell Analysis

Interactive laser cytometers facilitate detection and measurements of chromosomal damage and investigations of chemical-induced alterations in gap junction-mediated cell-to-cell communication in cell culture systems. They permit multiple measurements on the same cells without manipulation and are applicable for all anchored cell types and configurations. One application under consideration is the detection of tumor-promoting potential using human cells. The same fluorescent probes as are used with flow cytometers can

Table 7 Fluorescent Probes and Their Applications

Probe	Application
Antibodies and amines	Covalent labeling reagents
Hoechst 33342	DNA-RNA content
Propidium iodide	
Ethidium monoazide	
Acridine orange	
Rhodamine 123[a]	Membrane potential
Positively charged carbocyanines	
DiS-C_3	
Nile red	Liquid content and fluidity
BCECF[b]	pH
7-Hydroxycoumarins	
Fura-2	Calcium
Indo-1	
Fluo-3	
Rhod-4	
Propidium iodide	Cell viability
Carboxyfluorescein diacetate	
Fluorescent dextrans and flow, cell lineage	Endocytosis, tissue permeability
Biotinylated and lysine-modified dextrans	
Caged nucleotides	Regulatory processes
Acridine orange	Lysosomal integrity
Fluorescein dextran	

[a]Mitochondrial membrane.
[b]2′7′-Bis(2-carboxyethyl)-5(and 6)-carboxyfluorescein.
Source: Adapted from Ref. 69.

be incorporated for quantitating cystosolic Ca^{2+} and intracellular H^+ levels. Other applications include unscheduled DNA repair, free radical quantitation, membrane motility, in situ hybridization, mutant cell isolation, and quantitative confocal imaging, which is discussed further below.

Microscopy

The field of microscopy has advanced dramatically. Newer developments in the last few years are having a profound impact on biological (including toxicological) investigations. The key advances have progressed on a broad front in areas as diverse as the design of more efficient and stable fluorescent probes (noted above), the combining of computer and laser technology, development of monoclonal antibodies for toxicological studies, solid-state charge-coupled device imagers, biotin-conjugated DNA probes, and piezo-electric transducers among others (73). These innovations have contributed to unprecedented ability to examine the structure of cells, cell components, and biological macromolecules, and they function in an integrated fashion without the need for fixation or extra technical manipulations. Much of this progress is made possible by combining standard light microscopy or fluorescence imaging with video techniques for enhancing contrast.

Confocal microscopy is one example of such a technique. It offers distinct advantages over conventional microscopy by eliminating haze from out-of-focus structures, allowing researchers to see deep inside thick specimens without losing resolution (74). Quantitation of light emitted by fluorescent dyes is made more precise, allowing a three-dimensional view and improved resolution. Although primarily of interest in basic research, some of these applications may ultimately facilitate assays intended specifically to reduce animal use (e.g., improved assays to monitor disorganization of chromosomes within the nucleus when cells are between divisions or to detect a potential for interference with fertilization or development).

Video technology coupled with bright-field and fluorescence light microscopy is useful in many ways, including detection of low-contrast objects such as single unstained macromolecular complexes and weakly fluorescing objects, convenient image recording and retrieval, automated analysis of motion and geometrical parameters, image overlay and three-dimensional reconstruction, two-dimensional photometry and quantitative fluorescence microscopy, and ratio imaging for two-dimensional distributions of concentrations of H^+, Ca^{2+}, Mg^{2+}, and Na^+ (75). Terms often used to describe these techniques include video-enhanced contrast (to remove unwanted background), video-intensified contrast (to provide signal amplification for fluorescent probes), and differential interference contrast (for high contrast).

Multiparameter digitized video microscopy can offer a potentially valuable approach to screening when the objective is to acquire as much information as possible in time-lapsed format. Various fluorimetric probes are available for determining cytosolic Ca^{2+} levels (e.g., fura-2), plasma and mitochondrial membrane potentials (diS-C_3 and rhodamine 123, respectively), pH [2′7′-bis(2-carboxyethyl)-5(and 6)-carboxyfluorescein (BCECF)], cell viability (propidium iodide), lysosomal integrity (acridine orange and fluorescein dextran), and plasma membrane integrity (propidium iodide, fluorescein diacetate). The technology is applicable to both flow cytometric and anchor-dependent cell analyses.

Other Techniques

Many specialized techniques are proving advantageous, including patch clamping to assess the effects of irritants and inflammatory changes (e.g., in neuronal culture models) and the use of monoclonal antibodies and enzyme-linked immunosorbent assays (ELISAs) as well as improved (HPLC) methods (5), to characterize cell cultures, verify type and quality, and assess stability in extended cultures. Whole cell patch techniques are now being used to study the effects of toxicants on calcium channels (76). ^{19}F- and ^{31}P nuclear magnetic resonance (NMR) spectroscopy can be used at the cellular level to noninvasively quantitate fluorine-radiolabeled chelators of Ca^{2+} and the energy status of cells (77) and ^{23}Na NMR provides information of transmembrane transport (78). Other powerful biophysical techniques such as electron spin resonance (ESR) are applied to detect changes in membrane fluidity. For various reasons, not the least of which is the expense of the apparatus and the poor economics of its use for testing, many of these techniques will be limited to specialized applications in toxicology.

Among techniques not quite so sophisticated but no less interesting is a new approach that pairs a silicon-based biosensor with a respondent target cell to defect cytotoxic effects of chemicals by the changes they produce in intermediary metabolism (79). The beating rat heart cell culture technique has been applied to the study of solvent-induced arrhythmias (61). One biotechnology company has transfected human cytochrome P-450s and microsomal epoxide hydrolase cyclic DNAs (cDNAs) into human lymphoblastoid cells as part of an effort to develop a panel of cell lines for studying xenobiotic metabolism (80).

Automated Screens

Most of the bioanalytical instruments described above are sophisticated, expensive, and specialized in application, and they require special expertise. They can be valuable for mechanistic studies but are not so likely to find routine use in screening protocols. Much less expensive devices are now becoming available that facilitate automation, standardization, and reproducibility of test results in this area with simple assays. Adaptation of multiwell dish technology, previously the domain of medical technologists, to cytotoxicity screening has gained momentum (81,82). Microplate readers that are fully automated, have variable wavelengths, are suitable for generating kinetic profiles, and monitor multiple parameters virtually simultaneously are available from more than one supplier. These devices include scanning fluorimeters that perform automatic cell staining and separation for unbound or bound fluorescence in 96-well, unidirectional filtration plates and computerization for analysis of cytolytic end points such as Ca^{2+} flux and target cell proteins, pH change, and antiproliferative effects using 5-bromodeoxyuridine (BrdU) and anti-BrdU as indicators, among their features.

VALIDATION AND STANDARDIZATION

Almost any assay that is reproducible, easy to execute, and low cost can be considered a candidate for validation if a correlation is shown to exist between its in vitro results and an in vivo response for the same modest set of chemicals. This may be qualitative (+ or −), as in tests for mutagenicity or carcinogenicity, or quantitative, as in cytotoxicity screening data. In the latter case, data such as the chemical concentration needed to cause a 50% change in a particular measurable parameter, median effective concentration (EC_{50}) value, or some lower percentage may be acquired and used to rank the test chemicals for their intrinsic potential to produce that change. The value obtained is more or less sensitive to the cell type and experimental conditions used, but the relative potencies can be compared under a limited set of conditions to optimize the ranking order against in vivo potency. If there is a strong statistical correlation and a mechanistic similarity or basis for the comparison established with a subset from the chemicals being ranked, one would expect the assay to predict the relative potency of a previously untested chemical with an acceptable degree of certainty relative to other members of that class.

Validation of the assay in terms of whether the original test system gives a false-positive or false-negative result is of little relevance in this context. Classification into subgroups that differ in relative magnitude of the response is particularly useful, in validation with large data sets, to facilitate identification of chemical structures that show substantial discrepancy between in vitro and in vivo potency (e.g., differ by two classifications) and to attempt to explain that discrepancy. As long as the differences are relatively few and the assay exhibits high output (is economical to run) and reproducibility, it may be acceptable as either a limited or general screen for the specific effect being assessed.

Logically, the systems that might be expected to yield the best correlative results a priori would be primary cells or tissues from target organs, ideally from humans if these are available, because human risk from drug or chemical exposure is the central issue. Indeed, the use of animals as a source of tissue for in vitro assays remains controversial and is questioned by many on ethical and scientific grounds. The most direct way to gain insight into what effect a chemical will have on humans would be, apart from administering it directly, which is not ethically acceptable, to prescreen it in human-derived tissue.

There are serious drawbacks to this strategy, however. Most primary cells are difficult to maintain in culture; human tissue is a scarce resource and often yet more difficult to handle once available (83). The ability to form stable long-term cultures or to preserve human cells for convenient experimentation or transportation to user laboratories has not yet been mastered in most cases. In general, once isolated the cells must be used immediately. Immortalization techniques are being attempted with a variety of human cell types and human-derived tissues to overcome the problems of irregular supply and preservation, and a few cell types, as noted above, are commercially available. Because of the scarcity of human cells from normal donors, keratinocytes, for example, which, as noted above, are available commercially, are being evaluated as screens for several different applications, including eye and skin irritation and tumor promotion (84).

A single cell type would not be expected to accurately reflect toxic responses and record cytotoxic potentials in target tissues other than that from which it was derived, but this view may be overly restrictive. Most chemicals are acutely toxic because they disrupt function or integrity in key organelles or structures (mainly mitochondria or the plasma membrane). Several investigators have reported that in vitro data from nondifferentiated cells on a large number of randomly selected chemicals correlate well with human and animal lethal dosages for about 80% of cases (85). These results suggest that genuine organ- or cell-specific toxicity is a relatively rare event, and that screens for general cytotoxic potential may have an important position in the in vitro toxicology testing stratagem.

A relatively new program called the Multicenter Evaluation of In Vitro Cytotoxicity (MEIC), sponsored by the Scandinavian Society of Cell Toxicology, has emerged in Sweden partly on the basis of these observations. Its aim is to compare test results on a select group of reference compounds in various cell-based assays from different participating laboratories with available data on circulating or target tissue levels of the compounds known to cause acute toxicity in humans (86). From this survey MEIC hopes to find the best predictive test or battery of tests based on validation directly against human rather than animal data. Early results with the HeLa cell and hepatocytes from different laboratories are encouraging (87).

From an operational standpoint, if the assay is intended to assess cytotoxic potency and the in vivo response is related, some reasonably good preliminary results might be expected that justify closer scrutiny. Some assays appear somewhat exotic compared with the particular in vivo effect they are intended to predict. For example, among assays being evaluated for eye irritation potential are those based on monitoring for structural defects in the chorioallantoic membrane of chick eggs treated with the chemical, wound healing in rabbit corneal epithelial cells, *Tetrahymena* motility, corneal plasminogen activation, cytotoxicity in various cell lines (mouse Balb/c-3T3 cells, macrophages and fibroblasts, erythroleukemic cell line K-562, Chinese hamster V79, and canine kidney cells are diverse examples), and reactivity with matrix proteins in the Eytex assay (Chap. 7).

Responses in these systems are almost entirely dependent on the cytotoxic effects of chemicals or formulations and, therefore, exclude mechanisms of irritation such as those based on nonspecific inflammatory responses that are equally if not more important (e.g., Ref. 88). Indicators for noncytotoxic mechanisms are not yet at a state of practical application (89). A test battery accommodating different mechanisms may ultimately be required to screen for eye irritation potential alone. Considering the pressures to have some system in place reasonably soon, the aim is to find the best assay or assays from an operational standpoint to use now. Second-generation tests that improve on these will follow, but there is concern that once specific tests are accepted (in peer review and by regulators, users, and antivivisectionists), the urgency and momentum for developing and validating complementary or improved successor tests will be dramatically reduced.

Regardless of whether nonhuman or nonmammalian cell systems can substitute for human tissue in various assays, such as for acute cytotoxicity or eye irritation testing, there will be increased pressure and demand for human tissue as a complementary screen or basic research tool. Some examples of potential applications include (1) provision of biotransformation data on human and animal tissues for physiological-based pharmacokinetic models used for risk assessment, and (2) comparative toxicity and mechanistic investigations on quantitative and qualitative differences in response to chemicals in these tissues. This demand will be there well into the foreseeable future as regulatory agencies continue to rely heavily on whole animal tests for evaluating chemical handling and toxicity in the whole organism.

Short-term solutions to the problem of tissue scarcity are needed until cryopreservation or long-term culture and cell packaging techniques are developed for most target tissues of interest. One possible solution is the creation of human tissue research "centers" for chemical experimentation and screening. Such a facility for research on liver tissue was established at SRI International through funding from the NIDDK and NTP/NIEHS of the National Institutes of Health. This approach has both economic and ethical merit and ensures that organs generously given for research by next-of-kin are used to the fullest extent for that purpose.

FUTURE CONSIDERATIONS

In Vitro Versus In Vivo

It may be anticipated that testing chemicals in a single cell system or other in vitro screen will probably not yield results that correlate precisely with relative in vivo potency rankings for a specific effect. Few if any would expect otherwise. The limitations of some tests that were originally thought to be highly correlated with the in vivo response for complex processes like carcinogenicity are now well recognized and attempts are being made to refine and improve them. For example, one approach being evaluated is to complement in vitro tests for genotoxic potential with tests for nongenotoxic (promoter) mechanisms. Another is to use a combined in vivo-in vitro approach in which a limited number of animals are first treated with the test compound at different doses and treatment periods and prospective target tissues analyzed for indicator changes. Although the savings in animals is not so great as in a purely in vitro approach, correlations can be improved (90) and the new UK guidelines recognizing this situation specify that such options are acceptable (91). A negative result in such a test, of course, is no assurance that the screened-for effect would not be produced after longer exposure to the testing chemical or in a second species.

A different strategy employed by some laboratories is to incorporate genotoxic, reproductive, and biochemical assays, such as those for peroxisomal enzyme induction, in short-term repeated dose experiments with the chemical to assess the potential for a positive adverse effect if longer-term studies were conducted. If the results are positive, further animal testing of the chemical might be contraindicated. The result is a more cost-efficient use of the animal, foregoing long-term testing that will result in a waste of resources and time. The trend in this direction appears to be gaining momentum, leading some to predict that 2-year bioassays in the future will be conducted only in special cases instead of routinely for registration purposes (92).

The use of in vivo-in vitro tests or strictly in vivo tests of this kind for more general information, of course, is limited to those candidate chemicals in adequate supply. Drugs and other chemicals in the early stage of development, when only laboratory-scale quantities are available for testing, could more economically be screened first in purely in vitro systems. These considerations, among others, spur continued efforts to improve the predictivity of in vitro screens for specific chemical-induced injuries. Such screens will play their part in reducing animal usage and toxicity testing costs by allowing only those drugs and chemicals with increased probability of being "safe" at the anticipated human exposure levels to pass on to the animal-testing stage.

One possible way to advance the state of in vitro toxicology more rapidly and at the same time distribute the cost among the potential beneficiaries more evenly might be the organization of symposia and peer review panels for examination of validation results from industry or a requirement for provision of in vitro along with standard in vivo data at the time of submission of data packages to regulatory authorities. The latter approach would allow rapid accumulation of a large database on various tests and in vitro-in vivo comparisons to ascertain the predictive value of the in vitro data while protecting confidentiality. Initially, an approach like this would need to be specific for, says, irritancy or teratogenicity for its usefulness to be determined. Such a requirement would have to be carefully invoked to achieve its aim. The tests to be provided and the methodology to be used would have to be worked out and agreed upon with the contributors in advance. Furthermore, a designated agency would need to take the overall lead in a project of this nature.

Technical Developments

Molecular biological techniques applied to cell lines to make them more humanlike in response would seem to be very important to the future of in vitro toxicology. Some of the problems, such as low capability of cell lines to biotransform a wide variety of substrates, lend themselves to resolution by application of such techniques. These developments will not be easy to achieve, and it is not clear how practical this approach will be as a general one, but examples of apparently similiar applications are known. Such possibilities have been suggested by others in recent years (93,94). Thus, a worthwhile goal would be establishment of a continuously dividing cell line with a full complement of human biotransformation enzymes. These could be used in their own right or in coculture with other validated target cells, perhaps for organ-specific toxicity.

Continued development of specific test systems for particular toxic responses with well-defined endpoints is likely to provide valuable predictive information. This is particularly true for chemical classes for which the target organ may be inferred from other information in advance and from which newer members have been synthesized. The use of nonmammalian cells or cell lines will continue as a basic test system or for a reproducible response. The ultimate development of economical systems designed to facilitate metered delivery of test chemicals and removal of metabolites under simulated in vivo conditions should provide improved in vitro testing. Better cell preservation or culture techniques for human tissues and packaging of systems to supply human tissues to laboratories involved in in vitro toxicology are also expected in the future.

One area that probably requires more attention than others relates to predicting subchronic or chronic toxicity other than carcinogenicity. The idea of being able to determine a no-observed-effect level to set acceptable limits for repeated exposures to humans is not viewed as a viable proposition at this stage. Advances in both systems and endpoints will be needed before this aspect can be seriously entertained. Several important types of chemical-induced lesions associated with repeated exposures cannot yet be modeled in vitro, e.g., cirrhosis and host idiosyncratic reactions, but progress is also being made in these areas.

Conceptual Issues

While technical progress will continue, some fundamental issues remain to be resolved and are still being hotly debated; others will arise in the future. One fundamental question relates to validation. Should these systems be validated against animal data, as most involved organizations are attempting to do, or against human response directly, as, for example, in the MEIC approach for predicting acute systemic toxicity?

The scarcity of human data for validation purposes for most chemical-induced effects makes this a moot point but perhaps not for some endpoints like acute toxicity and eye and skin irritation. If it can be agreed from test data that one or more of these assays is reasonably predictive of human response, is further testing in a laboratory species necessary?

This is a particularly difficult and sensitive ethical and scientific problem for toxicologists and regulatory personnel. The current animal test methods have been in use for decades and practitioners rely upon them as their main line of defense against missing an unexpected toxic chemical action on a living organism before human exposure. No new in vitro method, no matter how good the concordance (predictivity) for a particular end point, can be expected to readily displace this historical advantage and familiarity whole animal testing offers, even though such testing has been shown in some cases to exhibit low concordance of commonly used species for man (e.g., rodent carcinogenicity) (95). If both in vitro (to assess species differences in response for man using human tissue) and in vivo testing are done on a chemical or drug and the test species is indicated to be more sensitive to it than man, would we be willing to continue its development? Situations now exist where human clinical experience was discounted in the safety evaluation of a new drug and animal data given greater weight. The use of in vitro approaches to provide data to bridge the species gap may encounter more serious resistance still among regulatory scientists in their development of safety dossiers.

This is a continually evolving situation. As validation exercises progress and we become more proficient and sophisticated in using in vitro methods intelligently to aid risk assessment, these problems may slowly be resolved. Animal testing will remain an integral part of that assessment process well into the foreseeable future. One important role for in vitro systems in safety evaluations is under intensive study; namely, coupling results from them using animal- and human-derived tissues, together with physiological based pharmacokinetic models to improve extrapolations of data from animal studies to humans and provide a mechanistic basis for any species difference observed. Often the reference drug and the test compound may be handled differently in humans and in the laboratory species, or they may involve toxic mechanisms with different susceptibilities in the two species. An example is methylene chloride, for which there is good evidence relating its carcinogenicity in mouse lung to the singularly high levels of glutathione transferase involved in metabolic activation of the chemical in target lung cells, compared in both humans and various laboratory species (96).

On the other hand, validating (we assume this will be possible eventually) a system composed of one cell type or a battery of cells against in vivo circulating or target tissue levels of drugs and chemicals implies that that assay can be used with confidence to predict in vivo toxic levels of compounds for which no previous human data are available. For some, the high interindividual variability in response to drugs and chemicals in humans makes such efforts unrealistic and futile (97). How then will it be possible to validate in vitro assays on the basis of in vivo data and apply test results in the system as directly extrapolatable to humans for establishing safe exposure levels with confidence?

These are not insurmountable problems. They may simply require the incorporation of safety factors into the in vitro test data, as is done in risk assessments using whole animal data. The problem of developing practical in vitro toxicology tests for predicting human toxicity, whether directly or as an aid in interpreting the significance of animal data, requires many specialists besides the cell biologist and dictates a team approach for success that individual laboratories do not usually employ.

CONCLUSIONS

In our view and in that of many others in the field, toxicologists must be sensitive to the issue of minimization or replacement of animals in toxicological testing with valid alternatives whenever possible and receptive to the actual economic and scientific benefits that well-validated in vitro systems can offer. It is commonly stated that in vitro and nonanimal techniques cannot replace whole animal testing but, as will be recalled from the Introduction, there are several instances in which that has already occurred. Animal use reduction brought about in part by shifting to in vitro test methodology is also a reality (98). While blanket replacement of animals in toxicity testing by alternative techniques is not a realistic expectation, the use of in vitro methods as prescreens, as models for detailed mechanistic studies, or as substitutes for whole animals in special cases will proceed and most certainly continue to increase in the future.

REFERENCES

1. Ashby, J. (1986). The prospects for a simplified and internationally harmonized approach to the detection of possible human carcinogens and mutagens. *Mutagenesis* **1**: 3-16.
2. Tennant, R. W., Margolin, B. H., Shelby, M. D., Zeiger, E., Haseman, J. K., Spalding, J., Caspary, W., Resnick, M., Stasiewicz, S., Anderson, B., and Minor, R. (1987). Prediction of chemical carcinogenicity in rodents from in vitro genetic toxicity assays. *Science* **236**: 933-941.
3. The Alternatives Report (1989). To test or not to test: Avon, Mary Kay, Noxell. Center for Animals and Public Policy, Grafton, Massachusetts, July/Aug. issue. See also Sept./Oct. issue, p. 1.

4. Klausner, A. (1987). Tissue culture for improved toxicology. *Biotechnology* **5**: 779-786.
5. Tretheway, J. (1986). Moving away from animal tests for the standardization of insulin formulations. *Trends Pharmacol. Sci.* **8**: 287-288.
6. Johnson, M. K. (1990). Organophosphates and delayed neuropathy—Is NTE alive and well? *Toxicol. Appl. Pharmacol.* **102**: 385-399.
7. Duffy, P. A. (1989). Irritancy testing—A cultured approach. *Toxicol. In Vitro* **3**: 157-158.
8. Rubinstein, L. V., Shoemaker, R. H., Paull, K. D., Simon, R. M., Tosini, S., Skehan, P., Scudiero, D. A., Monks, A. and Boyd, M. R. (1990). *J. Natl. Canc. Inst.* **82**: 1113-1118.
9. Mehlman, M. A., Pfitzer, E. A., and Scala, R. A. (1989). A report on methods to reduce, refine, and replace animal testing in industrial toxicology laboratories. *Cell Biol. Toxicol.* **5**: 349-358.
10. Wu. K., Bonin, A. M., Leslie, C. L., Baker, R. S. U., and Stacey, N. H. (1989). Genotoxicity and effects on rat liver drug-metabolizing enzymes by possible substitutes for 4,4′-methylene bis(2-chloroaniline). *Carcinogenesis* **10**: 2119-2122.
11. Johnson, M. K. (1977). Improved assay of neurotoxic esterase for screening organophosphates for delayed neurotoxicity potential. *Arch. Toxicol.* **37**: 113-115.
12. Babich, H., and Borenfreund, E. (1987). *In vitro* cytotoxicity of organic pollutants to bluegill sunfish (BF-2) cells. *Environ. Res.* **42**: 229-237.
13. Spanggord, R. J., Myers, C. J., Le Valley, S. E., Green, C. E., and Tyson, C. A. (1990). Structure-activity relationship for the intrinsic hepatotoxicity of dinitrotoluenes. *Res. Chem. Toxicol.* **3**: 551-558.
14. Andrews, L. S., and Snyder, R. (1986). Toxic effects of solvents and vapors. In *Casarett and Doull's Toxicology. The Basic Science of Poisons.* 3rd Ed. J. Doull, C. D. Klaassen, and M. O. Amdur (Eds.). Macmillan, New York, pp. 659-660.
15. Carrington, C. D., Carrington, M. N., and Abou-Donia, M. B. (1985). Neurotoxic esterase in cultured cells: An *in vitro* alternative for the study of organophosphorous compound-induced delayed neurotoxicity. In *Alternative Methods in Toxicology.* Vol. 3, *In Vitro Toxicology. A Progress Report from the Johns Hopkins Center for Alternatives to Animal Testing.* A. M. Goldberg (Ed.). Mary Ann Liebert, New York, pp. 455-465.
16. Goldberg, A. M. (1987). Approaches to the development of *in vitro* neurotoxicological methods. In *Model Systems in Neurotoxicology. Alternative Approaches to Animal Testing.* A. Shahar and A. M. Goldberg (Eds.). Liss, New York, pp. 1-11.
17. Lundberg, P., Cederberg, I., Wiklund, L., and Pettersson, B. (1983). Effects of waste incineration combustion emissions measured by some toxicity test systems. *Toxicol. Lett.* **19**: 97-107.
18. Mandel, L. J., Solthoff, S. P., and Brazy, P. C. (1986). Energy compartmentation and active transport in proximal kidney tubules. *Adv. Exp. Med. Biol.* **194**: 213-228.

19. Schiestl, R. H. (1989). Nonmutagenic carcinogens induce intrachromosomal recombination in yeast. *Nature* **337**: 285-288.
20. Tenenbaum, S., DiNardo, J., Morris, W. E., Wolf, B. A., and Schnetzinger, R. W. (1984). A quantitative *in vitro* assay for the evaluation of phototoxic potential of topically applied materials. *Cell Biol. Toxicol.* **1**: 1-9.
21. Silverman, J., and Pennisi, S. (1985). *Tetrahymena thermophila* (30377) as an indicator of ocular irritancy in rabbits. In *Alternative Methods in Toxicology.* Vol. 3. *In Vitro Toxicology. A Progress Report from The Johns Hopkins Center for Alternatives to Animal Testing.* A. M. Goldberg (Ed.). Mary Ann Liebert, New York, pp. 673-680.
22. Bruner, L. H., and Parker, R. D. (1990). Evaluation of six *in vitro* alternatives for ocular irritancy testing. The *Toxicologist* **10**: 258.
23. Grisham, J. W., and Smith, G. J. (1984). Predictive and mechanistic evaluation of toxic responses in mammalian cell culture systems. *Pharmacol. Rev.* **36**: 151S-168S.
24. Foliot, A., Glaise, D., Erlinger, S., and Guguen-Guillouzo, C. (1985). Long-term maintenance of taurocholate uptake by adult rat hepatocytes cocultured with a liver epithelial cell line. *Hepatology* **5**: 215-219.
25. Stammati, A. P., Silano, V., and Zucco, F. (1981). Toxicology investigations with cell culture systems. *Toxicology* **20**: 91-153.
26. Rowan, A. N., and Goldberg, A. M. (1985). Perspectives on alternatives to current animal testing techniques in preclinical toxicology. *Annu. Rev. Pharmacol. Toxicol.* **25**: 225-247.
27. Atterwill, C. K., and Steele, C. E. (1987). Conclusion. In *In Vitro Methods in Toxicology.* C. K. Atterwill and C. E. Steele (Eds.). Cambridge University Press, Cambridge, England, pp. 443-446.
28. Flint, O. P. (1988). *In vitro* toxicology: a commercial proposition? *Xenobiotica* **18**: 707-714.
29. Enger, M. D. (1988). Cellular toxicology. *Rev. Environ. Contam. Toxicol.* **102**: 79-115.
30. Atterwill, C. K., and Walum, E. (1989). Neurotoxicology *in vitro*: Model systems and practical applications. *Toxicol. In Vitro* **3**: 159-161.
31. Kotin, P. (1985). Chairman's summary: cell- and organ-specific responses. In *Alternative Methods in Toxicology.* Vol. 3. *In Vitro Toxicology. A Progress Report from The Johns Hopkins Center for Alternatives to Animal Testing.* A. M. Goldberg (Ed.). Mary Ann Liebert, New York, pp. 335-339.
32. Smith, P. F., Gandolfi, A. J., Krumdieck, C. L., Putnam, C. W., Zukoski, C. F., III, Davis, W. M., and Brendel, K. (1985). Dynamic organ culture of precision liver slices for *in vitro* toxicology. *Life Sci.* **36**: 1367-1375.
33. Ruegg, C. E., Wolfgang, G. H. I., Gandolfi, A. J., Krumdieck, C. L., and Brendel, K. (1987). Preparation of positional renal slices for study of cell-specific toxicity. *J. Pharmacol. Meth.* **17**: 111-123.
34. Bauer, M. F., and Herzog, V. (1988). Miniorgan culture of thyroid tissue: A new technique for maintaining the structural and functional integrity of thyroid tissue *in vitro. Lab. Invest.* **59**: 281-291.
35. Honegger, P., and Werffeli, P. (1988). Use of aggregating cell cultures for toxicological studies. *Experientia* **44**: 817-823.

36. Resau, J. H., Cottrell, J. R., Elligett, K. A., and Hudson, E. A. (1987). Cell injury and regeneration of human epithelium in organ culture. *Cell Biol. Toxicol.* **3**: 441-458.
37. Curvall, M., Enzell, C. R., and Pettersson, B. (1984). An evaluation of the utility of four *in vitro* short-term tests for predicting the cytotoxicity of individual compounds derived from tobacco smoke. *Cell Biol. Toxicol.* **1**: 173-193.
38. Oliver, G. J. A., Pemberton, M. A., and Rhodes, C. (1986). An *in vitro* skin corrosivity test—Modifications and validation. *Food Chem. Toxicol.* **24**: 507-512.
39. Delfino, G., Amerini, S., and Mugelli, A. (1988). Barium cardiotoxicity: Relationship between ultrastructural damage and mechanical effects. *Toxicol. In Vitro* **2**: 49-55.
40. Spencer, P. S., Crain, S. M., Bornstein, M. B., Peterson, E. R., and Van de Water, T. (1986). Chemical neurotoxicity: deduction and analysis in organotypic cultures of sensory and motor systems. *Food Chem. Toxicol.* **24**: 539-544.
41. Gautam, A., Ng, O. C., and Boyer, J. L. (1987). Isolated rat hepatocyte couplets in short-term culture: structural characteristics and plasma membrane reorganization. *Hepatology* **7**: 216-223.
42. Kucera, P., and Burnand, M. -B. (1988). Teratogenicity screening in standardized chick embryo culture: effects of dexamethasone and diphenylhydantoin. *Experientia* **44**: 827-833.
43. Cicurel, L., and Schmid, B. P. (1988). Postimplantation embryo culture for the assessment of the teratogenic potential and potency of compounds. *Experientia* **44**: 833-840.
44. Luepke, N. P. and Kemper, F. H. (1986). The HET-CAM test: An alternative to the Draize eye test. *Food Chem. Toxicol.* **24**: 495-496.
45. Lawrence, R. S., Groom, M. H., Ackroyd, D. M., and Parish, W. E. (1986). The chorioallantoic membrane in irritation testing. *Food Chem. Toxicol.* **24**: 497-502.
46. OTA Report. (1986). *Alternatives to Animal Use in Research, Testing, and Education.* Congress of the United States. Office of Technology Assessment, Washington, D.C., p. 119. Marcel Dekker, New York, 1988.
47. Stark, D. M., Shopsis, C., Borenfreund, E., and Babich, H. (1986). Progress and problems in evaluating and validating alternative assays in toxicology. *Food Chem. Toxicol.* **24**: 449-455.
48. Frazier, J. M., and Bradlaw, J. A. (1989). Technical Problems Associated with *In Vitro* Toxicity Testing Systems. A Report of the CAAT Technical Workshop, May 17-18. The Johns Hopkins Center for Alternatives to Animal Testing, Baltimore.
49. Jones, C. A., Huberman, E., Callahan, M. F., Tu, A., Halloween, W., Pallota, S., Sivak, A., Lubet, R. A., Avery, M. D., Kouri, R. E., Spalding, J., and Tennant, R. W. (1988). An interlaboratory evaluation of the Syrian hamster embryo cell transformation assay using 18 coded chemicals. *Toxicol. In Vitro* **2**: 103-116.
50. Kukongviriyapan, V., and Stacey, N. H. (1989). Comparison of uptake kinetics in freshly isolated suspensions and short-term primary cultures of rat hepatocytes. *J. Cell. Physiol.* **140**: 491-497.

51. Stacey, N. H., and Klaassen, C. D. (1981). Inhibition of lipid peroxidation without prevention of cellular injury in isolated rat hepatocytes. *Toxicol. Appl. Pharmacol.* **58**: 8-18.
52. Fariss, M. W., Pascoe, G. A., and Reed, D. J. (1985). Vitamin E reversal of the effect of extracellular calcium on chemically induced toxicity in hepatocytes. *Science* **227**: 751-754.
53. Benoit, J., Cormier, M., and Wepierre, J. (1987). Effect of proteins on the assessment of surfactant cytotoxicity by an *in vitro* test: Possible correlations with *in vivo* data. *Toxicol. In Vitro* **1**: 91-96.
54. Maier, P. (1988). Development of *in vitro* toxicity tests with cultures of freshly isolated rat hepatocytes. *Experientia* **44**: 807-817.
55. Stacey, N. H., Ottenwalder, H., and Kappus, H. (1982). CCl_4-induced lipid peroxidation in isolated rat hepatocytes with different oxygen concentrations. *Toxicol. Appl. Pharmacol.* **62**: 421-427.
56. Tyson, C. A., Dabbs, J. E., Cohen, P. M., Green, C. E., and Melnick, R. L. (1990). Studies of nephrotoxic agents in an improved renal proximal tubule system. *Toxicol. In Vitro* **4**: 403-408.
57. Kluwe, W. M., and Hook, J. B. (1981). Potentiation of acute chloroform nephrotoxicity by the glutathione depletor diethylmaleate and protection by the microsomal enzyme inhibitor piperonyl butoxide. *Toxicol. Appl. Pharmacol.* **59**: 457-466.
58. Guillouzo, A., Begue, J-M., Campion, J. -P., Gascoin, M-N., and Guguen-Guillouzo, C. (1985). Human hepatocyte cultures: a model of pharmacotoxicological studies. *Xenobiotica* **15**: 635-641.
59. Stacey, N. H., Cook, R., and Priestly, B. G. (1978). Comparative stability of alanine aminotransferase in rat plasma and hepatocyte suspensions. *Aust. J. Exp. Biol. Med. Sci.* **56**: 379-381.
60. Pounds, J. G., and Kodell, R. L. (1985). Statistical analysis for the characterization of the joint action of two chemicals in an *in vitro* test system. In *Alternative Methods in Toxicology*. Vol. 3. *In Vitro Toxicology. A Progress Report from The Johns Hopkins Center for Alternatives to Animal Testing*. A. M. Goldberg (Ed.). Mary Ann Liebert, New York, pp. 627-640.
61. Dunn, C. Y., Yarmush, M. L., Koebe, H. G., and Tompkins, R. G. (1989). Hepatocyte function and extracellular matrix geometry: long-term culture in a sandwich configuration. *FASEB J.* **3**: 174-177.
62. Reid, L. M., Narita, M., Fujita, M., Murray, Z., Liverpool, C., and Rosenberg, L. (1987). Matrix and hormonal regulation of differentiation in liver cultures. In *Isolated and Cultured Hepatocytes*. A. Guillouzo and C. Guguen-Guillouzo (Eds.). John Libbey Eurotext, Paris, pp. 225-258.
63. Van Buskirk, R. G., Gabriels, J., and Wagner, J. (1988). PC12 cells grown on cellulosic filters differentiate in response to NGF and exhibit a polarity not seen when they are grown on solid substrata. *In Vitro Cell. Develop. Biol.* **24**: 451-456.
64. Naughton, G. K., Jacob, L., and Naughton, B. A. (1989). A physiological skin model for *in vitro* toxicity studies. In *Alternative Methods in Toxicology*. Vol. 7. *In Vitro Toxicology: New Directions*. A. M. Goldberg (Ed.). Mary Ann Liebert, New York, pp. 183-189.

65. CAAT Newsletter. (1988). *Engineering Humanlike Tissues.* Vol. 6. The Johns Hopkins Center for Alternatives to Animal Testing, Baltimore, pp. 4-6.
66. Dagani, R. (1984). *In vitro* methods may offer alternatives to animal testing. *Chem. Eng. News,* November 12, pp. 215-28.
67. Simmons, S. J., Jumblatt, M. M., and Neufeld, A. H. (1987). Corneal epithelial wound closure in tissue culture: an *in vitro* model of ocular irritancy. *Toxicol. Appl. Pharmacol.* **88**: 13-23.
68. Gordon, V. C., Kelly, C. P., and Bergman, H. C. (1989). Applications of the Eyetex™ method for determination of the ocular irritation of surfactant formulations. In *Alternative Methods in Toxicology.* Vol. 7. *In Vitro Toxicology: New Directions.* A. M. Goldberg (Ed.). Mary Ann Liebert, New York, pp. 337-345.
69. Haugland, R. P. (1989). *Handbook of Fluorescent Probes and Research Chemicals.* Molecular Probes, Inc., Eugene, Oregon.
70. Lemasters, J. J., DiGuisippi, J., Nieminin, A. -L., and Herman, B. (1987). Blebbing, free Ca^{2+}, and mitochondrial membrane potential preceding cell death in hepatocytes. *Nature* **325**: 78-81.
71. Pounds, J. G., and Rosen, J. F. (1988). Cellular Ca^{2+} homeostasis and Ca^{2+}-mediated cell processes as critical targets for toxicant action: Conceptual and methodological pitfalls. *Toxicol. Appl. Pharmacol.* **94**: 331-341.
72. Trump, B. F., Berezesky, I. K., Smith, M. W., Phelps, P. C., and Elliget, K. A. (1989). The relationship between cellular ion deregulation and acute and chronic toxicity. *Toxicol. Appl. Pharmacol.* **97**: 6-22.
73. Agard, D. (1989). Introduction to advances in microscopy. Part 1. *BioTechniques* **7**: 154.
74. Taylor, R. (1989). Confocal microscopy sheds new light on the dynamics of living cells. *J. NIH Res.* **1**: 113-115.
75. Salmon, T., Walker, R. A., and Pryer, N. K. (1989). Video-enhanced differential interference contrast light microscopy. *BioTechniques* **7**: 624-633.
76. Borle, A. B., and Snowdowne, K. W. (1987). Methods for the measurement of intracellular ionized calcium in mammalian cells: Comparison of four classes of calcium (2^+) indicators. In *Molecular Biology: An International Series of Monographs and Textbooks.* Vol. VII. *Calcium Cell Function.* W. Y. Cheung (Ed.). Academic Press, New York, pp. 159-200.
77. Dowd, T. L., Schanne, F. A. X., Gupta, R. K., and Rosen, J. F. (1988). Fluorine-19 NMR detection of the effects of lead toxicity on intracellular calcium in osteoblastic bone cells. *Biophys. J.* **53**: 215A.
78. Kaplan, O., and Cohen, J. S. (1990). Magnetic resonance as a non-invasive tool to study metabolism in pharmacological research. *Trends Pharm. Sci.* **11**: 398-400.
79. Parce, J. W., Owicki, J. C., Kercso, K. M., Sigal, G. B., Wada, H. G., Muir, V. C., Bousse, L. J., Ross, K. L., Sikic, B. I., and McConnell, H. M. (1989). Detection of cell-affecting agents with a silicon biosensor. *Science* **246**: 243-247.
80. Crespi, C. L., and Penman, B. W. The development of a panel of human cell lines expressing specific human cytochrome P-450 cDNAs. In *Mutation and the Environment. Part B.* M. L. Mendelsohn and R. J. Albertini (Eds.), Wiley-Liss, New York, pp. 97-106.

81. Elliget, K. A., Berezeksy, I. K., and Trump, B. F. Normal rat kidney proximal tubule cell cultures for *in vitro* studies of nephrotoxicity. (1989). Presented at the CAAT Symposium: *In Vitro Toxicology: New Directions.* Baltimore, Apr. 4-5.
82. Chesne, C., Clere, C., Guyomard, C., Fautrel, A., and Guillouzo, A. (1989). Evaluation of various parameters in testing drug cytotoxicity in primary hepatocyte cultures. In *Alternative Methods in Toxicology: New Directions.* A. M. Goldberg (Ed.). Mary Ann Liebert, New York, pp. 191-196.
83. Frazier, J. M., Tyson, C. A., McCarthy, C., McCormick, J., Meyers, D., Powis, G., and Ducat, L. (1989). Potential use of human tissues for toxicity studies and testing—a minireview. *Toxicol. Appl. Pharmacol.* **97**: 387-397.
84. Wegener, P. T. (1988). Current uses of normal human epidermal keratinocytes in serum-free medium for *in vitro* toxicology. In *Alternative Methods in Toxicology.* Vol. 6. *Progress in In Vitro Toxicology.* A. M. Goldberg (ed.), Mary Ann Liebert, New York, pp. 333-338.
85. Ekwall, B. and Ekwall, K. (1988). Comments on the use of diverse cell systems in toxicity testing. *ATLA* **15**: 193-200.
86. Bondesson, I., Ekwall, B., Hellberg, S., Romert, L., Stenberg, K., and Walum, E. (1989). MEIC - A new international multicenter project to evaluate the relevance to human toxicity of *in vitro* cytotoxicity tests. *Cell Biol. Toxicol.* **5**: 331-347.
87. Ekwall, B., Bondesson, I., Castell, J. V., Gómez-Lechón, M. J., Hellberg, S., Högberg, J., Jover, R., Ponsoda, X., Romert, L., Stenberg, K., and Walum, E. (1989). Cytotoxicity evaluation for the first ten MEIC chemicals: Acute lethal toxicity in man predicted by cytotoxicity in five cellular assays and by oral LD_{50} in rodents. *ATLA* **17**: 83-100.
88. Kennah II, H. E., Albulescu, D., Hignet, S., and Barrow, C. S. (1989). A critical evaluation of predicting ocular irritancy potential from an *in vitro* cytotoxicity assay. *Fund. Appl. Toxicol.* **12**: 281-290.
89. Parish, W. E. (1989) Inflammatory mediators applied to *in vitro* toxicology: Studies on mediator release and two cell systems. Presented at the Second International Conference on Practical *In Vitro* Toxicology, Nottingham, England, July 23.
90. Mirsalis, J. C. (1987). *In vivo* measurement of unscheduled DNA synthesis and S-phase synthesis as an indicator of hepatocarcinogenesis in rodents. *Cell Biol. Toxicol.* **3**: 165-173.
91. DHSS (1989). *Guidelines for the Testing of Chemicals for Mutagenicity.* Report No. 35. Dept. of Health and Social Sciences. ISBN 0 11 32122 4. HMSO Publications Centre, London.
92. Moore, J. A. (1989). Presentation at the Toxicology Forum, Aspen, Colorado, July 16-21.
93. Greim, H., Andrae, U., Forster, U., and Schwarz, L. (1986). Application, limitations, and research requirements of *in vitro* test systems in toxicology. *Arch. Toxicol.* **9**: (Suppl.):225-236.
94. Knox, P. (1986). Cellular and *in vitro* techniques. In *The Future of Predictive Safety Evaluation.* A. N. Worden, D. V. Parke, and J. Marks (Eds.). MTP Press, Lancaster, England, pp. 171-180.

95. Young, S. S. (1989). A blind renanalysis of a random subset of NCI bioassay studies: agreement between rats and man. *Fund. Appl. Toxicol.* **12**: 189-190.
96. Green, T., and Provan, W. M. (1990). *In vitro* metabolic kinetics in risk assessment. In *Basic Science in Toxicology*. G. N. Volans, J. Sims, F. M. Sullivan, and P. Turner (Eds.). Taylor and Francis, New York, pp. 69-78.
97. Hüttenrauch, R., and Speiser, P. (1985). *In vitro-in vivo* correlation. An unrealistic problem. *Pharm. Res.* **3**: 97-107.
98. Goldberg, A. M. (1989). *Alternative Methods in Toxicology*. Vol. 7. *In Vitro Toxicology: New Directions*. Mary Ann Liebert, New York.

3

Hepatotoxicity

André Guillouzo

Hôpital de Pontchaillou, Institut National de la Santé et de la Recherche Médicale
Rennes, France

INTRODUCTION

Liver diseases constitute a major medical problem of worldwide proportions: They can be caused by a variety of agents, the most frequent being viruses, parasites, and toxins. In Africa and in Asia, the main causes of liver diseases are viruses and parasitic infections, whereas in Europe and North America the major cause is alcohol abuse. Approximately 200 million humans are infected with hepatitis B virus and probably at least the same number of individuals suffer from the consequence of alcohol abuse. Other xenobiotics and drugs are responsible for various liver lesions. More than 600 compounds are suspected of being possibly hepatotoxic (1). In Western countries, the percentage of acute hepatitis caused by drugs increases with age. In French adults, it represents 10% of cases of acute hepatitis while it raises to 50% or more in adults over 50 years (2). As a consequence, it is desirable to determine how the liver handles and responds to any new chemical.

Biotransformation of exogenous compounds is one of the major functions performed by the liver. This function is expressed by the hepatocytes, which represent about 65% of the total cell population and 90% of the volume of the organ. Hepatocytes are richly endowed with drug-metabolizing enzymes which are conveniently divided into two groups. Phase I reactions are generally oxidative, reductive, and hydrolytic processes; they provide the necessary functional group for phase II reactions, which are generally conjugations. If the overall effect of these enzymes is to convert chemicals to more water-soluble forms which can be secreted readily by the body, it appears that a number of compounds are metabolized to toxic metabolites.

In vivo studies make it difficult to distinguish the primary effects of a compound to those induced secondarily because liver functions are under the influence of various endogenous and exogenous factors which result in complex interactions with other organs. Moreover, most of our understanding of liver injury induced by drugs and other chemicals at a mechanistic level remains confined to experimental models. Since the rates and the routes of drug metabolism can vary greatly, particularly when comparisons involved laboratory animals and man, data obtained in animals cannot be extrapolated with certainty to the human situation. These drawbacks of in vivo animal studies explain why many investigators have turned to simpler experimental models for studying drug metabolism and the response of the organ or liver cells to potentially toxic agents.

This chapter will discuss the various liver lesions which can be induced by toxic compounds and then consider the current in vitro liver systems available for toxicity testing of xenobiotics. The advantages and the limitations of the isolated liver preparations will be analyzed with consideration to future developmental needs.

THE LIVER: A TARGET ORGAN FOR TOXIC DRUG-INDUCED LESIONS

Whatever the agent responsible for injury the reaction of the liver involves a common sequence of events which can be analyzed at the molecular, cellular and tissular levels. The physiological response to injury results in a variety of lesions which have been described by pathologists as necrosis, cholestasis, steatosis, inflammation, and fibrosis. These conditions lead to impaired liver functions; some markers have been identified for the different types of lesions (Table 1).

Table 1 Functional Markers of Liver Lesions Induced by Hepatotoxic Compounds

Lesion	Biological response
Necrosis	Serum transaminase increase
Inflammation	Overproduction of acute-phase proteins
Cholestasis	Alkaline phosphatase elevation
Steatosis	Fatty acid accumulation
Fibrosis/cirrhosis	Increased production and deposition of collagen

Clinicopathological Forms of Drug-Induced Lesions

Drugs and other chemicals can induce almost all types of lesions of the liver; the most frequent one being hepatitis. For the clinician, drug-induced lesions are classified as acute or chronic injury and are divided in different types—cytolytic hepatitis and cholestasis (2) (Table 2). Acute cytolytic hepatitis is characterized by more or less extended necrosis of liver lobules. Some areas may be preferentially affected. Thus, centrilobular hepatocytes are more sensitive than their periportal counterparts to various compounds. Increased levels of serum transaminases are usually observed. Cholestasis is predominantly found in centrilobular areas with limited cell necrosis, if any. It results from modulation of the secretion of bile. Serum bilirubin and alkaline phosphatase levels are increased. In a few cases, both cytolytic and cholestatic features are found (mixed hepatitis).

Prolonged exposure to certain hepatotoxic drugs can result in three types of chronic hepatitis: chronic active hepatitis, alcoholiclike hepatitis, and chronic cholestasis. Chronic active hepatitis is characterized by liver cell necrosis, inflammation, and a conspicuous increase in serum transaminases. Alcoholiclike hepatitis consists of lesions resembling those induced by chronic alcohol intoxication; they include hepatocyte death, steatosis, and fibrosis. Chronic cholestasis is an uncommon drug-induced injury characterized by changes in intralobular bile ducts and inflammatory infiltration.

Some drugs responsible for each of these lesions are listed in Table 2. The list of most hepatotoxic compounds and a brief description of the lesions induced by each of them are given in several reviews and books (1,3,4).

Liver lesions other that hepatitis include storage diseases (vitamin A, iron), vascular and sinusoidal alterations, and tumors (2).

Factors Influencing Drug Hepatotoxicity

Drug hepatotoxicity is influenced by various physiological, nutritional, and therapeutic factors. It can be modulated when exposure occurs in the presence of enzyme inducers. Fasting enhances the toxicity of acetaminophen, probably by decreasing glutathione content (5).

The higher percentage of hepatitis caused by drugs in the elderly may be explained by the higher consumption of drugs by this group, or possibly by a greater susceptibility of the subjects (2). In Western countries, 12-18% of the population is now over 65 years and this group consumes 30-40% of national drug budgets. Recent studies have shown that there is no increased susceptibility to the development of adverse drug reactions in aged subjects when frequency of drug prescriptions is taken into account (6,7) (Table 3).

Besides these factors, it is now recognized that drug toxicity can be genetically modulated. Oxidation by cytochrome P-450 enzymes and acetyla-

Table 2 Different Forms of Hepatitis Induced by Some Drugs Used in Medicine

Hepatitis form	Potentially toxic drugs
Acute injury	
acute cytolytic hepatitis	Halothane (particularly when readministered)
	Isoniazid (particularly when associated with rifampicin)
	Nonsteroidal inflammatory drugs
	Monoamine oxidase inhibitors
	Tienilic acid
	Valproic acid
	Dihydralazine
	Ketoconazole
	Isaxonine
	Amodiaquine
	Papaverine
	Clometacin
cholestatic hepatitis	Oral contraceptives
	Carbamazepine
	Chlorpromazine
	Macrolides
	Tricyclic antidepressants
	Ajmaline
mixed hepatitis	Phenylindanedione
	Ticlopidine
	Cholestatic drugs except for steroids
Chronic injury	
chronic active hepatitis	Clometacin
	Alpha-methyldopa
	Methotrexate
	Papaverine
alcoholiclike hepatitis	Perhexiline maleate
	Amiodarone
chronic cholestasis	Chlorpromazine
	Ajmaline
	Troleandomycin
	Tricyclic antidepressants

Source: Adapted from Ref. 2.

Table 3 Correlation Between the Percentages of Adverse Drug Reactions and of Prescriptions in Subjects Over 65 Years of Age

Drug	Adverse drug reactions (%)	Prescriptions (%)	Reactions/ prescriptions ratio
Zimelidine	24	24	1.00
Co-trimoxazole	40	34	1.18
Cimetidine	32	27	1.18
Sulindac	50	37	1.32
Carbamazipine	18	17	1.05
Nitrofurantoin	43	30	1.43
Chlorpromazine	20	32	0.63
Hydralazine	37	55	0.67
Phenytoin	12	23	0.52
Naproxen	37	37	1.00
Piroxicam	20	44	0.45
OVERALL	30	32	0.94

Source: Adapted from Ref. 7.

tion are metabolic pathways which are low or deficient in some subjects, making them more susceptible to the toxic effects of various drugs (8).

Mechanisms of Drug Hepatotoxicity

Drug toxicity can be induced by the compound itself, a stable metabolite, or a reactive metabolite. The formation of chemically reactive metabolites by oxidation mediated by cytochromes P-450 or in few cases by reduction may lead to three main initial molecular lesions: covalent binding to proteins and nucleic acids, covalent binding to lipids and lipid peroxidation produced by free radicals, or activated oxygen and glutathione depletion (9,10).

Most of the toxic agents induce liver damage in a predictable dose-dependent manner and can be considered as true (predictable) hepatotoxins. However, a few compounds produce hepatic injury only in unusually susceptible humans and have been named idiosyncrasy-dependent unpredictable toxins. Idiosyncrasy toxicity can be related either to an unusual metabolism or to an immunoallergic phenomenon (Table 4). It is observed in a very small proportion of the patients taking the drug. Metabolic idiosyncrasy is related to the conversion of the drug into a reactive metabolite produced by and directly toxic to hepatocytes. Susceptible individuals produce abnormally high levels of reactive metabolites from a given drug. This high concentration may result from various situations, including induction with a potent inducer as shown by the toxicity of isoniazid in patients receiving rifampicin (11).

Table 4 Features of Metabolic and Immunoallergic Idiosyncrasies

	Metabolic idiosyncrasy	Immunoallergic idiosyncrasy
Treatment with enzyme inducers	increased hepatotoxicity	no effect
Duration of administration	1 week - 12 months or more	1-5 weeks
Hypersensitivity treatment	absent	present
Delay after readministration	unchanged	reduced
Circulating autoantibodies	absent	present in some cases

Source: Adapted from Ref. 2.

Some features of immunoallergic hepatitis are given in Table 4. Supposedly, this type of hepatitis results from the formation of a complex between a reactive metabolite and a macromolecule, which behaves as a hapten and induces an immune reaction. In several instances, autoantibodies directed against normal cellular constituents are detected (12). In some cases autoantibodies recognize specifically the cytochrome P-450 enzyme responsible for oxidation of the toxic drug (13,14).

Mechanisms of Detoxication

Detoxication can be performed by endogenous and/or exogenous mechanisms (9,10,15,16). The different ways of protection include prevention of metabolic activation, interaction with receptor binding, supply of antioxidants and radical scavengers, and stabilization of membranes.

The hepatocyte possesses several mechanisms of defense against toxic compounds, which can act simultaneously: (1) autoinactivation of cytochrome P-450 enzymes, (2) inactivation of reactive epoxides by epoxide hydrolases or conjugation with glutathione, (3) reduction of lipid peroxidation by glutathione, glutathione peroxidase, glutathione S-transferases, and vitamins E and C.

A variety of exogenous compounds have been proposed as hepatoprotective agents. Many chemicals may function as inhibitors of cytochrome P-450-dependent monooxygenases. Some of them, like SKF-525A, piperonylbutoxide, and α-naphtoflavone are of limited interest because of their own toxicity. Others, however, like metyrapone, cimetidine, and disulfiram and its metabolite, diethyldithiocarbamate, can be used as an antidotal principle in human intoxications.

A number of naturally occurring or synthetic molecules have been tested as antioxidants in order to limit lipid peroxidation induced by hepatotoxic substances. Naturally occurring antioxidants include vitamins C and E, prostaglandins, and certain substances of plant origin such as flavonoids and silymarin. Synthetic antioxidants include butylated hydroxyanisole and butylated hydroxytoluene. During recent years, the protective effects of malotilate (diisopropyl-1,3-dithiol-2-ylidene malonate) have been reported in various experimental models, including hepatotoxicity due to paracetamol, galactosamine, and CCl_4 (17).

THE IN VITRO LIVER MODELS

The most frequently used isolated liver preparations include isolated perfused organ, tissue slices, subcellular fractions, and isolated and cultured liver cells.

Isolated Perfused Organ

The isolated perfused liver represents the closest in vitro model of the in vivo situation. The major advantages are that the tridimentional architecture is preserved and that bile flow can be collected and analyzed separately. However, this model system is delicate to handle; it must be oxygenated and the pH continuously recorded. A well-perfused liver has an homogeneous aspect and color and its physiological integrity and stability during perfusion can be evaluated by morphological, biochemical, and metabolic criteria. Functional integrity is retained for only a few hours and analysis of various experimental conditions is not possible from a single organ.

Tissue Slices

The liver slice was one of the first preparations used to study in vitro liver metabolism (18). In this system, tissue organization and cell-cell and cell-matrix interactions are maintained; however, bile secretion cannot be analyzed separately. Liver slices fell into relative disuse because of their major limitations owing to the release of cytolytic enzymes from damaged cells and the poor penetration of oxygen and nutrients to the center of the slice. Recently, this model system has regained interest owing to improved methods for its preparation and maintenance. Slices of consistent dimension and thickness with minimal tissue trauma can be prepared using a newly designed tissue slicer (19,20). Cell viability and function appear to be maintained for several hours. Biotransformation of halothane through both oxidative and reductive pathways by male guinea pig liver slices over a 6-hr period has been recently reported (21). This system could have a significant impact on the study of in vitro liver functions from human liver biopsies, provided that various functions are properly preserved for a prolonged period.

Subcellular Fractions

Homogenates, microsomes, and purified organelles can be prepared from whole organs or liver pieces. These models can be obtained from animals pretreated by inducers and are useful to study the mechanisms of hepatotoxicity. Microsomes are widely used to identify drug metabolic pathways, covalent binding, and lipid peroxidation induced by hepatotoxins. Isolated mitochondria are widely used in the study of the effects of toxicants on cellular energy transformation.

Liver Cells

Isolated and Cultured Hepatocytes

Liver cells were first obtained from explant cultures. However, the proliferating cell population was consistently a mixture of various cell types, with fibroblasts and undifferentiated epithelial cells being the most abundant when explants of adult liver tissue were put in culture (22).

A considerable step forward in obtaining intact adult hepatocytes was made by the introduction of collagenase and hyaluronidase as dissociating agents (23). Berry and Friend (24) established the basic protocol involving a two-step perfusion of the liver in situ, first with calcium-free buffer, followed by a calcium-supplemented buffer containing collagenase. This protocol primarily developed for the disaggregation of the adult rat liver is now used with slight modifications to isolate hepatocytes from various species, including man (25,26). These cells can be further separated into subpopulations. Perivenous or periportal hepatocytes can be obtained by selective destruction of the periportal or perivenous part of the microcirculation by digitonin perfusion before applying the basic collagenase method (27,28). Hepatocyte subpopulations according to their degree of ploidy are prepared by counterflow centrifugation (29,30). The two-step collagenase perfusion method yields large numbers of viable parenchymal cells, which retain responsiveness to signals to which they reacted prior to liver dissociation. Regarding adult human hepatocytes, a number of factors may be responsible for conspicuous individual variations in cellular functions. In addition to sex, age, liver diseases and genetic polymorphisms, premedication, and the nutritional status of the donor as well as the duration and the conditions of liver preservation before cell disruption may greatly influence the metabolic activities of freshly isolated human hepatocytes. Viable parenchymal cells can be obtained 10-20 h after hypothermic organ preservation in the University of Wisconsin solution (unpublished observations).

Dear Book or CD Buyer,

Thank you for your purchase from Research Triangle Books. We aim to provide a wide variety of books and CDs, give accurate descriptions, package items well, and ship quickly. Your satisfaction is our goal.

If you have any problems, please contact us via Amazon, and please check that our response is not in your Spam folder. Or you can contact us directly at researchtrianglebooks@gmail.com . You may also contact us directly if you have questions about other items that you are looking for. If you must return an item, please try to reuse the original shipping materials if possible.

Please note: New, sealed, CDs and DVDs cannot be returned after opening them, unless there is a manufacturing problem with them, so please make sure that you have the correct item before opening.

Lastly, we ask that you provide seller feedback when requested by Amazon, or you may do it now by clicking "My Account" and "Leave seller feedback".

Bob and MJ

The advantages of the use of freshly isolated hepatocytes are the homogeneity of the suspension, functional similarities with the in vivo state, and the ability to analyze multiple parameters from a single cell suspension. However, freshly isolated hepatocytes do not survive in suspension for more than a few hours. Moreover, their functional capacity is quite dependent on the composition of the incubation medium. In an amino acid-free medium, the cells are in a strongly negative nitrogen balance owing to the rate of protein synthesis which is 10 times lower than that of protein degradation (31). The protein anabolic state is maintained by using a medium containing a balanced mixture of amino acids (32). The survival of isolated hepatocytes is increased by immobilization in alginate gels (33) or by microencapsulation (34).

Hepatocyte Function in Conventional Culture Conditions To survive for prolonged periods parenchymal cells must be put in culture. A number of studies have shown that rodent hepatocytes survive for only a few days and are very unstable in conventional culture conditions, rapidly losing their most differentiated functions (35-37). Complete loss of some functions and attenuation of others occur within a few days. At the same time, the cells begin to express fetallike functions such as fetal isozymes and alpha-fetoprotein (38, 39). After 24 h in culture, the rates of transcription of liver-specific genes drop to between 1 and 10% of those found in the liver (40,41). Early phenotypic changes affect particularly cytochrome P-450 content and related enzymes. Cytochrome P-450 concentration decreases approximately 50% during the first 24-48 h in rodent hepatocytes (42-45). Several immunoblotting analyses have shown that cytochrome P-450 enzymes are differently affected and that changes are dependent on the composition of the culture medium (46-48). Even when decreased several cytochrome P-450 enzymes may respond to inducers in vitro (49-54). The response can, however, be different from that observed in vivo (55). Functional alterations occur later and are less dramatic in human hepatocytes than in their rodent counterparts (56, 57). More than 50% of the initial cytochrome P-450 content is still present after 1 week of culture and all cytochrome P-450 enzymes analyzed (i.e., IA, IIC, IIE, and IIIA) are expressed (57,58). Moreover, specific inductions were demonstrated with rifampicin, phenobarbital, 3-methylcholanthrene, and omeprazole (57,59,60). As found in vivo rifampicin controls expression of cytochrome P-450 IIIA at the transcriptional level (60).

A different profile is observed for glutathione S-transferases (GST) which catalyze the conjugation of electrophilic metabolites. After an initial decrease (61,62), GST activity remains relatively stable or shows a moderate or strong increase in rat hepatocytes, depending on the composition of the culture medium (61). These variations are associated with changes in the GST subunit profile (63-65). A much lower decrease, if any, was found by Croci and Williams (66) using different culture conditions. By contrast, no increase in

GST activity is observed after the initial decrease in cultured human hepatocytes (67).

Another way to demonstrate the preservation of functional drug-metabolizing enzymes in cultured hepatocytes is to identify metabolites formed from various drugs. The results are in accordance with investigations on drug-metabolizing enzyme activities. Short-term hepatocyte cultures retain their capability of metabolizing drugs through phase I and phase II pathways (68-75).

Factors Influencing Hepatocyte Function In Vitro In the early years, it was assumed that phenotypic changes resulting in preferential loss of the most differentiated functions represent adaptative responses of hepatocytes to an inappropriate environment. A number of studies have dealt with the definition of suitable culture conditions and have led to the conclusion that three groups of factors can affect cellular functions in vitro: soluble factors, extracellular matrix components, and cell-cell interactions. The influence of the different factors has been discussed in a recent review (76).

Exogenous Soluble Factors A variety of soluble factors have been tested, which comprises hormones, growth factors, and trace elements. Hormones have a beneficial effect on hepatocyte survival and function. Cell survival is increased several days in the presence of corticosteroids (77). Better preserved functions include drug-metabolizing enzymes (78) and plasma protein production (79). Improved functions probably result from messenger ribonucleic acid (mRNA) stabilization (80). Deoxyribonucleic acid (DNA) synthesis can be stimulated by various soluble factors, particularly in the presence of epidermal growth factor combined with insulin and pyruvate (81).

Various nonphysiological soluble factors also enhance hepatocyte survival and function in vitro. They include ligands such as metyrapone and isonicotinamide (82), drug inducers such as phenobarbital (83,84) and clofibrate (54,85), and solvents such as dimethyl sulphoxide (86). The most significant effects were obtained with this last compound added at a concentration of 2% (86,87).

Extracellular Matrix Components The influence of extracellular matrix components has been widely explored. The efficiency of attachment of hepatocytes and longevity of cultures are increased when the cells are cultured in plastic dishes coated with matrix proteins (88-90). However, in general, liver-specific functions are not well preserved. In fact, it is now clear that maintenance of hepatocellular functions requires the preservation of the globular cell shape (37,91,92).

The best ways hitherto proposed to preserve the shape of hepatocytes are the Matrigel support and the "sandwich" method. When seeded on Matrigel, a laminin-rich gel matrix isolated from a mouse sarcoma, rat hepatocytes retain a spherical shape and exhibit remarkably enhanced expression of various liver-specific functions (93-95). However, the significance of Matrigel effects is difficult to interpret, since contamination with hormones and/or growth factors cannot be ruled out with certainty. Rat hepatocytes also maintain a high albumin secretion rate for more than 40 days when cultured between two layers of type I collagen (96). It would be of interest to determine whether in this last model drug-metabolizing enzymes are preserved and whether other matrix proteins, particularly basement membranes, are more effective if used instead of type I collagen.

Cell-Cell Interactions The liver being an organ composed of many cell types, both homotypic and heterotypic interactions may influence hepatocellular functions (92). When placed in pure culture hepatocytes reaggregate but intercellular communication by way of gap junctions disappears within a few hours (97). Various functions are dependent upon cell density, but whether at low density or at high density hepatocytes show comparable survival times and exhibit phenotypic changes in standard culture conditions, indicating that homotypic interactions are not critical in the maintenance of specific functions in vitro.

The first attempts to coculture hepatocytes with other cell types, either sinusoidal cells (98) or human fibroblasts (99), were not convincing. A considerable step forward in long-term maintenance of functional hepatocytes was made by adding another liver epithelial cell type (100). Indeed, when cocultured with untransformed rat epithelial cells probably derived from biliary primitive cells, hepatocytes from various species, including man, and from adults and fetuses (100-104) survive for several weeks and retain high functional capacities (68,100,105-109). Cocultured hepatocytes retain the capability of transcribing specific genes (41) and of communicating by way of gap junctions (110,111). Coculturing parenchymal cells with various nonhepatic epithelial and mesenchymal cell lines has also been reported to favor in vitro maintenance of liver functions (112,113). Whether the primary signal which involves an integral plasma membrane glycoprotein present on both liver cell types (114) also exists when other cells are used instead of epithelial liver cells has not been investigated yet. Moreover, it would be important to determine whether hepatocytes can be easily separated from these different cell types as shown with liver epithelial cells (41). Specific functions are also better preserved in hepatocytes cultured in aggregates. These structures contain nonparenchymal cells, leading to the conclusion that they mimic the coculture system (115,116). Interestingly, an earlier deposition of matrix proteins is observed in coculture (100,101). In addition, medium composition may greatly affect liver functions. As a rule, some qualitative and quantitative changes still occur and the reappearance of fetallike functions is not totally prevented (65).

Liver Cell Lines

Liver cell lines can be obtained from hepatomas or transfected hepatocytes. However, none of the established liver cell lines has maintained all the liver-specific markers.

Hepatoma cell lines are difficult to establish from primary carcinomas and exhibit only some of the characteristics of normal liver. When present, foreign chemical-metabolizing activities are usually low. Moreover, their levels are depending on the composition of the medium and may vary with time in culture. However, some rat hepatoma cell lines after cloning have been reported to express phenobarbital-inducible cytochromes P-450 (117, 118).

Another approach is to immortalize liver cells by transfecting viral and cellular DNA. Cell lines have been obtained after transfection with the SV40 virus or adenovirus. Again, only some liver-specific functions are expressed and they are not stable in vitro (119).

USE OF IN VITRO LIVER MODELS IN TOXICITY TESTING

State of the Art

The use of in vitro liver systems for toxicity studies has received increased attention in recent years. The number of published investigations of a toxicological nature is probably over a thousand. Freshly isolated suspensions and primary cultures of hepatocytes represent the most popular models. These are used for comparing the relative toxicity of different classes of chemicals and studying mechanisms of action of hepatotoxins (120-125). Toxicity effects are assessed using various unspecific and/or specific endpoints.

Indicators of Cytotoxicity

As listed above (Table 1), hepatotoxic agents can reduce a variety of lesions. A wide array of morphological and biochemical markers are available for obtaining information at the cellular and molecular levels in order to detect and measure chemical-induced perturbations. They have been recently analyzed in detail by Tyson and Green (126), and will only be summarized here. The main cytotoxic indices are displayed in Table 5. They may be classified as unspecific and liver-specific parameters.

Unspecific criteria may monitor membrane integrity, subcellular perturbations, and metabolic activities. Indicators for membrane integrity include cell count, trypan blue exclusion, enzyme leakage, and membrane permeability for ions or small molecules. The trypan blue exclusion test is widely used, basically as an estimation of the percentage of viable cells in freshly isolated hepatocyte suspensions. Several enzymes are used for monitoring

Table 5 Quantitative Indicators for Cytotoxicity Evaluation

- Unspecific criteria
- Membrane integrity
  - cell viability
    - cell count,
    - trypan blue exclusion test
    - intracellular LDH content
    - enzyme leakage:
      - LDH; transaminases
  - membrane permeability perturbations
    - leakage of intracellular ions or small molecules:
      - K^+ content, Ca^{2+} flux
    - intracellular accumulation of external molecules:
      - ^{51}Cr; succinate
  - subcellular perturbations
      - mitochondria
      - MTT test: reduction of a formozan salt
      - ATP content
    - membrane-bound and free ribosomes
      - protein synthesis
    - lysosomes
      - neutral red uptake
  - metabolite competence
    - total protein synthesis
    - lactate/pyruvate ratio
    - glutathione content
    - lipid peroxidation
    - covalent binding
- Liver-specific criteria
  - protein synthesis: plasma proteins like albumin
  - urea synthesis
  - lipoprotein synthesis
  - peroxisome proliferation
  - cytochrome P-450 induction/inhibition
  - bile acids secretion

the loss of plasma membrane integrity. The percentage of lactate dehydrogenase (LDH) release correlates better than that of other enzymes with morphological changes observed by phase-contrast microscopy examination and cell viability assessed by trypan blue exclusion (127,128). This parameter is, however, often much less reliable and sensitive when human hepatocytes are concerned and measurement of intracellular LDH activity is preferred (129, 130) (Fig. 1). Intracellular LDH content is also used as an index of hepatocyte number (90,131). Increased plasma membrane permeability usually precedes loss of cell viability. K^+ release, and Ca^{2+} influx are sensitive endpoints but require more sophisticated techniques of measurement.

Subcellular alterations can be selectively visualized by electron microscopic examination. However, it is a time-consuming and expensive approach which should be used appropriately. The functional markers of organelle perturba-

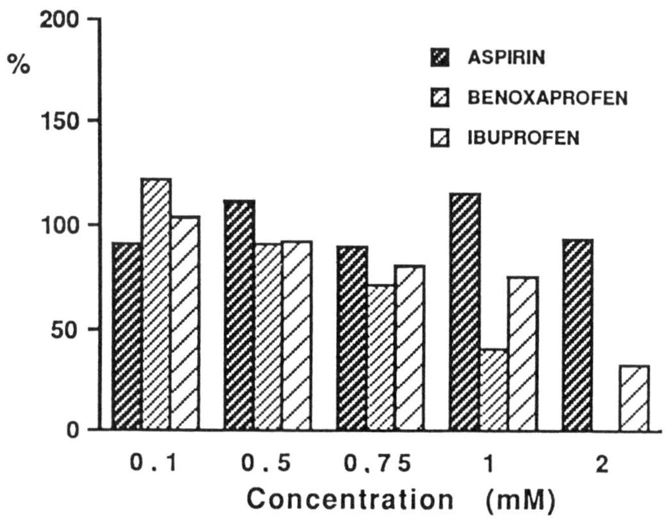

Figure 1 Effects of nonsteroidal antiinflammatory agents on intracellular LDH content of human hepatocyte cultures. The cells prepared by the two-step collagenase perfusion method were allowed to acclimate in culture for about 15 hrs before exposure to various concentrations of drugs. The three compounds were solubilized in dimethyl sulphoxide (final concentration of solvent: 0.5%). LDH content was measured in cell homogenates after a 24-h exposure. Aspirin, used a reference compound, was not toxic. Benoxaprofen, known to be more hepatotoxic than ibuprofen in vivo, was also more cytotoxic in vitro. The values are expressed as percent of controls; they are means of two independent experiments in duplicate.

tion include MTT reduction by mitochondrial dehydrogenases, neutral red uptake by lysosomes, and total protein synthesis which involves both mitochondria as energy producers, and free and bound ribosomes. MTT and neutral red tests are widely used as nonspecific endpoints, the latter being frequently more sensitive. Other metabolic indicators such as glutathione content, lipid peroxidation, and covalent binding are not organelle specific.

Liver-specific criteria may include production of plasma proteins like albumin and acute phase proteins, glycogen synthesis (132), urea synthesis (133), induction or inhibition of specific cytochrome P-450 enzymes (134), and proliferation of peroxisomes associated with the induction of the peroxisomal β-oxidation pathway (135). These criteria are usually more sensitive than unspecific endpoints; some of them can be assessed on living cultures (e.g., albumin secretion rate). However, there is no single indicator for metabolic competence. An example is given by protein synthesis and urea synthesis. Cycloheximide inhibits protein synthesis but not urea synthesis, whereas norvaline does the opposite (136).

Toxicity Studies

Screening of Toxic Chemicals Isolated hepatocytes, either in suspension or in culture, represent a unique experimental approach to screen various compounds at several concentrations using different criteria on the same cell suspension. Most of the tests can be carried out in 96-well plates with only around 30,000 cells per well while 4 to 6×10^8 and 10^9 or more viable hepatocytes can be obtained from a single rat or human liver, respectively (26, 137). Various tests can be miniaturized and automatized (138). Dose-response curves are calculated from the results obtained, then the results are summarized as IC^{50} values; i.e., the concentrations of test chemicals which modify the response of test wells by 50%. The IC^{50} value is considered to be the best indicator of in vitro cytotoxicity, since it is taken from the middle of the dose-response curve (139).

Most studies have been carried out over a short period of time not exceeding 24 h and the addition of a single dose of the test chemical. Comparison of the data obtained with hepatocytes in suspension or in monolayer culture with those obtained with nonhepatic cells like HeLa cells indicates that hepatocytes are usually more sensitive to compounds that require metabolic activation (140). Normal hepatocytes are also often more sensitive than hepatoma cells, which exhibit only some drug-metabolizing enzyme activities (138). In general, the in vitro-in vivo correspondence in discriminating between hepatotoxicants and nonhepatotoxicants is good. Tyson et al. (141) investigated 23 chemicals and found good correspondence for all but two, thioacetamide and allyl alcohol, using enzyme release to evaluate toxicity. Story et al. (127) came to the same conclusion by studying 34 compounds. Inconsistancies can be related to the nature of the chemical tested, the incubation conditions, and the endpoint selected.

Volatile and liposoluble compounds require appropriate culture conditions. Interestingly, the relative hepatotoxic potentials for five haloalkanes measured in hepatocyte suspensions and in vivo were ranked correctly if partition coefficients were factored into the data to reconcile the differences between solvent volatility and retention in the two systems (142).

The lack of extrahepatic release of toxic compounds and accumulation of compounds in the culture medium may cause major problems as emphasized by Paine and Hockin (143). These authors studied the effects of three groups of toxins on cultured rat hepatocytes maintained in conditions that resulted in either a low or a high concentration of cytochrome P-450. As predicted, toxins which are not metabolized by cytochrome P-450, i.e., ethionine and galactosamine, were equally toxic regardless of the cytochrome P-450 concentration. In contrast, the behavior of the two other groups of toxins was not predictable. Indeed, compounds that are activated by cytochrome P-450 (carbon tetrachloride, bromobenzene, cyclophosphamide, paracetamol) and those which are detoxifed by cytochrome P-450 (pentobarbital, strychnine) were also equally toxic regardless of the cytochrome P-450 content of the cells after a 24-h incubation. Only when the exposure was limited to 1-4 h and followed by a 20-h incubation in a toxin-free medium was carbon tetrachloride more toxic to cultured hepatocytes containing high levels of cytochrome P-450. The problem of accumulation of toxic metabolites into the culture medium could be overcome by coculturing rat hepatocytes with fibroblasts (144,145). The toxicity of cyclophosphamide to fibroblasts as judged by the 50% inhibition growth was obtained at a concentration of 16 μg/ml and > 500 μg/ml in the presence and absence of adult hepatocytes, respectively (120).

A single endpoint can be insufficient to evaluate xenobiotic cytotoxicity. Vonen and Morland (146) were unable to demonstrate in vitro inhibition of protein synthesis by oxytetracycline and proposed to select at least two endpoints; i.e., LDH release and protein synthesis to screen hepatotoxins. Arising from various studies there is now the consensus that for any one in vivo response no one test but a battery of two or more in vitro techniques, each reflecting one or two features of the in vivo changes, is likely to be necessary.

The presentation of biological data as numerical scores raises the problem of their interpretation. The suitability of in vitro hepatocyte preparations as a screen procedure early in drug development is certainly more convincing when structurally related chemicals are ranked. Each test has its own control substances, treated in exactly the same conditions, thereby overcoming the problem of variability of nearly all biological changes. Good examples from our laboratory include neuroleptic agents (128), macrolides (134), and nonsteroidal antiinflammatory agents (Fig. 1). It is interesting to note that drugs associated with human hepatotoxicity are generally more cytotoxic to rat or human hepatocytes in vitro.

However, short-term assays do not reflect the common in vivo situation in which drugs often induce liver damage after repeated administration for weeks or months. Hepatocyte cocultures have been used to mimic such a situation (147,148). Various drug concentrations can be tested, starting when cell confluency is reached and being renewed daily. The highest concentration used is the maximum nontoxic dose defined after a 24-h incubation of the drug with pure hepatocyte cultures. Since rat liver epithelial cells employed in coculture do not metabolize drugs, comparison of the effects of similar drug concentrations on pure cultures of these cells make it possible to determine whether a drug requires biotransformation in order to be cytotoxic. Depending on the compound tested, four different situations can be observed: (1) no cytotoxicity to both cell types; (2) only hepatocytes are damaged; (3) only rat liver epithelial cells are damaged; and (4) both cell types are sensitive to the drug (76). As found in acute toxicity testing, major differences in the sensitivity of endpoints can be observed (147).

Studies on Mechanisms of Action of Hepatotoxins The majority of toxicity studies have dealt with the aspects of the mechanisms of action of hepatotoxins and there is now a substantial body of evidence of similarity of response between in vivo and in vitro studies as far as intrinsic hepatotoxins are concerned (120-122,125,149). The major limitations of in vitro liver preparations for studying mechanisms of cytotoxicity have already been stated for screening studies. They are related to the differential unstability of drug-metabolizing enzymes and other liver-specific functions in vitro. Indeed, as seen in the first part of the chapter, the toxicity of a large number of xenobiotics is mediated through production of reactive metabolites. This production is dependent on a balance of activation and inactivation pathways.

The requirement for a metabolizing system for activation of chemicals has been met by use of a liver 9000-g supernatant fraction fortified with cofactors. The inhibition of cell division of an undifferentiated cell line (V-79 chinese hamster fibroblasts) which does not express P-450-related enzymes has been used as the endpoint of cytotoxicity (150,151). Several compounds that are converted to cytotoxic reactive metabolites have been evaluated in this coincubation system (151,152).

However, many investigators have preferred to use liver slices or isolated hepatocytes in an attempt to mimic more closely the metabolite pattern in vivo and so obtain a more realistic impression of the role of metabolism in cytotoxicity. Many examples have been reported showing similar toxin-induced biochemical changes in vivo and in vitro; these include toxicity induced by carbon tetrachloride (153), galactosamine (154), bromobenzene (155), thioacetamide (156), and paracetamol (157). Marked species differences in susceptibility to paracetamol have been reproduced in vitro (158).

The reactive metabolites are often strong electrophils, leading to irreversible alkylation of cellular macromolecules, which are the first events in a reaction cascade responsible for the acute direct hepatotoxic effects. Obviously, measurement of total covalent binding does not permit discrimination among potentially critical individual arylated protein targets. Up to now, the target molecules which interact with reactive metabolites have received little attention. Alkylation of proteins by reactive metabolites is, however, not random but highly selective. Thus, cysteine residues represent primary target sites for arylation by the electrophilic metabolite of paracetamol, suggesting that proteins rich in free thiols could be particularly vulnerable to paracetamol-induced cellular damage (159). Two proteins of 44 kD and 58 kD, respectively, have been identified to be covalently associated with paracetamol metabolites by using antibodies directed against paracetamol-bound proteins (160).

Studies of Idiosyncratic Toxins Since their drug metabolic equipment can be easily manipulated by exposure to inducers and inhibitors, in vitro systems are particularly useful to determine whether qualitative and/or quantitative alterations in the drug-metabolism profile, i.e., changes in the balance of activation/inactivation pathways, can affect the degree of drug cytotoxicity. Consequently, these models could be used to understand idiosyncratic drug reactions related to metabolism and drug interactions.

Whether in vitro liver preparations can also be used to study idiosyncratic drug toxicity related to the involvement of immune mechanisms may be questioned. A first approach was proposed, which consists in using hepatocytes from pretreated rabbits and in analyzing the cytotoxic effects of sera from patients with drug-induced hepatitis. Successful results were obtained with methyldopa (161) and halothane (162). Absorbed sera gave consistently negative results when tested with normal hepatocytes and frequent positive results when tested with cells previously exposed to the drug. These observations suggest that administration of methyldopa or halothane to rabbits could generate neoantigenic determinants on hepatocyte plasma membranes which are very similar, if not identical, to those generated in the patients with hepatitis induced by the corresponding drug (163). These antibodies appear to be remarkably specific, since negative results were obtained with sera from patients with hepatitis of other origin.

However, the use of nonhuman hepatocytes could have some limitation, since metabolic pathways are often different in humans. This led Siproudhis et al. (164) to use human hepatocytes to determine whether specific circulating antibodies from patients with drug-induced immunoallergic hepatitis could be involved in antibody-dependent cell-mediated cytotoxicity. Clometacin, a drug responsible for several immunologically induced hepatitis cases, was tested. Normal human hepatocytes were incubated with clometacin in the presence of autologous lymphoid cells and then with sera from patients with clometacin-induced hepatitis. Hepatocyte injury was consistently observed, characterized by morphological alterations and a decrease in intracellular cytosolic enzyme activity (Fig. 2). Since sera were preabsorbed with autologous normal hepatocytes, it is likely that the antigen recognized by circulating antibodies was a plasma membrane molecule modified by or linked to a metabolite of clometacin. All the studies suggest that in vitro liver systems could be a suitable tool to identify the nature of the antigen recognized in circulating autoantibodies in drug-induced immunoallergic hepatitis.

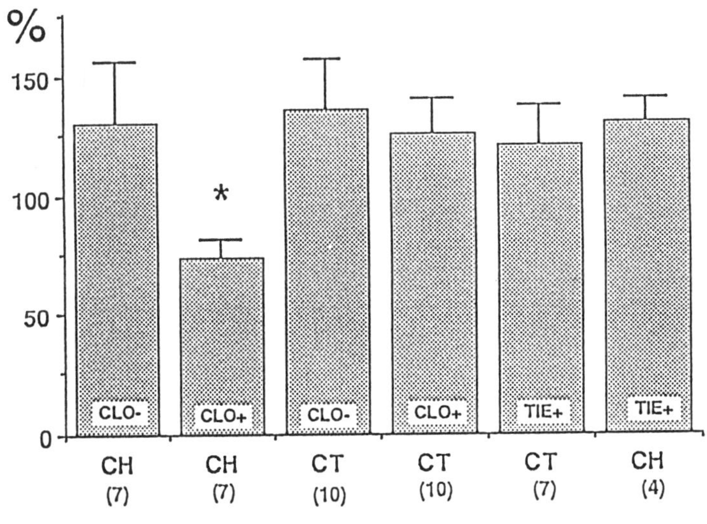

Figure 2 Cytotoxicity of sera with clometacin-induced immunoallergic hepatitis to human hepatocytes previously exposed in vitro to the drug in the presence of autologous lymphoid cells. Cytotoxicity effects were estimated by determination of intracellular LDH content. 100% correspond to LDH amount in control hepatocyte cultures. Addition of lymphoid cells resulted in an increase in LDH content (values > 100%). Cocultures of normal human hepatocytes and autologous lymphoid cells were pretreated (+) or not (−) with clometacin (CLO) or tienilic acid (TIE), another drug responsible for immunoallergic hepatitis. Addition of sera from clometacin-induced hepatitis (CH) but not sera from controls (CT) results in a decrease in intracellular LDH content. The values are mean ± SD (*$p < 0.05$). The number of sera tested is given in parentheses. (From Ref. 164.)

Studies of Genotoxic Compounds In vitro liver models have also long been used to assess the genotoxic potential of chemical and physical agents on the basis of their ability to covalently bind to and damage DNA, induce DNA repair responses, mutate specific genetic loci, induce phenotypically altered cells, or induce chromosome- or chromatid-level aberrations (165, 166). For chemicals, their metabolism of procarcinogens to a carcinogenic form is frequently a necessary prerequisite.

Since they can provide monooxygenase activity to metabolize chemicals to their genotoxic forms, cell-free systems such as liver 9000-g supernatant fractions or microsomal fractions supplied with NADPH-generating systems are widely recognized in in vitro mutagenicity testing (167, 168). However, intact cells are preferable, since they retain the critical activation/inactivation balance. This assumption is supported by the observations of Neis et al. (169), who compared the two systems. They studied mutagenicity of two structurally related carcinogenic arylamines, (i.e., benzidine and 4-aminobiphenyl) and found that the mutagenic responses with hepatocytes used for metabolic activation was more closely related to those obtained with animals. The difference was due to the lack of N-acetylation activity in the microsomal fraction.

Rodent hepatocytes have been extensively used. However, because of frequent xenobiotic metabolic differences between rodents and humans, human hepatocytes represent the most logical choice as an in vitro model for genotoxicity investigations. They are well suited for quantitation of DNA repair elicited by exposure to genotoxic agents. The unscheduled DNA synthesis (UDS) assay which requires small numbers of cells has been used to test a number of compounds (166,170,171). Various chemicals have been found to induce UDS in human hepatocytes; they include nitrosamines, 2-acetylaminofluorene, benzo(a)pyrene, aflatoxin B_1 and dinitropyrenes. Aflatoxin B_1, a suspected human hepatocarcinogen, induces an UDS response at or below 1 μM.

Surprisingly, the UDS response is usually quite similar in human and rat hepatocytes (172), whereas marked differences are found when human hepatocytes are compared to monkey, mouse, or hamster parenchymal cells (170, 172). Only a few chemicals, including cimetidine (173), b-naphthylamine (171), 2,6-diaminotoluene (171), and 5-methylchrysene (171), have been reported to give a qualitative different response between the rodent and human cells.

A major link interfering with the direct study of liver carcinogenesis in vitro is the lack of systems in which clonal growth of hepatocytes can be maintained. Consequently, direct mutagenesis assays are not possible. To obviate this difficulty, investigators have used cocultures of hepatocytes with human fibroblasts (174) or V-79 Chinese hamster fibroblasts (175). A dose-dependent induced mutagenesis was demonstrated for diethylnitrosamine by quantification of mutations at the hypoxanthine-guanine phosphoribosyltransferase locus of human skin fibroblasts (174). Moore and Gould (175) reported the mutagenic activation of benzo(a)pyrene by human hepatocytes in the presence of V-79 cells.

The hepatocyte-mediated induction of sister chromatin exchange was used by Green et al. (176). Dimethylnitrosamine induced significant sister chromatid exchange in V-79 or CHO cells cocultured with hepatocytes.

Assessment of Cytoprotection In Vitro Isolated hepatocytes either in suspension or in primary culture have been widely used to analyze the effects of hepatoprotective agents. Various antioxidants and scavengers of free radicals have been tested and found to act as described in vivo. During recent years in vitro preparations have also been used to evaluate new naturally occurring substances of plant origin and synthetic compounds (Table 6). These studies have led to the selection of the most active molecules and have shown that the beneficial effects could be dependent on the toxin. In addition, structure-activity correlations have been sometimes established and a few molecules have been reported to have their own toxicity (177,179,181). Species differences have been demonstrated. Thus (+)-cyanidanol-3 was effective on rat hepatocytes intoxicated by aflatoxin B_1 when added at least 5 min before the mycotoxin but was without effect on human hepatocytes (179). However, the significance of in vivo and in vitro experimental data to the human situation may be questioned. Indeed potential antidotes have to be added before or just after toxin administration to be effective. Such conditions do not always mimic the human situation. In vitro repeated exposure to the hepatoprotective agent should be more appropriate to test the drug effect on chronic liver diseases as expected with malotilate. This compound was reported to protect rats intoxicated with carbon tetrachloride (17,182) when administered before or simultaneously with the toxin, but it was without effect on rat or human hepatocytes even after repeated treatment in vitro (180). These in vitro observations were recently confirmed by a multicenter clinical trial that showed no significant improvement of active chronic hepatitis in alcoholic patients (personal communication). All these studies indicate that in vitro liver systems are very useful to screen hepatoprotective agents and to analyze their mechanism of action.

Future Developments

In Vitro Models

The advantages and limitations of the different in vitro liver preparations have been extensively illustrated and discussed above. It is likely that the perfused isolated organ and liver slices will remain marginal models. The

Table 6 Effects of Some Hepatoprotective Agents In Vitro

In vitro systems	Compound tested	Results	References
Rat hepatocytes after 24 h in primary culture exposed to CCl_4 or D-galactosamine (D-gal)	Titerpenoid saponins added with the toxin	After 60 min reduced toxicity of CCl_4; no effect on D-gal toxicity	177
Isolated rat hepatocytes $+CCl_4$	Cyranin incubated for 10 min with CCl_4	Decreased release of transaminases	178
Rat hepatocytes in primary culture + aflatoxin B_1 (AFB_1) for 24 h	(+)-Cyanidanol-3 added at least 5 min before AFB_1	Decreased release of LDH	179
Human hepatocytes in primary culture	(+)-Cyanidanol-3 on AFB_1 toxicity	No effect	179
Cocultures of rat or human hepatocytes	Malotilate added daily for 10-20 days	No effect on hepatocyte survival and albumin production; decrease in collagen synthesis	180
Rat hepatocytes after 24 h in primary culture exposed to CCl_4 or D-gal	Lignoids added with the toxin	Some lignoids reduce CCl_4 toxicity, others decrease D-gal toxicity	181

isolated liver is difficult to handle, but it is the model of choice to analyze bile secretion. However, the use of hepatocyte couplets obtained by partial collagenase digestion of the liver, which retain their structural and functional polarity, could increase studies on toxicity directed toward the hepatobiliary system (183). Hepatocyte couplets have been shown to extensively secrete fluorescent cholephils into sealed canalicular spaces (183,184). The advantage of liver slices will remain related to the fact that the cells express specific functions for several hours (20), and that this system is easily applicable to liver tissue available from biopsies, surgical resections, or whole organs. Further developments of in vitro models will concern mainly isolated normal hepatocytes and liver cell lines.

Isolated Normal Hepatocytes Whatever the culture conditions used, adult hepatocytes do not remain functionally stable in vitro. However, three groups of factors, i.e., soluble factors, extracellular matrix components, and cell-

cell interactions, have been found to improve in vitro maintenance of liver-specific functions. There is a need to devise new experimental conditions which limit decreased transcriptional activity of specific genes and qualitative and quantitative functional changes. Further research should allow significant progress, particularly in devising more suitable defined media.

Although adult hepatocytes do not divide actively, many recent investigations have demonstrated that under appropriate conditions more than 80% of hepatocytes undergo at least one round of replicative DNA synthesis (81, 185). The most active hepatotrophic factors include epidermal growth factor, insulin, and glucagon, factors present in serum from partially hepatectomized rats. The hepatocyte growth factor has been recently cloned and sequenced (186). Stimulated cells can go through mitosis, particularly at low seeding densities (187). Components of the basal medium, especially pyruvate, modulate the response of hepatocytes to growth stimuli in vitro (81). The better knowledge of environmental conditions for hepatocyte culture and the identification of the different factors involved in hepatocyte replication especially those acting at the prereplicative DNA step, should lead to prolonged maintenance of differentiated hepatocytes and more than one cycle of replication. Such improvements would be particularly advantageous to studies in liver toxicology and carcinogenesis.

Another critical problem is the availability of human hepatocytes and hepatocytes from large mammals as well as the preservation of the cells in excess obtained from a single perfusion. We have recently shown that viable cells can be isolated from rat livers stored for 48 h in a cold University of Wisconsin solution which is effective for long-term storage of organs before transplantation. Cell viability is reduced by only 15% compared to cells isolated from unstored organs. When put in culture, hepatocytes from hypothermically preserved organs exhibit only limited functional alterations (188). Similar results have been obtained from human livers stored for 10-20 h (unpublished observations). The University of Wisconsin solution is, however, much less effective in preserving isolated hepatocytes. After a 48-h hypothermic storage in this solution rat hepatocytes show a 30% decreased cell viability and no more than 3% attach to plastic. By contrast, the Leibovitz L-15 medium, a cell culture medium, is suitable for hypothermic preservation of suspensions of freshly isolated hepatocytes for 24 or 48 h (189).

Presently, the only way of storing viable cells for a prolonged period is cryopreservation (190). Most cryopreservation protocols have been devised for rat hepatocytes (191) and the few reports on parenchymal cells from other species, including man are more sensitive to freezing/thawing conditions than their rat counterparts (192-194). By using a well-defined protocol originally designed for rat hepatocytes, we found that more than 50% of animal or human hepatocytes able to attach on plastic and to survive in culture when plated just after isolation still possess these properties after freezing in liquid nitrogen (195). Thawed cells exhibited limited functional alterations (195) and survived for several weeks when maintained in coculture (196). Further studies should allow improvement of the freezing/thawing protocol and subsequent culture conditions following cryopreservation and to determine whether cell recovery results in a selection of hepatocyte subpopulations.

Liver Cell Lines The development of immortalized hepatocyte lines represents a promising alternative to nonreplicating normal hepatocytes. Further progress can be expected with new DNA constructs and more informations on the role of oncogenes in the regulation of growth and liver-specific functions of hepatocytes. Human hepatocyte lines would be the optimal choice, but to our knowledge all immortalized cell lines obtained transiently expressing liver functions are of animal origin.

Establishment of hepatocyte lines from transgenic mouse is a exciting approach. Immortalized fetal hepatocyte lines prepared from the liver before visible pathological changes are not transformed and retain differentiated functions for several months in appropriate culture conditions (197).

In Vitro Toxicity Tests

Interlaboratory validation schemes have been recently set up using common experimental conditions (138) or various in vitro assays (198). The first results indicate that no single protocol (i.e., one culture condition) can be used for testing every compound, and that problems of interpretation can be greatly magnified when tests involving different mechanisms of toxicity or endpoints are compared (199). Obviously, several criteria of cytotoxicity have to be measured simultaneously for cytotoxicity screens of new compounds. When using unspecific indicators some compounds are found to be less toxic in vitro than in vivo (138,200). However, because of its simplicity such an approach appears to be a very useful step in defining the concentration range of a drug that will be selected for further analysis using more specific tests. It must be kept in mind that hepatocytes are generally more sensitive than other cell types than do not significantly metabolize chemicals, and that differences in metabolism of xenobiotics attributable to species, sex, and age may account for much of the difference in the susceptibility to hepatotoxicants. In addition, chemicals can produce liver damage at several orders of magnitude lower than those that cause death (201). Therefore, cytotoxicity screens and studies of mechanisms of cytotoxicity must be performed on well-differentiated hepatocytes, whereas immortalized hepatocyte lines could be suitable to assess genotoxic potential. Moreover, it is obvious that further studies are needed to define more appropriate experimental conditions to test some types of chemicals like volatile ones and formulations.

Further improvements of the freezing/thaving protocol will lead to the establishment of a bank of frozen human hepatocytes, making it possible to analyze genetic polymorphism in vitro and effects of hepatotoxicants in both extensive and poor drug metabolizers. Moreover, since human hepatocytes in culture produce matrix proteins (202) and can be infected with sporozoites of plasmodia (203,204) and with hepatitis B virus (205), they represent a promising experimental model for the development of antifibrotic, antiviral, and schizontocidal drugs.

CONCLUSIONS

Over the last 2 decades in vitro liver preparations have been increasingly used for toxicological studies. Major progress has been made in the development of reproducible methods for the isolation and culture of differentiated hepatocytes from both animal and human origin. Numerous investigations have demonstrated the usefulness of isolated hepatocytes for drug metabolism and cytotoxicity studies using the cells either in suspension or in culture in various experimental conditions. However, some limitations still exist related to the fact that normal hepatocytes exhibit in vitro phenotypic changes and do not actively divide. The major challenges of the next years will include development of experimental conditions for prolonged in vitro maintenance of functionally stable hepatocytes, creation of immortalized, untransformed hepatocytes retaining specific functions, and in vitro testing of non-water-soluble chemicals.

ACKNOWLEDGMENTS

I wish to thank Dr. C. Guguen-Guillouzo for helpful suggestions and Mrs. A. Vannier for typing the manuscript. Studies performed by my colleagues and myself in the INSERM liver Unit in Rennes were supported by the Institut National de la Santé et de la Recherche Médicale, the Ministère de la Recherche, the Association de la Recherche contre le Cancer, the Ligue contre le Cancer, and the Fondation de la Recherche Médicale.

REFERENCES

1. Stricker, B. H. C. H., and Spoelstra, P. (1985). *Drug-Induced Hepatic Injury*. Elsevier, Amsterdam.
2. Benhamou, J. P. (1988). Drug-induced hepatitis: Clinical aspects. In *Liver Cells and Drugs*. A. Guillouzo (Ed.). Les Editions INSERM and John Libbey Eurotext, Paris, pp. 3-12.
3. Zimmerman, H. J. (1978). *Hepatotoxicity: The Adverse Effect of Drugs and Other Chemicals on the Liver*. Appleton-Century-Crofts, New York.
4. Biour, M., Poupon, R., Calmus, Y., Grangé, J. D., Hamel, J. D., Lévy, V. G., Bodin, F., and Cheymol, G. (1988). Hépatotoxicité des médicaments. Mise

à jour du fichier bibliographique des atteintes hépatiques et des médicaments responsables. *Gastroenterol. Clin. Biol.* **12**: 48-60.
5. Pessayre, D., Dolder, A. Artigou, J. Y., Wandscheer, J. C., Descatoire, V., Degott, C., and Benhamou, J. P. (1979). Effect of fasting on metabolite-mediated hepatotoxicity in the rat. *Gastroenterology* **77**: 264-271.
6. Woodhouse, K. W., Mortimer, O., and Wiholm, B. E. (1986). Hepatic adverse drug reactions. In *The Effect of Age in Liver and Aging.* K. Kitani (Ed.), Amsterdam, Elsevier, pp. 75-80.
7. James, O. F. W., Rawlins, M. D., Wynne, H., and Woodhouse, K. W. (1988). The liver, ageing and drugs. In *Liver Cells and Drugs.* A. Guillouzo (Ed.). Les Editions INSERM and John Libbey, Eurotext, Paris, pp. 13-21.
8. Larrey, D., and Pessayre, D. (1988). Genetic factors in hepatotoxicity. In *Liver Cells and Drugs.* A. Guillouzo (Ed.). Les Editions INSERM and John Libbey Eurotext, Paris, pp. 143-152.
9. Guengerich, F. P. (1985). Enzymatic activation of chemicals to toxic metabolites. *CRC Crit. Rev. Toxicol.* **14**: 259-307.
10. Pessayre, D., and Larrey, D. (1988). Mechanisms of drug-induced hepatitis. In *Liver Cells and Drugs.* A. Guillouzo (Ed.). Les Editions INSERM and John Libbey Eurotext, Paris, pp. 129-142.
11. Pessayre, D., Bentata, M., Degott, C., Nouel, O., Miguet, J. P., Rueff, B., and Benhamou, J. P. (1977). Isoniazid-rifampin fulminant hepatitis. A possible consequence of the enhancement of isoniazid hepatotoxicity by enzyme induction. *Gastroenterology* **72**: 284-289.
12. Homberg, J. C., Abuaf, N., Helmy-Khalil, S., Biour, M., Poupon, R., Islam, S., Darnis, F., Levy, V. G., Opolon, P., Beaugrand, M., Toulet, J., Danan, G., and Benhamou, J. P. (1985). Drug-induced hepatitis associated with anticytoplasmic organelle autoantibodies. *Hepatology* **5**: 722-727.
13. Beaune, P., Dansette, P. M., Mansuy, D., Kiffel, M., Finck, M., Amar, C., Leroux, J. P., and Homberg, J. C. (1987). Human antimicrosome antibodies appearing in a drug induced hepatitis are directed against cytochrome P-450 that hydroxylates the drug. *Proc. Natl. Acad. Sci. USA* **84**: 551-555.
14. Bourdi, M., Larrey, D., Nataf, J., Bernuau, J., Pessayre, D., Iwasaki, M., Guengerich, F. P., and Beaune, P. H. (1990). Anti-liver endoplasmic reticulum autoantibodies are directed against human cytochrome P-450IA2. A specific marker of dihydralazine-induced hepatitis. *J. Clin. Invest.* **85**: 1967-1973.
15. Siegers, C. P. (1988). Modifiers of metabolic toxication and detoxication. In *Liver Drugs from Experimental Pharmacology to Therapeutic Application.* B. Testa and D. Perrissoud (Eds.). CRC Press, Boca Raton, pp. 15-25.
16. Guillouzo, A., Clerc, C., Mallédant, Y., Chesné, C., Ratanasavanh, D., and Guguen-Guillouzo, C. (1989). Modèles d'étude de la cytoprotection hépatique. *Gastroenterol. Clin. Biol.* **13**: 725-730.
17. Dumont, J. M., Maignan, M. F., Janin, B., Herbage, D., and Perrissoud, D. (1986). Effect of malotilate on chronic liver injury induced by carbon tetrachloride in the rat. *J. Hepatol.* **3**: 260-268.
18. Campbell, A. K., and Hales, C. N. (1971). Maintenance of viable cells in an organ culture of mature rat liver. *Exp. Cell Res.* **68**: 33-42.

19. Smith, P. F., Krack, G., McKee, K. L., Johnson, D. G., Gandolfi, A. J., Hruby, V. J., Krumdieck, C. L., and Brendel, K. (1986). Maintenance of adult rat liver slices in dynamic organ culture. *In Vitro Cell. Devel. Biol.* **22**: 706-712.
20. Brendel, K., Gandolfi, A. J., Krumdieck, C. L., and Smith, P. F. (1987). Organ slices revisited. *Trends Pharmacol. Sci.* **8**: 11-15.
21. Ghantous, H. N., Fernando, J., Gandolfi, A. J., and Brendel, K. (1990). Biotransformation of halothane in guinea pig liver slices. *Drug Metab. Disp.* **18**:514-518.
22. Guillouzo, A., Oudea, P., Le Guilly, Y., Oudea, M. C., Lenoir, P., and Bourel, M. (1972). An ultrastructural study of primary cultures of adult human liver tissue. *Exp. Mol. Path.* **16**: 1-15.
23. Howard, R. B., Christensen, A. K., Gibbs, A. F., and Pesch, L. A. (1967). The enzymatic preparation of isolated intact parenchymal cells from rat liver. *J. Cell Biol.* **35**: 675-684.
24. Berry, M. N., and Friend, D. S. (1969). High-yield preparation of isolated rat liver parenchymal cells. A biochemical and fine structural study. *J. Cell. Biol.* **43**: 506-520.
25. Seglen, P. O. (1975). Preparation of isolated rat liver cells. *Meth. Cell Biol.* **13**: 29-83.
26. Guguen-Guillouzo, C., and Guillouzo, A. (1986). Methods for preparation of adult and fetal hepatocytes. In *Isolated and Cultured Hepatocytes.* A. Guillouzo and C. Guguen-Guillouzo (Eds.). Les Editions INSERM, and John Libbey, Eurotext, Paris, pp. 1-12.
27. Quistorff, B., Grunnet, N., and Cornell, N. W. (1985). Digitonin perfusion of rat liver. A new approach in the study of intracellular compartmentation in the liver. *Biochem. J.* **226**: 2189-2197.
28. Lindros, K. O., and Penttilä, K. E. (1985). Digitonin-collagenase perfusion for efficient separation of periportal and perivenous hepatocytes. *Biochem. J.* **228**: 560-575.
29. Bernaert, D., Wanson, J. C., Mosselmans, R., De Parmentier, F., and Drochmans, P. (1979). Separation of adult rat hepatocytes into distinct subpopulations by centrifugation elutriation. Morphological, morphometrical and biochemical characterization of cell fractions. *Biol. Cell.* **34**: 159-174.
30. Le Rumeur, E., Guguen-Guillouzo, C., Beaumont, C., Saunier, A., and Guillouzo, A. (1983). Albumin secretion and protein synthesis by cultured diploid and tetraploid rat hepatocytes separated by elutriation. *Exp. Cell Res.* **147**: 247-254.
31. Seglen, P. O. (1977). Protein-catabolic state of isolated rat hepatocytes. *Biochim. Biophys. Acta* **496**: 182-191.
32. Seglen, P. O., Solheim, A. E., Grinde, B., Gordon, P. B., Schwarze, P. E., Gjessing, R., and Poli, A. (1980). Amino acid control of protein synthesis and degradation in isolated rat hepatocytes. *Ann. N.Y. Acad. Sci.* **349**: 1-7.
33. Miura, Y., Akimoto, T., Kanazawa, H., and Yagi, K. (1986). Synthesis and secretion of protein by hepatocytes entrapped within calcium alginate. *Artificial Organs* **10**: 460-465.
34. Cai, Z., Shi, Z., Sherman, M., and Sun, A. M. (1989). Development and evaluation of a system of microencapsulation of primary rat hepatocytes. *Hepatology* **10**: 855-860.

35. Bissell, D. M., and Guzelian, P. S. (1980). Phenotypic stability of adult rat hepatocytes in primary monolayer culture. *Ann. N.Y. Acad. Sci.* **349**: 85-98.
36. Sirica, A. E., and Pitot, H. C. (1980). Drug metabolism and effects of carcinogens in cultured hepatic cells. *Pharmacol. Rev.* **31**: 205-228.
37. Guguen-Guillouzo, C., and Guillouzo, A. (1983). Modulation of functional activities in cultured rat hepatocytes. *Mol. Cell Biochem.* **53/54**: 35-56.
38. Guguen C., Gregori, C., and Schapira, F. (1975). Modifications of pyruvate kinase isozymes in prolonged primary cultures of adult rat hepatocytes. *Biochimie* **57**: 1065-1071.
39. Sirica, A. E., Richards, W., Tsukada, C., Sattler, C., and Pitot, H. C. (1979). Fetal phenotypic expression by adult rat hepatocytes on collagen gel/nylon meshes. *Proc. Natl. Acad. Sci. USA* **114**: 307-315.
40. Clayton, D. F., and Darnell, J. E. (1983). Changes in liver-specific compared to common gene transcription during primary culture of mouse hepatocytes. *Mol. Cell Biol.* **3**: 1552-1561.
41. Fraslin, J. M., Kneip, B., Vaulont, S., Glaise, D., Munnich, A., and Guguen-Guillouzo, C. (1985). Dependence of hepatocyte specific gene expression on cell-cell interactions in primary culture. *EMBO J.* **4**: 2487-2491.
42. Guzelian, P. S., Bissell, D. M., and Meyer, U. A. (1977). Drug metabolism in adult rat hepatocytes in primary monolayer culture. *Gastroenterology* **72**: 1232-1239.
43. Fahl, W. E., Michalopoulos, G., Sattler, G. L., Jefcoate, C. R., and Pitot, H. C. (1979). Characteristics of microsomal enzyme controls in primary cultures of rat hepatocytes. *Arch. Biochem. Biophys.* **192**: 61-72.
44. Maslansky, C. J., and Williams, G. M. (1982). Primary cultures and the levels of cytochrome P-450 in hepatocytes from mouse, rat, hamster and rabbit liver. *In Vitro* **18**: 663-693.
45. Bégué, J. M., Guguen-Guillouzo, C., Pasdeloup, N., and Guillouzo, A. (1984). Prolonged maintenance of active cytochrome P-450 in adult rat hepatocytes co-cultured with another liver cell type. *Hepatology* **4**: 839-842.
46. Steward, A. R., Dannan, G. A., Guzelian, P. S. and Guengerich, F. P. (1985). Changes in the concentration of seven forms of cytochrome P-450 in primary cultures of adult rat hepatocytes. *Mol. Pharmacol.* **27**: 125-132.
47. Daujat, M., Pichard, L., Dalet, C., Larroque, C., Bonfils, C., Pompon, D., Li, D., Guzelian, P. S., and Maurel, P. (1987). Expression of five forms of microsomal cytochrome P-450 in primary cultures of rabbit hepatocytes treated with various classes of inducers. *Biochem. Pharmacol.* **36**: 3597-3606.
48. Namiki, M., Degawa, M., Masuki, T., and Hashimoto, Y. (1989). Changes in the quantity and activity of cytochrome P-450 isozymes in primary cultured rat hepatocytes. *Jap. J. Cancer Res.,* **80**: 126-131.
49. Elshourbagy, N. A., Barwick, J. L., and Guzelian, P. S. (1981). Induction of cytochrome P-450 by pregnenolone-16-α-carbonitrile in primary monolayer cultures of adult rat hepatocytes and in a cell-free translation system. *J. Biol. Chem.* **256**: 6060-6068.
50. Newman, S., and Guzelian, P. S. (1982). Stimulation of de novo synthesis of cytochrome P-450 by phenobarbital in primary nonproliferating cultures of adult rat hepatocytes. *Proc. Natl. Acad. Sci. USA* **79**: 2922-2926.

51. Pasco, D. S., Boyum, K. W., Merchant, S. N., Chalberg, S. C., and Fagan, J. B. (1988). Transcriptional and post-transcriptional regulation of the genes encoding cytochrome P-450c and P-450d in vivo and in primary hepatocyte cultures. *J. Biol. Chem.* **263**: 8671-8676.
52. Silver, G., and Krauter, K. S. (1988). Expression of cytochrome P-450c and P-450d mRNAs in cultured rat hepatocytes. *J. Biol. Chem.* **263**: 11802-11807.
53. Turner, N. A., Wilson, N. M., Jefcoate, C. R., and Pitot, H. C. (1988). The expression and metabolic activity of cytochrome P-450 isozymes in control and phenobarbital-induced primary cultures of rat hepatocytes. *Arch. Biochem. Biophys.* **263**: 204-215.
54. Perrot, N., Chesné, C., de Waziers, I., Conner, J., Beaune, P., and Guillouzo, A. Expression of cytochrome P-450 enzymes and epoxide hydrolase in cultures and co-cultures of rat hepatocytes: Effects of ethanol and clofibrate. *Eur. J. Biochem.* In press.
55. Watkins, P. B., Wrighton, S. A., Schuetz, E. G., Maurel, P., and Guzelian, P. S. (1986). Macrolide antibiotics inhibit the degradation of the glucocorticoid-responsive cytochrome P-450p in rat hepatocytes in vivo and in primary monolayer culture. *J. Biol. Chem.* **261**: 6264-2671.
56. Guillouzo, A., Beaune, P., Gascoin, M. N., Bégué, J. M., Campion, J. P., Guengerich, F. P., and Guguen-Guillouzo, C. (1985). Maintenance of cytochrome P-450 in cultured adult human hepatocytes. *Biochem. Pharmacol.* **34**: 2991-2995.
57. Morel, F., Beaune, P., Ratanasavanh, D., Flinois, J. P., Yang, C. S., Guengerich, F. P., and Guillouzo, A. (1990). Expression of cytochrome P-450 enzymes in cultured human hepatocytes. *Eur. J. Biochem.* **191**: 437-444.
58. Ratanasavanh, D., Beaune, P., Baffet, G., Rissel, M., Kremers, P., Guengerich, F. P., and Guillouzo, A. (1986). Immunocytochemical evidence for the maintenance of cytochrome P-450 isozymes, NADPH cytochrome c reductase and epoxide hydrolase in pure and mixed primary cultures of adult human hepatocytes. *J. Histochem. Cytochem.* **34**: 527-533.
59. Diaz, D., Fabre, I., Daujat, M., Saint Laurent, B., Bories, P., Michel, H., and Maurel, P. (1990). Omeprazole is an aryl hydrocarbon-like inducer of human hepatic cytochrome P-450. *Gastroenterology* **99**: 737-747.
60. Daujat, M., Fabre, I., Diaz, D., Pichard, L., Fabre, G., Fabre, J. M., Saint-Aubert, B., and Maurel, P. (1991). Inducibility and expression of class IA and IIIA cytochromes P-450 in primary cultures of adult human hepatocytes. *Life Sci.* In press.
61. Vandenberghe, Y., Ratanasavanh, D., Glaise D., and Guillouzo, A. (1988). Influence of medium composition and culture conditions on glutathione S-transferase activity in adult hepatocytes during culture. *In Vitro Cell Devel. Biol.* **24**: 281-288.
62. Abramovitz, M., Ishigaki, S., and Listowsky, I. (1989). Differential regulation of glutathione S-transferase in cultured hepatocytes. *Hepatology* **9**: 235-239.
63. Vandenberghe, Y., Glaise, D., Meyer, D. J., Guillouzo, A., and Ketterer, B. (1988). Glutathione transferase isoenzymes in cultured rat hepatocytes. *Biochem. Pharmacol.* **37**: 2482-2485.
64. Morel, F., Vandenberghe, Y., Pemble, S., Taylor, J. B., Ratanasavanh, D., Rogiers, V., Ketterer, B., and Guillouzo, A. (1989). Regulation of glutathione

S-transferase subunits 3 and 4 in cultured rat hepatocytes. *FEBS Lett.* **258**: 99-102.
65. Vandenberghe, Y., Morel, F., Pemble, S., Taylor, J. B., Rogiers, V., Ratanasavanh, D., Vercruysse, A., Ketterer, B., and Guillouzo, A. (1990). Changes in expression of mRNA coding for glutathione S-transferase subunits 1-2 and 7 in cultured rat hepatocytes. *Mol. Pharmacol.* **37**: 372-376.
66. Croci, T., and Williams, G. M. (1985). Activities of several phase I and phase II xenobiotic transformation enzymes in cultured hepatocytes from male and female rats. *Biochem. Pharmacol.* **34**: 3029-3035.
67. Vandenberghe, Y., Ratanasavanh, D., Rogiers, V., and Guillouzo, A. (1988). Glutathione S-transferase activity in cultured human hepatocytes. *Cell Biol. Int. Rep.* **34**: 449-460.
68. Bégué, J. M., Le Bigot, J. F., Guguen-Guillouzo, C., Kiechel, J. R., and Guillouzo, A. (1983). Cultured human adult hepatocytes: A new model for drug metabolism studies. *Biochem. Pharmacol.* **32**: 1643-1646.
69. Gee, S. J., Green, C. E., and Tyson, C. A. (1984). Comparative metabolism of tolbutamide by isolated hepatocytes from rat, rabbit, dog and squirrel monkey. *Drug Metab. Dispos.* **12**: 174-178.
70. Paine, A. J., Maurer, G., and Von Wartburg, B. R. (1984). The application of hepatocyte culture to the identification of pathways of drug metabolism. Studies with pindolol and fluperlapine. *Biochem. Pharmacol.* **33**: 3111-3114.
71. McQueen, C. A., Miller, M. J., and Williams, G. M. (1986). Sex differences in the biotransformation of 2-acetyl-aminofluorene in cultured rat hepatocytes. *Cell Biol. Toxicol.* **2**: 271-281.
72. Chenery, R. J., Ayrton, A., Oldham, H. G., Standing, P., Norman, S. J., Seddon, T., and Kirby, R. (1987). Diazepam metabolism in cultured hepatocytes from rat, rabbit, dog, guinea pig and man. *Drug. Metab. Dispos.* **15**: 312-317.
73. Le Bigot, J. F., Bégué, J. M., Kiechel, J. R., and Guillouzo, A. (1987). Species differences in metabolism of ketotifen in rat, rabbit and man: Demonstration of similar pathways in vivo and in cultured hepatocytes. *Life Sci.* **40**: 883-890.
74. Guillouzo, A., Bégué, J. M., Maurer, G., and Koch, P. (1988). Identification of metabolic pathways of pindolol and fluperlapine in adult human hepatocyte cultures. *Xenobiotica* **18**: 131-139.
75. Rahmani, R., Richard, B., Fabre, G., and Cano, J. P. (1988). Extrapolation of preclinical pharmacokinetic data to therapeutic drug use. *Xenobiotica* **18**: 71-88.
76. Guillouzo, A., Morel, F., Ratanasavanh, D., Chesné, C., and Guguen-Guillouzo, C. (1990). Long-term culture of functional hepatocytes. *Toxicol. In Vitro* **4**: 415-427.
77. Guguen, C., Guillouzo, A., Boisnard, M., Le Cam, A., and Bourel, M. (1975). Etude ultrastructurale de monocouches d'hépatocytes de rat adulte cultivés en présence d'hémisuccinate d'hydrocortisone. *Biol. Gastroenterol.* **8**: 223-231.
78. Decad, G. M., Hsieh, D. P. H., and Byard, J. L. (1977). Maintenance of cytochrome P-450 and metabolism of aflatoxin B_1 in primary hepatocyte cultures. *Biochem. Biophys. Res. Commun.* **78**: 279-287.
79. Enat, R., Jefferson, D. M., Ruiz-Opazo, N., Gatmaitan, Z., Leinwand, L. A., and Reid, L. M. (1984). Hepatocyte proliferation in vitro: Its dependence on

the use of serum-free hormonally defined medium and substrata of extracellular matrix. *Proc. Natl. Acad. Sci. USA* **81**: 1411-1415.
80. Jefferson, D. M., Clayton, D. F., Darnell, J. E., and Reid, L. M. (1984). Post-transcriptional modulation of gene expression in cultured rat hepatocytes. *Mol. Cell Biol.,* **4**: 1929-1934.
81. McGowan, J. A. (1986). Hepatocyte proliferation in culture. In *Isolated and Cultured Hepatocytes.* A. Guillouzo and C. Guguen-Guillouzo (Eds.). Les Editions INSERM and John Libbey Eurotext, Paris, pp. 13-38.
82. Paine, A. J. (1990). The maintenance of cytochrome P-450 in rat hepatocyte culture: Some applications of liver cell cultures to the study of drug metabolism, toxicity and the induction of the P-450 system. *Chem. Biol. Interact.* **74**: 1-31.
83. Guillouzo, A., Guguen-Guillouzo, C., Boisnard, M., Bourel, M., and Benhamou, J. P. (1978). Smooth endoplasmic reticulum proliferation and increased cell multiplication in cultured hepatocytes of the newborn rat in the presence of phenobarbital. *Exp. Mol. Pathol.* **28**: 1-9.
84. Miyazaki, M., Handa, Y., Oda, M., Yabe, T., Miyano, K., and Sato, J. (1985). Long-term survival of functional hepatocytes from adult rat in the presence of phenobarbital in primary culture. *Exp. Cell Res.* **159**: 176-190.
85. Lake, B. G., Gray, T. J. B., Stubberfield, C. R., Beamand, J. A., and Gangolli, S. D. (1983). Induction of lauric acid hydroxylation and maintenance of cytochrome P-450 content by clofibrate in primary cultures of rat hepatocytes. *Life Sci.* **33**: 249-254.
86. Isom, H. C., Secott T., Georgoff I., Woodworth, C., and Mummaw, J. (1985). Maintenance of differentiated rat hepatocytes in primary culture. *Proc. Natl. Acad. Sci. U.S.A.* **82**: 3252-3256.
87. Isom, H., Georgoff, I., Salditt-Georgieff, M., and Darnell, J. E. (1987) Persistence of liver-specific messenger RNA in cultured hepatocytes: Different regulatory events for different genes. *J. Cell Biol.* **105**: 2877-2885.
88. Michalopoulos, G. and Pitot, H. C. (1975). Primary culture of parenchymal liver cells on collagen membranes. *Exp. Cell Res.* **94**: 70-78.
89. Rojkind, M., Gatmaitan, Z., Mackensen, S., Giambrone, M. A., Ponce, P., and Reid, L. M. (1980). Connective tissue biomatrix: Its isolation and utilization for long-term cultures of normal rat hepatocytes. *J. Cell Biol.,* **87**: 255-263.
90. Guguen-Guillouzo, C., Seignoux, D., Courtois, Y., Brissot, P., Marceau, N., Glaise, D., and Guillouzo, A. (1982). Amplified phenotypic changes in adult rat and baboon hepatocytes cultured on a complex biomatrix. *Biol. Cell.* **46**: 11-20.
91. Ben-Ze'ev, A., Robinson, G. S., Bucher, N. L. R., and Farmer, S. R. (1988). Cell-cell and cell-matrix interactions differentially regulate the expression of hepatic and cytoskeletal genes in primary cultures of rat hepatocytes. *Proc. Natl. Acad. Sci. USA* **85**: 2161-2165.
92. Guguen-Guillouzo, C. (1986). Role of homotypic and heterotypic cell interactions in expression of specific functions by cultured hepatocytes. In *Isolated and Cultured Hepatocytes.* A. Guillouzo and C. Guguen-Guillouzo (Eds.). Les Editions INSERM and John Libbey Eurotext, Paris, pp. 271-296.
93. Bissell, D. M., Arenson, D. M., Maher, J. J., and Roll, F. J. (1987). Support of cultured hepatocytes by a laminin-rich gel. *J. Clin. Invest.* **79**: 801-812.

94. Schuetz, E. G., Li, D., Omiecinski, C. J., Muller-Eberhard, U., Kleinman, H. K., Elswick, B., and Guzelian, P. S. (1988). Regulation of gene expression in adult rat hepatocytes cultured on a basement membrane matrix. *J. Cell Physiol.* **134**: 309-323.
95. Sinclair, P. R., Schuetz, E. G., Bement, W. J., Haugen, S. A., Sinclair, J. F., May, B. K., Li, D., and Guzelian, P. S. (1990). Role of heme in phenobarbital induction of cytochromes P-450 and 5-aminolevulinate synthase in cultured rat hepatocytes maintained on an extracellular matrix. *Arch. Biochem. Biophys.* **282**: 386-392.
96. Dunn, J. Y., Yarmush, M. L., Koebe, H. G., and Tompkins, R. G. (1989). Hepatocyte function and extracellular matrix geometry: Long-term culture in a sandwich configuration. *FASEB J.* **3**: 174-177.
97. Spray, D. C., Fujita, M., Saez, J. C., Choi, H., Watanabe, T., Hertzberg, E., Rosenberg, L. C., and Reid, L. M. (1987). Proteoglycans and glycosaminoglycans induce gap junction synthesis and function in primary liver cultures. *J. Cell Biol.* **105**: 541-551.
98. Wanson, J. C., Mosselmans, R., Brouwer, A., and Knook, D. L. (1979). Interaction of adult rat hepatocytes and sinusoidal cells in co-culture. *Biol. Cell* **56**: 7-16.
99. Michalopoulos, G., Russel, F., and Biles, C. (1979). Primary cultures of hepatocytes on human fibroblasts. *In Vitro* **15**: 796-806.
100. Guguen-Guillouzo, C., Clément, B., Baffet, G., Beaumont, C., Morel-Chany, E., Glaise, D. and Guillouzo, A. (1983). Maintenance and reversibility of active albumin secretion by adult rat hepatocytes co-cultured with another liver epithelial cell type. *Exp. Cell Res.* **143**: 47-54.
101. Clément, B., Guguen-Guillouzo, C., Campion, J. P., Glaise, D., Bourel, M., and Guillouzo, A. (1984). Long-term co-cultures of adult human hepatocytes with rat liver epithelial cells: Modulation of active albumin secretion and accumulation of extracellular material. *Hepatology* **4**: 373-380.
102. Guguen-Guillouzo, C., Clément, B., Lescoat, G., Glaise, D., and Guillouzo, A. (1984). Modulation of human fetal hepatocyte survival and differentiation by interactions with a rat liver epithelial cell line. *Dev. Biol.* **105**: 211-220.
103. Lescoat, G., Thézé, N., Clément, B., Guillouzo, A., and Guguen-Guillouzo, C. (1985). Control of albumin and α-fetoprotein secretion by fetal and neonatal rat hepatocytes maintained in co-culture. *Cell Diff.* **16**: 259-268.
104. Fourel, I., Gripon, P., Hantz, O., Cova, L., Lambert, V., Jacquet, C., Watanabe, K., Fox, J., Guillouzo, C., and Trepo, C., (1989). Prolonged duck hepatitis B virus replication in duck hepatocytes co-cultivated with rat epithelial cells: A useful system for antiviral testing. *Hepatology* **10**: 186-191.
105. Guillouzo, A., Clément, B., Bégué, J. M., and Guguen-Guillouzo, C. (1984). Long-term production of acute-phase proteins by adult rat hepatocytes co-cultured with another liver cell type in serum-free medium. *Biuochem. Biophys. Res. Commun.* **120**: 311-317.
106. Foliot, A., Glaise, D., Erlinger, S., and Guguen-Guillouzo, C. (1985). Long-term maintenance of taurocholate uptake by adult rat hepatocytes co-cultured with a liver epithelial cell line. *Hepatology* **5**: 215-219.
107. Angius, L. (1988). Metabolic interactions of parenchymal hepatocytes and

dividing epithelial cells in co-culture. *Biochem. J.* **252**: 23-28.
108. Conner, J., Vallet-Collom, I., Daveau, M., Delers, F., Lebreton, J. P., and Guillouzo, A. (1990). Acute phase response induction in rat hepatocytes co-cultured with rat liver epithelial cells. *Biochem. J.* **266**: 683-688.
109. Schrode, W., Mecke, D., and Gebhardt, R. (1990). Induction of glutamine synthetase in periportal hepatocytes by co-cultivation with a liver epithelial cell line. *Eurp. J. Cell Biol.* **53**: 35-41.
110. Mesnil, M., Fraslin, J. M., Piccoli, C., Yamasaki, H., and Guguen-Guillouzo, C. (1987). Cell contact but not junctional communication (dye coupling) with biliary epithelial cells is required for hepatocytes to maintain differentiated functions. *Exp. Cell Res.* **173**: 524-533.
111. Gleiberman, A. S., Kudrjavtseva, E. I., Sharovskaya, U. Y., and Abelev, G. I. (1989). Synthesis of alpha-fetoprotein in hepatocytes is coordinately regulated with cell-cell and cell-matrix interactions. *Mol. Biol. Med.* **6**: 95-107.
112. Morin, O., and Normand, C. (1986). Long-term maintenance of hepatocyte functional activity in co-culture: Requirements for sinusoidal endothelial cells and dexamethasone. *J. Cell Physiol.* **129**: 103-110.
113. Donato, M. T., Castell, J. V., and Gomez-Lechon, M. J. (1990). Prolonged expression of biotransformation activities of rat hepatocytes co-cultured with established cell lines. *Toxicol. In Vitro* **4**: 461-466.
114. Corlu, A., Lhadi, C., Kneip, B., Leray, G., Glaise, D., Baffet, G., Bourel, D., and Guguen-Guillouzo, C. (1991). A plasma membrane protein innvolved in the cell contact-mediated regulation of tissue-specific genes in adult hepatocytes. *J. Cell Biol.* **115**: In press.
115. Landry, J., Bernier, D., Quellet, C., Goyette, R., and Marceau, N. (1985). Spheroidal aggregate culture of rat liver cells: histotypic reorganization, biomatrix deposition, and maintenance of functional activities. *J. Cell Biol.* **101**:914-923.
116. Guigoz, Y., Werffeli, P., Favre, D., Juillerat, M., Wellinger, R., and Honegger, P. (1987). Aggregate cultures of foetal rat liver cells: Development and maintenance of liver gene expression. *Biol. Cell* **60**: 163-172.
117. Wiebel, F. J., Keifer, F. and Murdia U.S. (1984). Phenobarbital induces cytochrome P-450-and cytochrome P-448-dependent monooxygenases in rat hepatoma cells. *Chem. Biol. Interact.* **52**: 151-162.
118. Corcos, L., and Rousset, J. P. (1988). Phenobarbital induces cytochrome P-450 mRNAs and enhances aflatoxin B1 toxicity in rat hepatoma cells. In *Liver Cells and Drugs*. A. Guillouzo (Ed.). Les Editions INSERM and John Libbey Eurotext, Paris, pp. 445-449.
119. Isom, H. C., and Georgoff, I. (1984). Quantitative assay for albumin-producing liver cells after simian virus 40 transformation of rat hepatocytes maintained in chemically defined medium. *Proc. Natl. Acad. Sci. U.S.A.* **81**: 6378-6382.
120. Fry, J. R. and Bridges, J. W. (1979). Use of primary hepatocyte cultures in biochemical toxicology. *Rev. Biochem. Toxicol.* **1**: 201-247.
121. Grisham, J. W. (1979). Use of hepatic cell cultures to detect and evaluate the mechanisms of action of toxic chemicals. *Int. Rev. Exp. Pathol.* **20**: 123-210.
122. Klaassen, C. D. and Stacey, N. H. (1982). Use of isolated hepatocytes in toxicity assessment. In *Toxicology of the Liver*. G. Plaa and W. R. Hewitt (Eds.). Raven Press, New York, pp. 147-179.

123. Zimmerman, H. J. (1982). Chemical hepatic injury and its detection. In *Toxicology of the Liver.* G. Plaa and W. R. Hewitt (Eds.). Raven Press, New York, pp. 1-45.
124. Bridges, J. W., Benford, D. J., and Hubbard, S. A. (1983). Mechanisms of toxic injury. *Ann. N.Y. Acad. Sci.* **407**: 42-63.
125. Guillouzo, A. (1986). Use of isolated and cultured hepatocytes for xenobiotic metabolism and cytotoxicity studies. In *Isolated and Cultured Hepatocytes.* A. Guillouzo and C. Guguen-Guillouzo. (Eds.). Les Editions INSERM and John Libbey, Eurotext, Paris, pp. 313-332.
126. Tyson, C. A. and Green, C. E. (1987). Cytotoxicity measures: Choices and methods. In *The Isolated Hepatocyte: Use in Toxicology and Xenobiotic Biotransformations.* E. J. Rauckman and G. M. Padilla (Eds.). Academic Press, Orlando, Florida, pp. 119-158.
127. Story, D. L., Gee, S. J., Tyson, C. A., and Gould, D. H. 1983). Response of isolated hepatocytes to organic and inorganic cytotoxins. *J. Toxicol. Environ. Health* **11**: 483-501.
128. Ratanasavanh, D., Riché, C., Bégué, J. M., and Guillouzo, A. (1988). Les hépatocytes en culture: Utilisation en pharmacotoxicologie. In *Méthodes in vitro en pharmacotoxicologie.* Vol. 170. M. Adolphe and A. Guillouzo (Eds.). Les Editions INSERM pp. 11-16.
129. Le Bot, M. A., Bégué, J. M., Kernaleguen, D., Robert, J., Ratanasavanh, D., Airiau, J., Riché, C., and Guillouzo, A. (1988). Different cytotoxicity and metabolism of doxorubicin, daunorubicin, epirubicin, esorubicin and idarubicin in cultured human and rat hepatocytes. *Biochem. Pharmacol.* **37**: 3877-3887.
130. Mallédant, Y., Siproudhis, L., Tanguy, M., Clerc, C., Chesné, C., Saint-Marc, C., and Guillouzo, A. (1990). Effects of halothane on human and rat hepatocyte cultures. *Anesthesiology* **72**: 526-534.
131. Rubin, K., Oldberg, A., Hook, M., and Obrink, B. (1978). Adhesion of rat hepatocytes to collagen. *Exp. Cell Res.* **117**: 165-177.
132. Goethals, F., Krack, G., Deboyser, D., Vossen, P., and Roberfroid, M. (1984). Critical biochemical functions of isolated hepatocytes as sensitive indicators of chemical toxicity. *Fund. Appl. Toxicol.* **4**: 441-450.
133. Santone, K. S., and Acosta, D. (1982). Measurement of functional metabolic activity as a sensitive parameter of cytotoxicity in cultured hepatocytes. *J. Tissue Cult. Meth.* **7**: 137-142.
134. Villa, P., Bégué, J. M., and Guillouzo, A. (1984). Effects of erythromycin derivatives on cultured rat hepatocytes. *Biochem. Pharmacol.* **33**: 4098-4101.
135. Reddy, J. K., and Lalwani, N. D. (1983). Carcinogenesis by peroxisome proliferators: Evaluation of the risk of hypolipidaemic drugs and industrial plasticizers to humans. *CRC Crit. Rev. Toxicol.* **12**: 1-58.
136. Hensgens, H. E. S. J., and Meijer, A. J. (1979). The interrelationship between ureogenesis and protein synthesis in isolated rat liver cells. *Biochim. Biophys. Acta* **582**: 525-532.
137. Cano, J. P., Rahmani, R., Fabre, G., Richard, B., Lacarelle, B., Boré, P., Bertault-Peres, P., de Sousa, G., Fabre, I., Placidi, M., Coulange, C., Ducros,

M., and Rampal, M. (1988). Human hepatocytes as an alternative model to the use of animals in experiments. In *Liver Cells and Drugs*. A. Guillouzo (Ed.). Les Editions INSERM and John Libbey Eurotext, Paris, pp. 301-308.

138. Fautrel, A., Chesné, C., Guillouzo, A., De Sousa, G., Placidi, M., Rahmani, R., Braut, F., Pichon, J., Hoellinger, H., Vintezou, P., Diarte, I., Melcion, C., Cordier, A., Lorenzon, G., Benicourt, M., Vannier, B., Fournex, R., Peloux, A. F., Bichet, N., Gouy, D., Cano, J. P., and Lounes, R. (1991). A multicentre study of acute in vitro cytotoxicity in rat liver cells. *Toxicol. In Vitro*. **5**: In press.
139. Riddell, R. J., Panacer, D. S., Wilde, S. M., Clothier, P. H., and Balls, M. (1986). The importance of exposure period and cell type in in vitro cytotoxicity tests. *ATLA* **14**: 86-92.
140. Ekwall, B., and Acosta, D. (1982). In vitro comparative toxicity of selected drugs and chemicals in Hela cells, Chang liver cells and rat hepatocytes. *Drug. Chem. Toxicol.* **5**: 219-231.
141. Tyson, C. A., Mitoma, C., Kalivoda, J. (1980). Evaluation of hepatocytes isolated by a nonperfusion technique in a prescreen for cytotoxicity. *J. Toxicol. Environ. Health* **6**: 197-205.
142. Tyson, C. A., Hawk-Prather, C., Story, D. L., and Gould, D. H. (1983). Correlations of in vitro and in vivo hepatotoxicity for five haloalkanes. *Toxicol. Appl. Pharmacol.* **70**: 289-302.
143. Paine, A. J., and Hockin, L. J. (1982). The maintenance of cytochrome P-450 in liver cell culture: Recent studies on P-450-mediated mechanisms of toxicity. *Toxicology* **25**: 41-45.
144. Fry, J. R. and Bridges, J. W. (1977). A novel mixed hepatocyte-fibroblast culture system and its use as a test for metabolism-mediated cytotoxicity. *Biochem. Pharmacol.* **26**: 969-973.
145. Acosta, D., and Mitchell, D. B. (1981). Metabolic activation and cytotoxicity of cyclophosphamide in primary cultures of postnatal rat hepatocytes. *Biochem. Pharmacol.* **30**: 3225-3230.
146. Vonen, B., and Morland, J. (1984). Isolated rat hepatocytes in suspension: Potential hepatotoxic effects of six different drugs. *Arch. Toxicol.* **56**: 33-37.
147. Ratanasavanh, D., Baffet, G., Latinier, M. F., Rissel, M., and Guillouzo, A. (1988). Use of hepatocyte co-cultures in assessment of drug toxicity from chronic exposure. *Xenobiotica* **18**: 765-771.
148. Grislain, L., Ratanasavanh, D., Moquard, M. T., Raquillet, L., Bégué, J. M., Du Vignaud, P., Génissel, P., Guillouzo, A., and Bromet, N. (1988). Primary cultures of rat and human hepatocytes as a model system for the evaluation of cytotoxicity and metabolic pathways of a new drug S-3341. In *Liver Cells and Drugs*. A. Guillouzo (Ed.). Les Editions INSERM and John Libbey Eurotext, Paris, pp. 357-363.
149. Suolinna, E. M. (1982). Isolation and culture of liver cells and their use in the biochemical research of xenobiotics. *Med. Biol.* **60**: 237-254.
150. Fry, J. R. (1982). Activation systems in tissue culture toxicity systems. *Toxicology* **25**: 1-12.

151. Borenfreund, E., and Puerner, J. A. (1987). Short-term quantitative in vitro cytotoxicity assay involving an S-9 activating system. *Cancer Lett.* **34**: 243-248.
152. Fry, J. R., Garle, M. J., and Hammond, A. H. (1990). Competiting pathways in metabolism-mediated cytotoxicity in vitro. *Toxicol. In Vitro* **4**: 467-473.
153. Long, R. M., and Moore, L. (1988). Biochemical evaluation of rat hepatocyte primary cultures as a model for carbon tetrachloride hepatotoxicity: Comparative studies in vivo and in vitro. *Toxicol. Appl. Pharmacol.* **92**: 295-306.
154. Tran-Thi, T. A., Phillips, J., Falk, H., and Decker, K. (1985). Toxicity of D-galactosamine for rat hepatocytes in monolayer culture. *Exp. Mol. Pathol.* **42**: 89-116.
155. Thor, H., Moldeus, P., Kristofenson, A., Hogberg, J., Reed, D. J., and Orrenius, S. (1978). Metabolic activation and hepatotoxicity: Metabolism of bromobenzene in isolated hepatocytes. *Arch. Biochem. Biophys.* **188**: 114-121.
156. Gudzinowicz, M., and Neal, R. A. (1979). Biochemical effects and metabolism of thiocetamide (TAA) and thioacetamide-S-oxide (TAAO) by isolated rat liver cells. *Pharmacologist* **21**:186.
157. Harman, A. W., and Fischer, L. J. (1983). Hamster hepatocytes in culture as a model for acetaminophen toxicity: studies with inhibitors of drug metabolism. *Toxicol. Appl. Pharmacol.* **71**: 330-341.
158. Moldeus, P. (1978). Paracetamol metabolism and toxicity in isolated hepatocytes from rat and mouse. *Biochem. Pharmacol.* **27**: 2859-2863.
159. Hoffmann, K. J., Streeter, A. J., Axworthy, D. B., and Barllie, T. A. (1985). Identification of the major covalent adduct formation in vitro and in vivo between acetaminophen and mouse liver proteins. *Mol. Pharmacol.* **27**: 566-573.
160. Bartolome, J. B., Birge, R. B., Sparks, K., Cohen, S. D., and Khairalla, E. A. (1988). Immunochemical analysis of acetominophen covalent binding to proteins. Partial characterization of the major acetominophen binding liver proteins. *Biochem. Pharmacol.* **37**: 4763-4774.
161. Neuberger, J., Kenna, J. G., Nouri Aria, K., and Williams, R. (1985). Antibody mediated hepatocyte injury in methyldopa induced hepatotoxicity. *Gut* **26**: 1233-1239.
162. Vergani, D., Mieli-Vergani, G., Alberti, A., Neuberger, J., Eddleston, A. L. W. F., Davis, M., and Williams, R. (1980). Antibodies to surface altered rabbit hepatocytes in patients with severe halothane associated hepatitis. *N. Engl. J. Med.* **303**: 66-71.
163. Kenna, J. G., Neuberger, J., and Williams, R. (1987). Specific antibodies to halothane-induced liver antigens in halothane-associated hepatitis. *Br. J. Anaesthiol.* **59**: 1286-1290.
164. Siproudhis, L., Beaugrand, M., Malledant, Y., Brissot, P., Guguen-Guillouzo, C., and Guillouzo, A. (1991). Use of adult human hepatocytes in primary culture for the study of clometacin-induced immunoallergic hepatitis. *Toxicol. In Vitro* **5**: In press.
165. Michalopoulos, G. K., Strom, S. C., and Jirtle, R. L. (1986). Use of hepatocytes for studies of mutagenesis and carcinogenesis. In *Isolated and Cultured Hepatocytes.* A. Guillouzo and C. Guguen-Guillouzo (Eds.). Les Editions INSERM and John Libbey, Paris, Eurotext, pp. 333-352.

166. Strom, S. C., Monteith, D. K., Manoharan, K., and Novotny, A. (1987). Genotoxicity studies with human hepatocytes. In *The Isolated Hepatocyte: Use in Toxicology and Xenobiotic Biotransformations.* E. J. Rauckman and G. M. Padilla (Eds.). Academic Press, Orlando, Florida, pp. 265-280.
167. Ames, B. N., McCann, J., and Yamasaki, E. (1975). Methods for detecting carcinogens and mutagens with the Salmonella/mammalian-microsome mutagenicity test. *Mutat. Res.* **31**: 347-364.
168. Maron, D. M., and Ames, B. N. (1983). Revised methods for the salmonella mutagenicity test. *Mut. Res.* **113**: 173-215.
169. Neis, J. M., Van Gemert, P. J. L., Roelofs, H. M. J., Bos, R. P., and Henderson, P. T. (1984). Mutagenicity of benzidine and 4-aminobiphenyl after metabolic activation with isolated hepatocytes and the 9 000 x g liver supernatant from rat, hamster and guinea pig. *Mutat. Res.* **129**: 13-18.
170. Steinmetz, K. L., Spak, D. K., Green, C. E., and Mirsalis, J. C. (1985). Induction of unscheduled DNA synthesis in primary cultures of hamster, rat, mouse and human hepatocytes. *Toxicologist* **5**: 20.
171. Butterworth, B. E., Smith-Oliver, T., Earle, L., Loury, D. J., White, R. D., Doolittle, D. J., Working, P. K., Cattley, R. C., Jirtle, R., Michalopoulos, G., and Strom, S. (1989). Use of primary cultures of human hepatocytes in toxicology studies. *Cancer Res.* **49**: 1075-1084.
172. Strom, S. C., Jirtle, R. L., and Michalopoulos, G. (1983). Genotoxic effects of 2-acetylaminofluorene on rat and human hepatocytes. *Environ. Health Perspect.* **49**: 165-170.
173. Martelli, A., Robbiano, L., Ghia, M., Giuliano, L., Angelini, G., and Brambilla, G. (1986). A study of the potential genotoxicity of cimetidine using human hepatocyte primary cultures: Discrepancy from results obtained in rat hepatocytes. *Cancer Let.* **30**: 11-16.
174. Strom, S. C., Novicki, D. L., Novotny, A., Jirtle, R., and Michalopoulos, G. (1983). Human hepatocyte-mediated mutagenesis and DNA repair activity. *Carcinogenesis* **4**: 683-686.
175. Moore, C. J., and Gould, M. N. (1984). Metabolism of benzo(a)pyrene by cultured human hepatocytes from multiple donors. *Carcinogenesis* **5** 1577-1582.
176. Green, C. E., Tyson, C. A., Mirsalis, J. C., and Blazak, W. F. (1985). Comparative metabolism and toxicity assessments using human hepatocytes. *Toxicologist* **5**: 224.
177. Hikino, H., Ohsawa, T., Kiso, Y., and Oshima, Y. (1984). Analgesic and antihepatotoxic actions of dianosides, titerpenoid saponins of Dianthus superbus var longicalycinus Herbs. *Planta Med.* **50**: 353-355.
178. Adzet, T., Camarasa, J., and Laguma, J. C. (1987). Hepatoprotective activity of polyphenolic compounds from cyanarascolymus against CCl_4 toxicity in isolated rat hepatocytes. *J. Natl. Prod.* **50**: 612-617.
179. Bégué, J. M. Baffet, G., Campion, J. P., and Guillouzo, A. (1988). Differential response of primary cultures of human and rat hepatocytes to aflatoxin B_1-induced cytotoxicity and protection by the hepatoprotective agent (+)-cyanidanol-3. *Biol. Cell.* **63**: 327-333.

180. Clément, B., Dumont, J. M., Ratanasavanh, D., Latinier, M. F., Brissot, P., and Guillouzo, A. (1988). Effects of malotilate on human and rat hepatocytes in short-term and long-term primary culture. In *Liver Cells and Drugs*. A. Guillouzo (Ed.). Les Editions INSERM and John Libbey Eurotext, Paris, pp. 417-421.
181. Hikino, H., Kiso, Y., Taguchi, H., and Ikeya, Y. (1984). Antihepatotoxic actions of lignoids from Schizandra chinesis fruits. *Planta Med.* **50**: 213-218.
182. Igarashi, S., Hatahara,T., Nagai, Y., Hori, H., Sakakibara, K., Katoh, M., Sakai, A., and Sugimoto, T. (1986). Anti-fibrotic effect of malotilate on liver fibrosis induced by carbon tetrachloride in rats. *Jpn. J. Exp. Med.* **56**: 235-245.
183. Gautam, A., Ng, O. C., and Boyer, J. L. (1987). Isolated rat hepatocyte couplets in short-term culture: Structural characteristics and plasma membrane reorganization. *Hepatology* **7**: 216-223.
184. Fentem, J. H., Foster, B., Mills, C. O., Coleman, R., and Chipman, J. K. (1990). Biliary excretion of fluorescent cholephiles in hepatocyte couplets: An in vitro model for hepatobiliary and hepatotoxicity studies. *Toxicol. In Vitro* **4**: 452-457.
185. Luetteke, N. C., and Michalopoulos, G. K. (1987). Control of hepatocyte proliferation in vitro. In *The Isolated Hepatocyte: Use in Toxicology and Xenobiotic Biotransformations*. E. J. Rauckman and G. M. Padilla (Eds.). Academic Press, Orlando, Florida, pp. 93-118.
186. Nakamura, T., Nishizawa, T., Higiya, M., Seki, T., Shimonishi, M., Sugimura, A., Tashiro, K., and Shimizi, S. (1989). Molecular cloning and expression of human hepatocyte growth factor. *Nature* **342**: 440-443.
187. Michalopoulos, G., Cianciulli, H. D., Novotny, A. R., Kligerman, A. D., Strom, S. C., and Jirtle, R. L. (1982). Liver regeneration studies with rat hepatocytes in primary culture. *Cancer Res.* **42**: 4673-4682.
188. Guyomard, C., Chesné, C., Meunier, B., Fautrel, A., Clerc, C., Morel, F., Rissel, M., Campion, J. P., and Guillouzo, A. (1990). Primary culture of adult rat hepatocytes after 48 hour preservation of the liver with cold UW solution. *Hepatology* **12**: 1329-1336.
189. Poullain, M. G., Fautrel, A., Guyomard, C., Chesné, C., Grislain, L. and Guillouzo, A. (1991). Viability and primary culture of rat hepatocytes after hypothermic preservation: The superiority of the Leibovitz medium over the UW solution for cold storage. *Hepatology* In press.
190. Guillouzo, A., Chesné, C., Ratanasavanh, D., Campion, J. P., and Guguen-Guillouzo, C. (1987). In *Drug Metabolism from Molecules to Man*. D. J. Benford, J. W. Bridges, and G. G. Gibson (Eds.). Taylor & Francis, London, pp. 423-435.
191. Chesné, C. and Guillouzo, A. (1988). Cryopreservation of isolated rat hepatocytes: A critical evaluation of freezing and thawing conditions. *Cryobiology* **25**: 252-330.
192. Rijntjes, P. J. M., Moshage, H. J., Van Gemert, P. J. L., De Waal, R., and Yap, S. H. (1986). Cryopreservation of adult human hepatocytes. The influence of deep freezing storage on the viability, cell seeding survival, fine structure and albumin synthesis in primary cultures. *J. Hepatol.* **3**: 7-18.

193. Powis, G., Santone, K. S., Melder, D. C., Thomas, L., Moore, D. J., and Wilke, T. J. (1987). Cryopreservation of rat and dog hepatocytes for studies of xenobiotic metabolism and activation. *Drug Metab. Dispos.* **15**: 826-832.
194. Taylor, J., Mason, W., Summers, J., Goldberg, J., Aldrich, C., Coates, L., Gerin, J. and Gowans, E. (1987). Regulation of human hepatitis Delta virus in primary cultures of woodchuck hepatocytes. *J. Virol.* **61**: 2891-2895.
195. Chesné, C., Gripon, P. and Guillouzo, A. (1988). Primary culture of cryopreserved rat hepatocytes. In *Liver Cells and Drugs.* A. Guillouzo (Ed.). Les Editions INSERM and John Libbey Eurotext, Paris, pp. 343-350.
196. Chesné, C., Guyomard, C., Grislain, L., Clerc, C., Fautrel, A., and Guillouzo, A. (1991). Use of cryopreserved animal and human hepatocytes for cytotoxicity studies. *Toxicol. In Vitro* **5**: In press.
197. Paul, D., Höhne, M., Pinkert, C., Piasecki, A., Ummelmann, E., and Brinster, R. L. (1988). Immortalized differentiated hepatocyte lines derived from transgenic mice harboring SV 40 T-antigen genes. *Exp. Cell Res.* **175**: 354-362.
198. Ekwall, B., Bondesson, I., Castell, J. V., Gomez-Lechon, M. J., Hellberg, S., Högberg, J., Jover, R., Pondoda, X., Romert, L., Stenberg, K., and Walum, E. (1989). Cytotoxicity evaluation of the first ten MEIC chemicals: Acute lethal toxicity in man predicted by cytotoxicity in five cellular assays and by oral LD50 tests in rodents. *ATLA* **17**: 83-100.
199. Clothier, R. H. and Balls, M. (1990). Validation of alternative toxicity tests: Principles, practices and cases. *Toxicol. in Vitro* **4**: 692-693.
200. Tyson, C. A. (1987). Correspondence of results from hepatocyte studies with in vivo response. *Toxicol. Ind. Health* **3**: 459-478.
201. Plaa, G. L. (1976). Quantitative aspects in the assessment of liver injury. *Environ. Health Perspect.* **15**: 39-46.
202. Clement, B., Rissel, M., Guerret-Stocker, S., Grimaud, J. A. and Guillouzo, A. (1986). Demonstration of collagens and fibronectin production by adult human hepatocytes in culture. In *Modern Trends in Aging Research.* Y. Courtois, B. Faucheux, B. Forette, D. Knook, and J. A. Treton. (Eds.). Les Editions INSERM and John Libbey Eurotext, Paris, pp 199-205.
203. Mazier, D., Landau, I., Druilhe, P., Miltgen, F., Guguen-Guillouzo, C., Baccam, D., Baxter, J., Chigot, J. P., and Gentilini, M. (1984). Cultivation of the liver forms of *Plasmodium vivax* in human hepatocytes. *Nature* **307**: 367-369.
204. Mazier, D., Beaudoin, R. L., Mellouk, S., Druilhe, P., Texier, B., Trosper, J., Miltgen, F., Landau, I., Paul, C., Brandicourt, O., Guguen-Guillouzo, C., Langlois, P. and Gentilini, M. (1985). Complete development of hepatic stages of *Plamodium falciparum in vitro. Science* **227**: 440-442.
205. Gripon, P., Diot, C., Thézé, N., Fourel, I., Loréal, O., Bréchot, C. and Guguen-Guillouzo, C. (1988). Hepatitis B virus infection of adult human hepatocytes cultures in the presence of dimethylsulfoxide. *J. Virol.* **62**: 4136-4143.

4

An Evaluation of In Vitro Models for Assessing Nephrotoxicity

Patricia D. Williams

American Cyanamid Company
Pearl River, New York

Glenn F. Rush

Eli Lilly and Company
Greenfield, Indiana

INTRODUCTION

Renal Toxicity In Vitro

Physiological Considerations

A clear understanding of the mechanisms and characteristics of chemical-induced damage in the kidney is key in evaluating and designing effective in vitro models for nephrotoxicity. A number of physiological considerations are worthy of mention in this regard. For several reasons, the kidney is a prime pharmacokinetic target for toxic insults. First, unlike other organs, the kidney is exposed to a variety of xenobiotics, since the majority of endogenous as well as exogenous substances are eliminated (or conserved) by the kidney. Second, presumably by virtue of its physiological role in maintaining fluid and electrolyte balance, the kidney receives an impressive blood flow, representing approximately 25% of the resting cardiac output. Considering the relative weight of the kidney with respect to total body mass (<1%), the kidney is, therefore, exposed to proportionately higher levels of circulating xenobiotics than the majority of other organs.

Within the kidney itself, certain functional characteristics also contribute to the susceptibility of this organ to foreign substances. One such characteristic is the reabsorptive function occurring along the nephron, which, while preserving and conserving body fluids and electrolytes, also serves to concentrate substances in the luminal compartment of the nephron. Renal cells may, therefore, be exposed to very high concentrations of xenobiotics.

Another important function of the kidney relates to its ability to extract substances from the blood and luminal surfaces of the renal cell by active secretion or reabsorption of endogenous substances such as amino acids, sugars, and organic ions. The renal transport systems which have evolved to secrete or reabsorb endogenous substances may also transport structurally similar xenobiotics. Beta-lactam antibiotics, such as the penicillins and cephalosporins, for example, are known to accumulate within the proximal tubular epithelium via the organic ion transport system.

When one considers the pharmacokinetic factors of susceptibility in concert with the specialized transport features of the kidney, it comes as no surprise that the kidney is a frequent site of toxic insult due to drug and chemical exposure in man. Broad classes of drugs, as well as industrial chemicals, are implicated in nephrotoxic reactions, including antibiotics, antitumor agents, analgesics, metals, hydrocarbons, and organic solvents.

Pathological Considerations

The kidney is a heterogeneous structure composed of distinct cell types in the proximal and distal tubules, descending and ascending limbs of the loop of Henle, and the collecting ducts. Coupled with the heterogeneity of chemical/drug classes that can alter renal structure and function, it is not surprising that very different patterns of nephrotoxicity can occur. Aminoglycoside antibiotics, for example, predominately damage the convoluted portion of the proximal tubule (1,2), whereas the site of action of the antifungal agent, amphotericin, is the distal convoluted tubule of the nephron (3). Ultrastructural patterns of renal injury also tend to possess a fingerprint quality for many nephrotoxins. Aminoglycosides, for example, induce a prominent increase in secondary lysosomal structures (myeloid bodies) in the cellular cytoplasm (4,5). Amphotericin, on the other hand, is an ionophore which produces characteristic pores in the plasma membrane, presumably through an interaction with membrane-associated cholesterol (6,7).

The timing of a nephrotoxic insult also varies considerably between classes of nephrotoxins. Whereas some nephrotoxins can induce damage following a single exposure, others may require multiple dosing to produce a chronic insult. Analgesic nephropathy, for example, is a chronic phenomenon observable after weeks to months of high-dose exposure in laboratory animals and man (8,9). Mercuric chloride nephrotoxicity, on the other hand, is observable within hours after a single dose exposure (10,11).

Requirements for In Vitro Models

The importance of the above physiological considerations in in vitro model development and evaluation is twofold. On one hand, the specialized transport features of the renal cell in vivo may be critical for the accumulation of a particular nephrotoxin and subsequent expression of nephrotoxicity. Thus, a representative in vitro model should retain those characteristic functions known to play an important role in in vivo reactions to nephrotoxins. Keeping the pharmacokinetic aspects in mind, one must also be prepared to (1) potentially utilize high concentrations of nephrotoxins in vitro to mimic in vivo exposure, and (2) recognize that renal tissue may not be exclusively sensitive to xenobiotics relative to other tissues in vitro.

With respect to pathological considerations, the identity of the cellular population present in any particular in vitro model is critical to providing an accurate "surrogate" of in vivo reactions. With isolated renal cellular models it is particularly important to determine cell identity prior to examining site-specific nephrotoxins. In vitro models, having fulfilled site-specific functional and structural criteria, should also exhibit morphological and biochemical reactions to nephrotoxins similar to effects observed in vivo. Morphologically, toxins will produce characteristic patterns, or "fingerprints," of cellular injury discernible at the light or electron microscopic level of examination. Perhaps most importantly, establishing a correlation between biochemical mechanisms of injury in vivo and in vitro affords a significant level of confidence that in vitro results will accurately predict in vivo nephrotoxic potential. Last, in vitro models should be selected based upon their ability to adequately provide the timing necessary for nephrotoxic reactions to occur in vivo. Thus, nephrotoxins that require chronic dosing in vivo would appropriately be tested in longer term in vitro models rather than in preparations having a working life span of several hours.

To summarize, in vitro models for nephrotoxicity testing should, from physiological, mechanistic, and pathological perspectives, correlate as closely as possible with what is known regarding the individual nephrotoxin to be examined. The shortcomings and unknown aspects of the in vitro systems selected must be carefully considered as the model selection as well as the data interpretation stages.

RENAL MODELS IN VITRO

The use of various in vitro models in studying renal toxicology is well documented in the literature (12-17). Each model system possesses its own advantages and disadvantages and all have demonstrated their usefulness and application in renal toxicology. A representative listing of the models to be discussed in this chapter as well as their respective advantages and disadvantages is provided in Table 1.

Isolated Perfused Kidney

As the name implies, the isolated perfused kidney consists of the intact organ maintained in a tissue bath apparatus. An excellent review of the methods

Table 1 In Vitro Models for Studying Renal Toxicity

Model	Advantages	Disadvantages
Isolated perfused kidney	Morphologically identical to kidney in vivo Can monitor renal function	Short-term use In the process of degenerating
Kidney slices	Maintenance of renal architecture and heterogeneity Ease of preparation Nonsterile procedures	Short-term use (h) Inaccessible brush border surface In the process of degenerating Anoxic
Isolated tubules	Tubular structure intact	Short-term use Limited access to brush border surface
Renal cells	Long-term use (days-months) Long-term storage Bidirectional exposure feasible Cell-specific events can be monitored	Dedifferentiation Sterile conditions required for culture
Cultures		
cell lines	Easily obtained and subcultured	Origin often ill-defined Greater dedifferentiation
primary cultures	Closely related to fresh tissue Origin identified	More difficult to prepare and maintain
Suspensions	Do not require culture conditions and equipment	Short-term use Nonpolarized orientation

involved in preparing this model has been published by Newton and Hook (18). The most difficult aspect of the preparation is the surgery which takes advantage of the rat anatomy by a retrograde cannulation of the mesenteric artery. This permits cannulation of the renal artery without any interruption of flow, which is critical for a high-quality, functioning perfused kidney (18). The kidney is then perfused in a closed recirculating system for determination of electrolyte and inulin clearances as well as drug-induced changes in renal function. Sodium reabsorption can be maintained as high as 95% or greater for a period of up to 90 min. With respect to functional integrity of the model, proximal tubule transport processes such as glucose uptake (19), protein reabsorption (20), and amino acid uptake (21) have been shown to be maintained.

The isolated perfused rat kidney has been used to examine the transport and metabolism of a variety of endogenous and exogenous compounds (18, 22-27). While this model has been used widely to examine renal physiological and drug disposition issues, it has not been extensively utilized as a toxicological tool (28). Cojocel et al. (29) have used the isolated perfused rat kidney to examine the mechanisms of proteinuria induced by various aminoglycosides. Using lysozyme as a model protein, these authors were able to determine that netilmicin had no effect on lysozyme reabsorption, whereas gentamicin and tobramycin caused a significant reduction in the tubular reabsorption of lysozyme. Lysozyme degradation, estimated as the release of tyrosine into the perfusate, was also reduced by gentamicin and tobramycin (29). Several other investigators have studied brush border and the basolateral aspects of renal accumulation and toxic reactions to aminoglycosides in the isolated perfused kidney (30,31). In another series of investigations, Newton et al. (32,33) examined the metabolism of acetaminophen in relationship to the nephrotoxicity of this agent. These authors hypothesized that *para*-aminophenol, a metabolite of acetaminophen, was the chemical species actually responsible for acetaminophen-induced nephrotoxicity. Using the isolated perfused kidney, they were able to show that the kidney was capable of metabolizing acetaminophen to *para*-aminophenol (32). In addition to these studies, Newton et al. (33) were also able to demonstrate metabolic activation of acetaminophen to electrophilic intermediates capable of depleting glutathione (GSH). They postulated that the reactive intermediate may be responsible for the nephrotoxicity.

The advantage of the isolated perfused rat kidney over other in vitro model is that the functional integrity of the tissue is intact. Thus, one can measure renal functional and hemodynamic changes in kidneys isolated from drug-treated rats (ex vivo) or after direct drug exposure (in vitro). These experiments can be performed without the complications of neural innervation or extrarenal hemodynamic changes. Perhaps one of the key advantages of the isolated perfused kidney model is the ability to evaluate and compare the contribution(s) of the peritubular (basolateral) surface of the kidney in the accumulation and toxicity of agents relative to the luminal (brush border) surface. This is accomplished by measuring parameters of interest in filtering (luminal and peritubular exposure) and nonfiltering (peritubular exposure only) preparations (34).

There are also some striking disadvantages of the isolated perfused kidney. The model is often markedly vasodilated, which results in an unusually high flow through the organ resulting in a concentration defect. Thus, the isolated perfused kidney is incapable of establishing a high concentration gradient as is observed in vivo. In addition, the model is stable for only a relatively short period of time (up to 120 min), thus limiting the exposure period. Last, the technique requires considerable skill to master, and is time consuming. Despite these disadvantages, the isolated perfused rat kidney continues to be a valuable, and sometimes the only, tool in which to study certain aspects of renal function.

Kidney Slices

Renal tissue slice technology has been extensively exploited for renal pharmacology and toxicology assessments. This methodology involves the removal of longitudinal sections of kidney tissue of varying thickness and weight with a razor guided either "free hand" or through the use of an apparatus known as a Stadie-Riggs microtome (35). Kidney slices from virtually all species can be prepared; however, rat and rabbit have been the most frequently utilized models. While cortical slices are primarily studied, medullary tissue can also be obtained (36,37). Renal slices maintain the architecture and cellular heterogeneity of the intact kidney with tubular segments and surrounding interstitial and vascular elements present. Functionally, renal slices also exhibit organic ion transport, gluconeogenesis, and active maintenance of cellular sodium and potassium balance through the enzymatic activity of Na^+, K^+-ATPase (38,39).

Typically, the functional and morphological integrity of renal slices has a relatively short life span of approximately 2 h. However, one laboratory has succeeded in prolonging the viability of tissue slices for as long as 24 h (40).

It is contended that the renal slice technique measures primarily basolateral uptake of substrates or nephrotoxins based upon histological evidence of collapsed tubular lumens. This results in the inaccessibility of brush border surfaces for reabsorptive transport (41,42). This observation limits the ability of this model to accurately reflect reactions to nephrotoxins which occur as the result of brush border accumulation of an injurious agent. Ultrastructurally, a number of alterations, particularly in the plasma membrane and mitochondrial compartments, have been shown to occur over a 2-h incubation period (43). This deterioration in morphology is very likely a consequence of the insufficient diffusion of oxygen, metabolic substrates, and waste products in the innermost regions of the kidney slice (42). Such factors also limit the use of slices in studying renal metabolism and transport functions.

The use of renal cortical slices has been applied to the study of numerous nephrotoxins, including gentamicin (44,45), cisplatin (46-48), cephaloridine (49,50), chloroform (15,36), potassium dichromate (14,51), and the mycotoxin citrinin (39,52), to name a few. While congruence between biochemical effects of nephrotoxins on in vitro and ex vivo renal slice function has been achieved, correlations of morphological features of nephrotoxin-induced damage in kidney slices with in vivo effects are largely lacking.

Isolated Tubules

Isolated renal proximal tubule segments are most commonly prepared from either rats or rabbits by collagenase digestion of the kidneys followed by dispersion of the tissue into an appropriate buffer and filtration through sieves. Although this technique yields a tubule suspension that is highly contaminated with cellular debris, glomeruli, and distal tubules, the preparation can be further purified in a number of ways (53). Proximal tubule-"enriched" suspensions can be prepared by infusing magnetic iron oxide along with the collagenase which lodges in the glomerular capillary network. The glomeruli can then be selectively removed with a magnet and the resulting tubule suspension washed and centrifuged repeatedly to remove the cellular debris (54,55). This preparation is, however, still contaminated by a significant number of distal tubule fragments and cellular debris. Recently, Hatzinger and Stevens (55) have reported on a simple settling procedure that removed distal tubular fragments (as indicated by the marker enzyme hexokinase), whereas the proximal tubular marker fructose-1,6-diphosphatase remained high. This technique can result in an eightfold purification of proximal tubular fragments (Table 2) and has the advantage of being quick (in our experience the total preparation time is approximately 1.5 h) and relatively nonstressful to the tubules. Balaban et al. (53) have reported a method of layering tubules on a cushion of 25% Ficoll (400,000 MW). Tubules prepared in this manner have open lumina and carry out ouabain-sensitive transepithelial transport functions. Vinay et al. (56) reported on the preparation of a homogeneous population of proximal tubules (at least with regard to gluconeogenesis and transport of *para*-aminohippurate) by Percoll density gradient centrifugation. Microscopy and analysis of the enzymatic tubular markers (57) within the different fragments can then pinpoint the band containing pure proximal tubules.

Of all techniques listed above, that described by Hatzinger and Stevens (54) appears to be the most useful for toxicology applications in that they can be prepared quickly and appear to survive longer. These tubules can be maintained for prolonged periods of time with only minimal changes in the morphology or the biochemical function. Suspensions of rabbit proximal tubules can be incubated for up to 8 h while still maintaining greater than 85% viability and a relatively normal morphological appearance. Longer

Table 2 Purification of Suspensions of Isolated Rat Kidney Proximal Tubules by Gravity Sedimentation

Tubules	Hexokinase	Fructose-1,6-diphosphatase
Unpurified	1.6 ± 0.5	40 ± 7
Purified	0.2 ± 0.2	42 ± 8
Ratio	8.0	1.0

Source: Enzyme activities expressed nmol/min mg protein. Data from Ref. 55.

incubations (up to 24 h) have been performed (R. G. Schnellman, personal communication).

Renal tubular fragments appear to retain most of their in vivo functions and morphology. Balaban et al. (53) reported that less than 3% of the tubular cells had any structural pathology except for the removal of the basement membrane. An important feature of this preparation was that the tubular lumina were open (53). Functionally, isolated proximal tubular fragments transport *para*-aminohippurate, tetraethylammonium, α-methylglucoside, phosphate, and ^{86}Rb in a fashion similar to that reported in vivo demonstrating functional integrity of membrane processes of the preparation (56,58-60). With respect to renal cortical glutathione (GSH), the kidney normally has 18-25 nmol GSH/mg protein (61). In the absence of any amino acids, isolated tubules are approximately 50-70% GSH depleted when compared to control tissue. After 4 h of incubation, they contain only 510 nmol/mg protein (Fig. 1). However, suspensions of isolated rabbit tubules will synthesize GSH from its constituent amino acids, glutamate, cysteine, and glycine. None of the amino acids alone or methionine alone will support GSH synthesis. Furthermore, the disulfide cystine (the prevalent form of cysteine in plasma), is equally effective in supporting GSH synthesis in the presence of glycine and glutamate as was cysteine. The synthesis of GSH occurs at an estimated rate of approximately 10 nmol/h/mg protein in suspensions of proximal tubules incubated with glycine, cystine, and glutamate (see Fig. 1). There is also apparently no feedback regulation of GSH synthesis under these in-

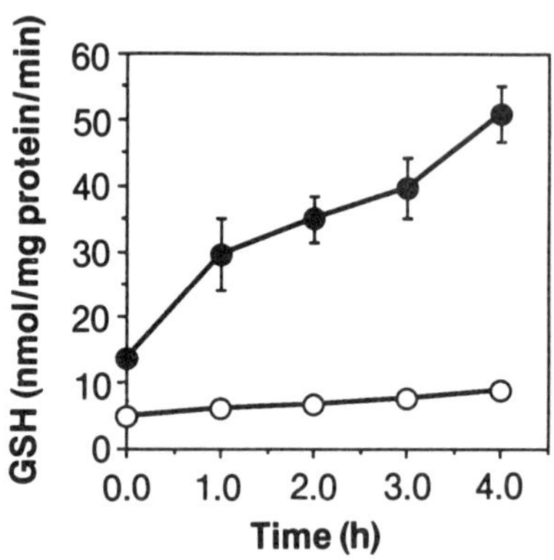

Figure 1 The effect of cystine, glutamate, and glycine on glutathione synthesis in suspensions of isolated rabbit proximal tubules. Amino acids were all present at 1.0 mM. Open and closed circles represent tubule GSH content in the absence and presence of amino acids, respectively.

cubation conditions, as total tubule GSH content reached 50 nmol/mg protein (compared to 18 nmol/mg protein in vivo). This is important to note, since the "GSH loading" that occurs upon incubation of tubules with amino acids may have an impact on studies with nephrotoxicants like cephaloridine which are potentiated by GSH depletion (62).

The technique of suspensions of isolated proximal tubules has been primarily adapted to the study of physiological studies of tubule function. Only recently have some investigators applied this technology to the study of mechanisms of nephrotoxicity. Isolated proximal tubules have, thus, been utilized to study the mechanisms of nephrotoxicity induced by antibiotics (63,64), radiocontrast dyes (65), metals (66), anoxia (67,68), cellular oxidants (61), cysteine conjugates (66,69,70), and a variety of nephrotoxic bromobenzene metabolites (70,71). Since this in vitro method has not been used historically as a toxicological tool, there has been little attempt to correlate the toxicological findings in isolated proximal tubules with in vivo toxicity. This clearly is an area which deserves some attention in future studies with this technique.

The advantages and disadvantages in using suspensions of isolated proximal tubules in toxicology studies are summarized in Table 1. One advantage is that the tubules can be prepared quickly and in large quantities such that a number of treatment groups from a single animal can be obtained. The environmental conditions of the experiments can be strictly controlled. Suspensions of isolated renal tubules also offer advantages over other in vitro renal techniques. For example, Balaban et al. (53) have elegantly demonstrated some the advantages of the tubule preparation over renal cortical slices. First, the oxygen consumption (QO_2) of the slice preparation was dependent on the bath PO_2, whereas the tubule QO_2 remained constant until near anoxia, indicating the presence of nonrespiring areas within the tissue slice. Second, in renal cortical slices, cytochrome a(a_3) was reduced ~50%, and became increasingly suppressed as bath PO_2 dropped, whereas cytochrome a(a_3) from isolated proximal tubules was only 6% reduced and essentially independent of bath PO_2, again demonstrating the anoxic condition of the slices (53).

There are distinct disadvantages to the use of tubule suspensions as well. They are essentially a dying preparation, and determining when the preparation becomes unusable is always a challenge, as with other short-term in vitro models. Finally, the tubules are only useful for relatively short-term toxicity (<24 h) testing and are of little use for studying chronic mechanisms of nephrotoxicity. Despite these disadvantages, the use of suspensions of proximal tubules is a valuable technique that is being used with increasing frequency as a tool to investigate mechanisms of toxicity to the renal proximal tubule.

Renal Cells

A variety of isolated cellular models exist for studying renal function and injury. These models can generally be divided into two categories: models derived from permanent renal cell lines and cellular models derived from freshly isolated renal tissue.

Cell Lines

Cell lines, derived from tissue of various species, are commercially available from tissue culture banks. These cell populations are "immortalized" in that they possess the capacity to permanently proliferate in culture. Several examples of renal cell lines are shown in Table 3. Such cellular models can be studied in short-term suspension (hours) or longer-term monolayer culture (days, weeks, months). Since cell lines have been extensively cultured or passaged for multiple generation, the degree of retention (or loss) of kidney-specific morphology and function is an important limitation which is not thoroughly addressed for a number of renal cell lines. Two renal cell lines which have been relatively well characterized are the pig kidney cell line LLC-PK_1, and the dog kidney cell line MDCK.

The MDCK (Madin-Darby Canine Kidney) cell line (83) is proposed to possess features predominantly of the distal tubule or collecting duct, including the expression of furosemide-sensitive Na^+, K^+, Cl^- transport and an amiloride-sensitive Na^+ channel (84). The LLC-PK_1 (porcine kidney) cell line (73), on the other hand, exhibits a range of morphological and functional properties of proximal tubule epithelium. For example, Na^+-dependent glucose and amino acid transport have been demonstrated in LLC-PK_1 cells (85-88). LLC-PK_1 cells have also demonstrated the ability to transport organic cations such as tetraethylammonium (TEA) (89), but do not appear to possess the capacity for organic anion transport (90). Morphologically, both MDCK and LLC-PK_1 cells have been shown to be polarized with apical

Table 3 Renal Cell Lines

Cell designation	Cell origin	References
LLC-RK_1	Rabbit kidney	72
LLC-PK_1	Porcine kidney	73
MDCK	Madin-Darby canine kidney	74
MDBK	Madin-Darby bovine kidney	75
RK-13	Rabbit kidney	76
LLC-MK-2	Rhesus monkey kidney	77,78
Vero	African green monkey kidney	79,80
RCC	Human renal cell carcinoma	81
TRKE-1	Rat kidney transformed cell line	82

microvilli, apical junctional complexes, desmosomes, and basolateral infoldings (91,92), which are typical of transporting epithelial cells. The expression of brush border morphology is most striking in LLC-PK_1 cells, although the amount of brush border is less than that observed in the proximal tubule in vivo (Fig. 2). High activities of proximal tubule brush border membrane enzymes have also been observed in LLC-PK_1 cells (93-95). Both MDCK and LLC-PK_1 cells possess significant levels of the basolateral enzyme marker, Na^+, K^+-ATPase, which is thought to result in the formation of fluid-filled "blisters" or domes in monolayer culture via transepithelial sodium and water transport (94,96).

Renal cell lines have been utilized to a limited extent for evaluating nephrotoxins. A rabbit kidney cell line (LLC-RK_1) has been utilized for evaluating nephrotoxic antibiotics (97-99). LLC-PK_1 cells have by far been the most widely employed cell line for studying drug-induced nephrotoxicity, specifically in the evaluation of aminoglycoside antibiotics (100-103). The morphological alterations induced by aminoglycosides in LLC-PK_1 cells correlate well with in vivo historical findings in the kidney, including the formation of secondary lysosomal inclusions referred to as myeloid bodies.

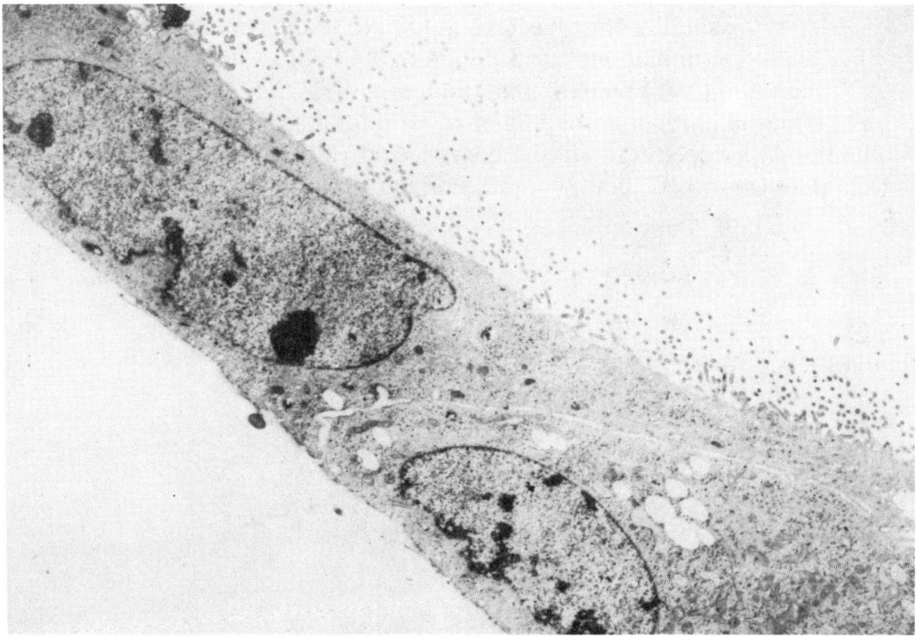

Figure 2 Electron micrograph of LLC-PK_1 cells in culture exhibiting polarized morphology and the presence of brush border microvilli ($\times$ 2500).

Primary Cells

Cells from freshly isolated renal tissue can be obtained by explant cultures, cultures of isolated renal tubules discussed in the previous section, and by digestion and isolation of individual renal cells. Cultures of isolated renal fragments such as the proximal tubule (104) and collecting tubule (105-107) have been the most extensively characterized models to date. Primary cultures of proximal tubules have been isolated from the rabbit (108), dog (109), rat (55,110), and human kidney (111-113). Primary cultures prepared from rabbit proximal tubules have been shown to exhibit polarity and transport characteristics consistent with proximal tubule function. As with certain renal cell lines such as the LLC-PK_1 and MDCK, primary cultures also possess tight junctions and basolateral Na^+, K^+-ATPase activity which results in the formation of fluid-filled "blisters" or domes in monolayer culture. Transport functions, including phlorizin-sensitive Na^+-glucose uptake (8) and organic anion and cation transport (114,115), have also been reported in rabbit primary cultures. Primary cultures of rabbit proximal tubules have also been shown to be responsive to parathyroid hormone (108,116), maintain cellular glutathione levels (117) and exhibit brush border enzyme activity (118). A representative listing of the types of renal primary cell culture systems developed is shown in Table 4.

Primary renal cell culture has been utilized to study a number of nephrotoxic agents, including mercuric chloride (117,119), cadmium (121), lead (120), cisplatin (16), aminoglycoside antibiotics (98,122,123), and cyclosporin (124). Studies reported by Tay et al. (16) in rabbit proximal tubule cell cultures with cisplatin revealed biochemical effects upon deoxyribonucleic acid (DNA) synthetic activity which correlated with in vivo histochemical

Table 4 Primary Renal Cell Culture Models

Method of preparation	Source	References
Isolated tubules	Rabbit:cortex	108
	Rabbit:microdissected tubules	116
		106
		107
	Rat:cortex	55
	Dog:cortex	109
	Human:microdissected tubules	112
Isolated cells	Rat:cortex	119
		120
		121
Explant cultures	Human:cortex	111

effects of this antitumor agent in animals. With respect to studies involving mercuric chloride and aminoglycoside antibiotics in primary renal cultures, light and electron microscopy revealed similar patterns of cellular pathology in vitro as compared to in vivo exposure in animals (117,123).

Suspensions rather than cultures of renal cell lines and primary cells are also available for short-term evaluations. Procedures for the isolation and purification of specific renal cell types include density gradient centrifugation, flow cytometry, free flow electrophoresis, enzymatic digestion, and monoclonal antibodies (125-130). While primary renal cell suspensions possess the advantage of being freshly isolated and derived from intact kidney tissue, a major disadvantage is their lack of cellular polarity which is exhibited with cells in culture. Relatively few reports of renal suspension cultures being used in nephrotoxic evaluations are in the literature at this time (102).

Several advantages and disadvantages of renal cell lines and primary cells as models for nephrotoxicity evaluations are listed in Table 1. One of the unique advantages of renal cell culture rests in the ability to study the directional aspects of drug exposure and cellular injury which operate in vivo. This potential provides the opportunity to study compounds which interact or accumulate within the renal tubular epithelium in vivo via tubular reabsorption from the luminal surface or extraction from the basolateral or blood surface. Preliminary data involving the directional aspects of antibiotic toxicity to LLC-PK_1 cells has recently been obtained. The data, summarized in Figure 3, indicate that LLC-PK_1 cells are significantly more sensitive to the nephrotoxin cephaloridine when the antibiotic was applied to the basolateral surface of the kidney cell. These data are consistent with the evidence that cephaloridine is accumulated in renal cells predominantly through basolateral transport. This cellular accumulation is then proposed to precipitate cellular injury and death.

Biochemical Systems

In addition to the isolated organ, tubule, and cellular models described above, biochemical systems derived from renal tissue represent valuable resources for in vitro evaluations of nephrotoxins. Particularly, the use of isolated cellular organelles such as mitochondria and plasma membranes has been applied to the study of nephrotoxins (131-134). The examination of mechanisms of accumulation of nephrotoxins in the kidney has been accomplished utilizing purified renal brush border and basolateral membrane vesicles for aminoglycosides (132,135), cephalosporins (136,137), and cisplatin (131). Williams and coworkers (135) reported that the affinity for renal membrane binding sites correlated well with the nephrotoxic potential for aminoglycosides (Fig. 4). Thus, this membrane model could be utilized to assess the

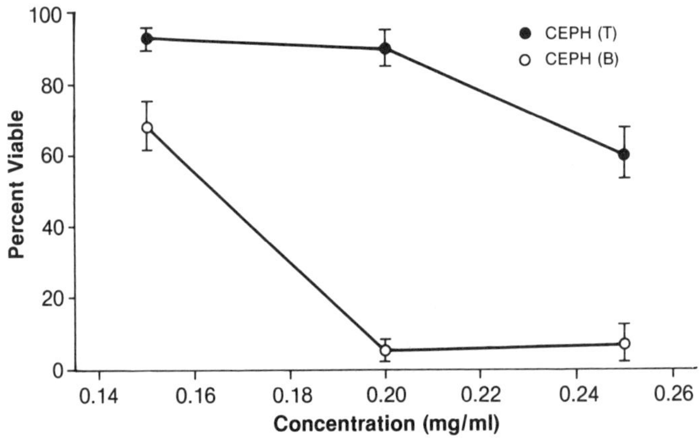

Figure 3 Toxicity of cephaloridine to LLC-PK_1 cells exposed from the top (T) or bottom (B) compartment of a cellulose acetate filter insert. Toxicity was assessed 48 hs after exposure to cephaloridine by nigrosin dye exclusion. The percent of viable cells is expressed relative to control cultures. The mean ± S.E. of 6-12 determinations is shown.

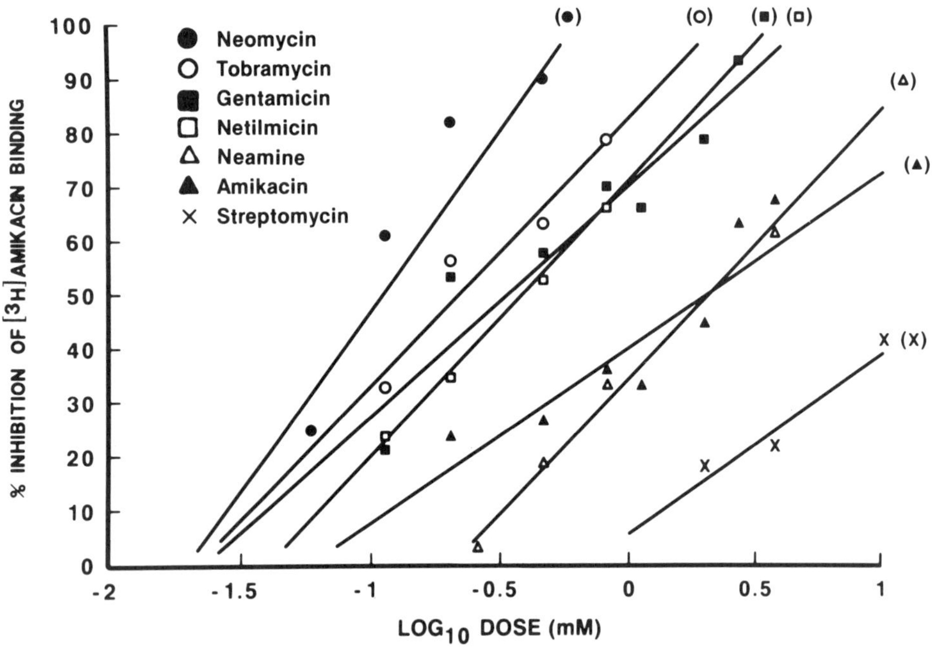

Figure 4 Inhibition of [^{3}H]amikacin binding to renal brush border membranes by the aminoglycosides neomycin, tobramycin, netilmicin, gentamicin, neamine, amikacin, and streptomycin.

relative nephrotoxic potential of new aminoglycosides. Furthermore, isolated renal membranes were successfully employed in the identification of in vivo nephrotoxicity inhibitors for aminoglycosides (138).

THE ROLE OF IN VITRO SYSTEMS IN RISK ASSESSMENT OF NEPHROTOXINS

In vitro renal methods can contribute in several ways to the safety evaluation of new chemical or pharmaceutical entities. At the early stages of compound identification, in vitro systems can serve to compare a new entity for nephrotoxic potential relative to agents with known liabilities or safety. This type of early evaluation permits the selection from a series of chemical analogs those agents that possess reduced nephrotoxic potential. The use of the various in vitro renal models in the evaluation of agents such as cephalosporin and aminoglycoside antibiotics is widely recognized, as described in the previous sections. Such preliminary screening can greatly enhance the probability of success of new agents in in vivo nephrotoxicity studies. Second, the use of in vitro techniques in investigating mechanisms of drug- or chemical-induced renal damage can contribute to the risk assessment process in two ways. First, as safety issues arise in the preclinical or clinical phases of drug development, the study of mechanisms of toxic action can aid in the resolution of these issues, particularly in determining the potential risk to man. Second, knowledge of the basic mechanisms of nephrotoxicity which may be disclosed in drug or chemical safety studies plays an important role in designing agents with improved safety profiles.

Since the development of safe as well as effective products is the ultimate goal not only of the toxicologist, but of the corporate and regulatory communities involved in marketing chemicals or drugs, the role that in vitro models can play in the design of new agents and improvement of existing ones is particularly exciting. Specifically, in vitro systems permit toxicologists as well as biochemists and chemists to study structure-activity relationships involved in toxic reactions. With respect to existing products, the modeling of toxic reactions in vitro, particularly at the mechanistic level, provides avenues for designing strategies to ameliorate or prevent injury at the target organ level. An example of the contribution in vitro renal models can play in drug discovery involves the identification of nephrotoxicity inhibitors of aminoglycoside antibiotics. Utilizing isolated renal cell membranes, large numbers of chemicals were screened for their potential to inhibit aminoglycoside binding to kidney membranes. This screening effort resulted in the discovery of several potent agents that effectively blocked the nephrotoxocity associated with this class of antibiotics (138).

As previously discussed, the ultimate value of in vitro models, regardless of their specific application, is dependent upon the degree of physiological and pathological correlation with in vivo aspects of the class of nephrotoxins to be studied. Specifically, the following questions should be asked prior to the use and interpretation of data from the in vitro models previously described:

Does the in vitro model exhibit the transport function(s) associated with the accumulation of the specific nephrotoxin in vivo?
Does the histopathological pattern of injury in vitro resemble what is observed in the kidney following in vivo exposure to this nephrotoxin?
Are biochemical pathways known to be involved in the expression or modulation of nephrotoxicity in vivo present in the in vitro model?
How do the concentrations in vitro relate to kidney or plasma levels achieved in vivo?
How does the duration of exposure used in vitro correlate with the timing of the nephrotoxic insult in vivo?

Only by answering this types of questions can the results of in vitro studies be properly interpreted in terms of their limitations as well as strengths in supporting our hypotheses and conclusions.

FUTURE DIRECTIONS

The immediate availability and utility of various in vitro renal models is apparent. Each system has its advantages and limitations as outlined in Table 1. Challenges for the future involve the continued development of current in vitro models to provide physiological and morphological characteristics which correlate more closely with the kidney in vivo. These challenges will include defining media constituents that will facilitate the retention of renal-metabolizing capabilities in cell culture, for example. In addition, the maintenance of normal kidney morphology poses an interesting challenge in in vitro model development. Last, and perhaps most challenging, is the need to establish in vitro systems that reproduce the dynamic features of the nephron in vivo. The kidney, like other organs, exists in a dynamic rather than static environment. The fluid dynamics and vasculature of the renal nephron most certainly play a role in the sensitivity of the kidney both in terms of dose and time response to nephrotoxins.

With the development of in vitro models more closely representing kidney function and dynamics, the ability to accurately predict nephrotoxic reactions in vivo will be enhanced. As time and experience build scientific confidence and validation of these in vitro models, one can envision the ability to utilize in vitro models more extensively in the assessment of nephrotoxicity. However, for the present, the utilization of in vivo models is imperative for responsible risk assessment of nephrotoxins. At the same time, the use of the described in vitro renal models can serve as valuable adjuncts to these in vivo assessments, not only reducing the number of animals used in risk assessment, but providing unique information and possibilities for scientists involved in the drug discovery and development process.

ACKNOWLEDGMENT

The authors wish to thank Mrs. Ann Laverty for her patience and expertise in preparing this manuscript.

REFERENCES

1. Hottendorf, G. H., and Williams, P. D. (1986). Aminoglycoside nephrotoxicity. *Toxicol. Pathol.* **14**: 66-72.
2. Kaloyanides, G. J. (1984). Aminoglycoside-induced functional and biochemical defects in the renal cortex. *Fund. Appl. Toxicol.* **4**: 930-943.
3. Burgess, J. L., and Birchall, R. (1972). Nephrotoxicity of amphotericin B, with emphasis on changes in tubular function. *Am. J. Med.* **53**: 77-84, 1972.
4. Kosek, J. C., Mazze, R. I., and Cousins, M. J. (1974). Nephrotoxicity of gentamicin. *Lab. Invest.* **30**: 48-57.
5. Luft, F. C., Yum, M. N., Walker, P. D., and Kleit, S. A. (1977). Gentamicin gradient patterns and morphological changes in human kidneys. *Nephron* **18**: 167-174.
6. Weissman, G., Hirschhorn, R., Pras, M., Sessa, G., and Bevans, V. (1967). Studies of lysosomes-VIII: The effects of polyene antibiotics on lysosomes. *Biochem. Pharm. acol.* **16**: 1057-1069.
7. Houslay, M. D., and Stanley, K. K. (1982). Dynamic membrane-associated processes. In *Dynamics of Biological Membranes.* Wiley, pp. 281-325.
8. Kincaid-Smith, P., Saker, B. M., McKenzie, I. F. C., and Muriden, K. D. (1968). Lesions in the blood supply of the papilla in experimental analgesic nephropathy. *Med. J. Aust.* **1**: 203-206.
9. Saker, B. M., and Kincaid-Smith, P. (1969). Papillary necrosis in experimental analgesic nephropathy. *Br. Med. J.* **1**: 161-162.
10. Ganote, C. E., Reimer, K. A., and Jennings, R. B. (1974). Acute mercuric chloride nephrotoxicity. An electron microscopic and metabolic study. *Lab. Invest.* **31**: 633-647.
11. Ware, R. A., Burkholder, P. M., and Chang, L. W. (1975). Ultrastructural changes in renal proximal tubules after chronic organic and inorganic mercury intoxication. *Environ. Res.* **10**: 121-140.
12. Hassall, C. D., Gandolfi, A. J., and Brendel, K. (1983). Correlation of the *in vivo* and in vitro renal toxicity of S-(1,2-dichlorovinyl)-L-cysteine. *Drug Chem. Toxicol.* **6**: 507-520.
13. Hook, J. B., and Hewitt, W. R. (1986). Toxic responses of the kidney. In *Casarett & Doull's Toxicology. The Basic Science of Poisons.* 3rd Ed. C. D. Klaassen, M. O. Amdur, and J. Doull, (Ed.). Macmillan, New York: pp. 310-329.

14. Kacew, S., and Hirsch, G. H. (1981). Evaluation of nephrotoxicity of various compounds by means of *in vitro* techniques and comparison to *in vivo* methods. In *Toxicology of the Kidney*. J. B. Hook (Ed.). Raven Press, New York, pp. 77-98.
15. Smith, J. H., and Hook, J. B. (1983). Mechanism of chloroform nephro-toxicity. II. *In vitro* evidence for renal metabolism of chloroform in mice. *Toxicol. Appl. Pharmacol.* **70**: 480-485.
16. Tay, L. K., Bregman, C. L., Masters, B. G., and Williams, P. D. (1988). Effects of cis-diamminedichloroplatinum (II) on rabbit kidney *in vivo* and on rabbit renal proximal tubule cells in culture. *Cancer Res.* **48**: 2538-2543.
17. Williams, P. D. (1989). The application of renal cells in culture in studying drug-induced nephrotoxicity. *In Vitro* **25**: 800-805.
18. Newton, J. F., and Hook, J. B. (1981). Isolated Perfused Rat Kidney. In *Methods in Enzymology*. Vol. 77. W. B. Jacoby (Ed.). Academic Press, New York.
19. Bowman, R. H., and Maack, T. (1972). Glucose transport by the isolated perfused rat kidney. *Am. J. Physiol.* **222**: 1499-1504.
20. Maack, T. (1975). Renal handling of low molecular weight proteins. *Am. J. Med.* **58**: 57-64.
21. De Mello, G., and Maack, T. (1976). Nephron function of the isolated perfused rat rat kidney. *Am. J. Physiol.* **231**: 1699-1707.
22. Trimble, M. E. (1982). Long chain fatty acid transport by the perfused rat kidney. *Renal Physiol.* **5**: 136-142.
23. Fonteles, M. C., Ganapathy, V., Pashley, D. H., and Leibach, F. H. (1983). Dipeptide Metabolism in the Isolated Perfused Rat Kidney. *Life Sci.* **33**: 431-436.
24. Besseghir, K., Pearce, L. B., and Rennick, B. (1981). Renal tubular transport and metabolism of organic cations by the rabbit. *Am. J. Physiol.* **241**: F308-F314.
25. Ormstad, K., Lastbom, T., and Orrenius, S. (1982). Evidence for different localization of glutathione oxidase and γ-glutamyltransferase activities during extracellular glutathione metabolism in isolated perfused rat kidney. *Biochim. Biophys. Acta* **700**: 148-153.
26. Acara, M., Gessner, H., Greizerstein, H., and Trudnowski, R. (1981). Renal N-oxidation of meperidine by the perfused kidney of the rat. *Drug Metab. Dispos.* **9**: 75-79.
27. Rocci, M. L., Szefler, S. J., Acara, M., and Jusko, W. J. (1981). Prednisolone metabolism and excretion in the isolated perfused rat kidney. *Drug Metab. Dispos.* **9**: 177-182.
28. Bekersky, I. (1983). The isolated perfused kidney as a pharmacological tool. *TIBS* **4**: 6-7.
29. Cojocel, C., Dociu, N., Maita, K., Sleight, S. D., and Hook, J. B. (1983). Effects of aminoglycosides on glomerular permeability, tubular reabsorption, and intracellular catabolism of the cationic low molecular weight protein lysozyme. *Toxicol. Appl. Pharmacol.* **68**: 96-109.

30. Collier, V., Lietman, P., and Mitch, W. (1979). Evidence for luminal uptake of gentamicin in the perfused rat kidney. *J. Pharmacol. Exp. Ther.* **210**: 247-251.
31. Williams, P. D., Trimble, M. E., Crespo, L., Holohan, P. D., Freedman, J. C., and Ross, C. R. (1984). Inhibition of renal Na^+, K^+-adenosine triphosphatase by gentamicin. *Pharmacal. and Exp. Ther.,* **231**(2): 1984.
32. Newton, J. F., Kuo, C.-H., Gemborys, M. W., Mudge, G. H., and Hook, J. B. (1982). Nephrotoxicity of p-aminophenol, a metabolite of acetaminophen, in the Fischer 344 rat. *Toxicol. Appl. Pharmacol.* **65**: 336-344.
33. Newton, J. F., Braselton, W. E., Kuo, Kluwe, W. M., C.-H., Gemborys, M. W., Mudge, G. H. and Hook, J. B. (1982). Metabolism of acetaminophen by the isolated perfused kidney. *J. Pharmacol. Exp. Therp. 221*: 76-79.
34. Johnson, V., and Maack, T. (1977). Renal extraction, filtration, absorption, and catabolism of growth hormone. *Am. J. Physiol.* **233**(3): F185-F196.
35. Stadie, W. C., and Riggs, B. C. (1944). Microtome for the preparation of tissue slices for metabolic studies of tissues *in vitro*. *J. Biol. Chem.* **154**: 687-690.
36. Smith, J. H., Maita, K., Sleight, S. D., and Hook, J. B. (1983). Mechanism of chloroform nephrotoxicity. I. Time course of chloroform toxicity in male and female mice. *Toxicol. Appl. Pharmacol.* **70**: 467-479.
37. Rapp, N. S., Zenser, T. V., Brown, W. W., and Davis, B. B. (1980). Metabolism of benzidine by a prostaglandin-mediated process in renal inner medullary slices. *J. Pharmacol. Exp. Ther.* **215**: 401-406.
38. Cross, R. J., and Taggart, J. L. (1950). Renal tubular transport: Accumulation of p-aminohippurate by rabbit kidney slices. *Am. J. Physiol.* **161**: 181-190.
39. Berndt, W. O., Hayes, A. W., and Baggett, J. M. (1984). Effects of fungal toxins on renal slice calcium balance. *Toxicol. Appl. Pharmacol.* **74**(1): 78-85.
40. Ruegg, C. E., Gondolfi, A. J., Brendel, K., Nagle, R. B., and Krumdieck, C. L. (1987). Preparation of positional renal slices for study of cell-specific toxicity. *J. Pharmacol. Meth.* **17**: 111-123.
41. Burg, M. B., and Orloff, J. (1969). *Para*-aminohippurate uptake and exchange by separated renal tubules. *Am. J. Physiol.* **217**: 1064-1068.
42. Cohen, J. J., and Kamm, D. E. (1976). Renal metabolism: Relation to renal function. In *The Kidney*. B. M. Brenner and F. C. Rector. (Eds.). Saunders, Philadelphia, pp. 126-214.
43. Martel-Pelletier, J., Guerette, D., and Bergeron, M. (1977). Morphologic changes during incubation of renal slices. *Lab. Invest.* **36**(5): 509-518.
44. Kluwe, W. M., and Hook, J. B. (1978). Functional nephrotoxicity of gentamicin in the rat. *Toxicol. Appl. Pharmacol.* **45**: 163-175.
45. Hsu, C. H., Kurtz, T. W., and Weller, J. M. (1977). In vitro uptake of gentamicin by rat renal cortical tissue. *Antimicrob. Agents Chemother.* **12**: 192-194.
46. Phelps, J. S., Gandolfi, A. J., Brendel, K., and Dorr, R. T. (1987). Cisplatin nephrotoxicity: In vitro studies with precision-cut rabbit renal cortical slices. *Toxicol. Appl. Pharmacol.* **90**: 501-512.
47. Goldstein, R. S., Noordewier, B., Bond, J. T., Hook, J. B., and Mayor, G. H. (1981). Cis-diaminedichloroplatinum nephrotoxicity: Time course and dose

response of renal functional impairment. *Toxicol. Appl. Pharmacol.* **60**: 163-175.
48. Safirstein, R., Miller, P., Dikman, S., Lyman, S., and Shapiro, C. (1981). Cisplatin nephrotoxicity in rats. *Kidney Int.* **25**: 753-758.
49. Goldstein, R. S., Contardi, L. R., Pasino, D. A., and Hook, J. B. (1987). Mechanisms mediating cephaloridine inhibition of renal gluconeogenesis. *Toxicol. Appl. Pharmacol.* **87**(2): 297-305.
50. Goldstein, R. S., Pasino, D. A., Hewitt, W. R., and Hook, J. B. (1986). Biochemical mechanisms of cephaloridine nephrotoxicity: Time and concentration dependence of peroxidative injury. *Toxicol. Appl. Pharmacol.* **83**(2): 261-70.
51. Ruegg, C. E., Gandolfi, A. J., Nagle, R. B., and Brendel, K. (1987). Differential patterns of injury to the proximal tubule of renal cortical slices following in vitro exposure to mercuric chloride, potassium dichromate or hypoxic conditions. *Toxicol. Appl. Pharmacol.* **90**: 261-273.
52. Baggett, J. M., and Berndt, W. O. (1984). Interactin of potassium dichromate with the nephrotoxins, mercuric chloride and citrinin. *Toxicology* **33**(2): 157-169.
53. Balaban, R. S., Soltoff, S. P., Storey, J. M., and Mandel, L. J. (1980). Improved renal cortical suspension: Spectrophotometric study of O_2 delivery. *Am. J. Physiol.* **238**: F50-F59.
54. Taub, M. (1984). Growth of primary and established kidney cell cultures in serum-free media. In *Methods for Serum-Free Culture of Epithelial and Fibroblastic Cells.* D. W. Barnes, D. A. A. Sirbasku and G. H. Sato (Eds.). Liss, New York, pp. 3-24.
55. Hatzinger, P. B., and Stevens, J. L. (1989). Rat kidney proximal tubule cells in defined medium: The roles of cholera toxin, extracellular calcium and serum in cell growth and expression of γ-glutamyltransferase. *In Vitro Cell. Devel. Biol.* **25**(2): 205-212.
56. Vinay, P., Gougoux, A., and Lemieux, G. (1981). Isolation of a pure suspension of rat proximal tubules. *Am. J. Physiol.* **241**: F403-F411.
57. Schmidt, U., and Guder, G. (1976). Sites of enzyme activity along the nephron. *Kidney Int.* **9**: 233-242.
58. Tessitore, N., Sakhrani, L. M., and Massry, S. G. (1986). Quantitative requirement for ATP for active transport in isolated renal cells. *Am. J. Physiol.* **251**: C120-C127.
59. Dantzler, W. H., Brokl, O. H., and Wright, S. H. (1989). Brush-border TEA transport in intact proximal tubules and isolated membrane vesicles. *Am. J. Physiol.* **256**: F290-F297.
60. Dantzler, W. H., and Brokl, O. H. (1984). Effects of low $[Ca^{2+}]$ and La^{3+} on PAH transport by isolated perfused renal tubules. *Am. J. Physiol.* **246**: F175-F187.
61. Messana, J. M., Cieslinski, D. A., O'Connor, R. P., and Humes, H. D. (1988). Glutathione protects against exogenous oxidant injury to rabbit renal proximal tubules. *Am. J. Physiol.* **255**: F874-F884.

62. Kuo, C.-H., and Hook, J. B. (1982). Depletion of renal glutathione content and nephrotoxicity of cephaloridine in rabbits, rats and mice. *Toxicol. Appl. Pharmacol.* **63**: 292-302.
63. Sina, J. F., Bean, C. L., Noble, C., and Bradley, M. O. (1985). An in vitro nehprotoxicity assay utilizing proximal tubule suspensions from rabbit kidney. In *In Vitro Toxicology.* Vol. 3, Maryann Liebert, New York, pp. 683-693.
64. Sina, J. F., Bean, C. L., Bland, J. A., MacDonald, J. J., Noble, C., Robertson, R. T., and Bradley, M. O. (1986). An in vitro assay for cytotoxicity to proximal tubule suspensions from rabbit kidney. *In Vitro Toxicol.* **1**(1): 13-22.
65. Humes, H. D., Hunt, D. A., and White, M. D. (1987). Direct toxic influence of the radiocontrast agent diatrizoate on renal proximal tubule cells. *Am. J. Physiol.* **252**: F246-F255.
66. Rylander, L. A., Gandolfi, A. J., and Brendel, K. (1985). Inhibition of organic acid/base transport in isolated rabbit renal tubules by nephrotoxins. In *In Vitro Toxicology: A progress report from The Johns Hopkins Center for Alternatives to Animal Testing.* Vol. 3. A. M. Goldberg. (Ed.) Mary Ann Liebert, New York, pp. 235-247.
67. Weinberg, J. M. (1985). Oxygen deprivation-induced injury to isolated rabbit kidney tubules. *J. Clin. Invest.* **76**: 1193-2108.
68. Weinberg, J. M., Davis, J. A., Abarzua, M., and Rajan, T. (1987). Cytoprotective effects of glycine and glutathione against hypoxic injury to renal tubules. *J. Clin. Invest.* **80**: 1446-1454.
69. Zhang, G., and Stevens, J. L. (1989). Transport and activation of S-(1,2-dichlorovinyl)-L-cysteine and N-acetyl-S-(1,2-dichlorovinyl)-L-cysteine in rat kidney proximal tubules. *Toxicol. Appl. Pharmacol.* **100**: 51-61.
70. Schnellman, R. G., Lock, E. A., and Mandel, L. J. (1987). A Mechanism of S-(1,2,3,4,4-Pentachloro-1,3-butadienyl)-L-cysteine Toxicity to Rabbit Proximal Tubules. *Toxicol. Appl. Pharmacol.* **90**: 513-521.
71. Schnellman, R. G., and Mandel, L. J. (1986). Cellular toxicity of bromobenzene and bromobenzene metabolites to rabbit proximal tubules: The role and mechanism of 2-bromohydroquinone. *J. Pharmacol. Exp. Ther.* **237**: 456-461.
72. Hull, R. N., Dwyer, A. C., Cherry, W. R., and Tritch, O. J. (1965). Development and characteristics of the rabbit kidney cell strain, LLC-RK_1. *Proc. Soc. Exp. Biol. Med.* **118**: 1054-1059.
73. Hull, R. N., Cherry, W. R., and Weaver, G. W. (1976). The origin and characteristics of a pig kidney cell strain LLC-PK_1. *In Vitro* **12**: 670-677.
74. Saier, M. (1981). Growth and differentiated properties of a kidney epithelial cell line (MDCK). *Amer. J. Physiol.* **240**: C106-C109.
75. Bracken, W. M., and Sharma, R. P. (1985). Biochemical responsiveness of a bovine kidney cell line to inorganic mercury. *Archs. Envir. Contam. Toxicol.* **14**: 509-515.
76. Szmigielski, S., Janiak, M., Mollby, R., Wadstrom, T., and Jeljaszwicz, J. (1978). Metabolism of rabbit kidney cells incubated in vitro with phospholipase c from staphylococcus aureus and clostridium perfringens. *Toxicon.* **16**: 567-574.

77. Abrahamson, I. A., and Kloetzel, J. K. (1980). Presence of *Trypanosoma cruzi* antigen on the surface of both infected and uninfected cells in tissue culture. *Parantol.* **80**: 147-152.
78. Middlebrook, J. L. (1981). Effect of energy inhibitors on cell surface diphtheria toxin receptor numbers. *J. Biol. Chem.* **256**: 7898-7904.
79. McLane, B. A., and McDonel, J. L. (1979). The effect of *Clostridium perfringens* enterotoxin on morphology, viability and macromolecular synthesis in Vero cells. *J. Cell. Physiol.* **99**: 191-200.
80. Speirs, J. I., Stavric, S., and Konowalchuk, J. (1977). Assay of *Escherichia coli* heat-labile enterotoxin with Vero cells. *Infect. Immunity.* **16**: 617-622.
81. Moon, T. D., Morley, J. E., Vessella, R. L., Levine, A. S., Peterson, G., and Lange, P. M. (1983). The role of calmodulin in human renal carcinoma. *Biochem. Biophys. Res. Commun.* **114**: 843-849.
82. Hard, G. C., and Brown, C. H. (1980). Isolation of a morphologically transformed epithelial cell line from rat kidney following an in vivo dose of dimethylnitrosamine. *Cancer Lett.* **10**: 277-283.
83. Abaza, N. A., Leighton, J., and Schultz, S. G. (1974). Effects of ouabain on the function and structure of a cell line (MDCK) derived from canine kidney. I. Light microscopic observations of monolayer growth. *In Vitro* **10**: 172-179.
84. Taub, M., and Saier, M. H. (1979). Regulations of ^{22}Na transport by calcium in an established kidney epithelial cell line. *J. Biol. Chem.* **254**: 11440-11444.
85. Misfeldt, D. S., and Sanders, M. J. (1981). Transepithelial transport in cell culture: D-glucose transport by a pig kidney cell line (LLC-PK_1). *J. Membr. Biol.* **59**: 13-18.
86. Rabito, C. A., and Ausiello, D. A. (1980). Na^+-dependent sugar transport in a cultured epithelial cell line from pig kidney. *J. Membr. Biol.* **54**: 31-38.
87. Rabito, C. A., and Karish, M. V. (1982). Polarized amino acid transport by an epithelial cell line of renal origin (LLC-PK_1). The basolateral systems. *J. Biol. Chem.* **257**: 6802-6808.
87a. Rabito, C. A., and Karish, M. V. (1983). Polarized amino acid transport by an epithelial cell line of renal origin (LLC-PK). The apical systems. *J. Biol. Chem.* **258**: 2543-2547.
88. Sakhrani, L. M., Badie-Dezfooly, B., Trizna, W., Mikhails, N., Lowe, A., Taub, M., and Fine, L. G. (1984). Transport and metabolism of glucose by renal proximal tubular cells in primary culture. *Am. J. Physiol.* **246**: F757-F764.
89. Inui, K., Saito, H., and Hori, R. (1985). H^+ gradient-dependent active transport of tetraethylammonium cation in apical-membrane vesicles isolated from kidney epithelial cell line LLC-PK_1. *Biochem. J.* **227**: 199-203.
90. Rabito, C. A. (1986). Occluding junctions in a renal cell line (LLC-PK_1) with characteristics of proximal tubular cells. *Am. J. Physiol.* **250**: F734-F743, 1986.
91. Cereijido, M., Ehrenfeld, J., Meza, I., and Martinez-Palomo, A. (1980). Structural and functional membrane polarity in cultured monolayers of MDCK cells. *J. Membr. Biol.* **52**: 147-159.
92. Cereijido, M., Robbins, E. S., Dolan, W. J., Rotunno, C. A., and Sabatini, D. D. (1978). Polarized monolayers formed by epithelial cells on a permeable and translucent support. *J. Cell Biol.* **77**: 853-880.

93. Perantoni, A., and Berman, J. J. (1979). Properties of Wilms' tumor line (TuWi) and pig kidney line ($LLC-PK_1$) typical of normal kidney tubular epithelium. *In Vitro* **15**: 446-454.
94. Gstraunthaler, G., Pfaller, W., and Kotanko, P. (1985). Biochemical characterization of renal epithelial cell cultures ($LLC-PK_1$ and MDCK). *Am. J. Physiol.* **248** (Renal Fluid Electrolyte Physiol. **17**) F536-F544, 1985.
95. Sepulveda, F. V., Burton, K. A., and J. D. Pearson. (1982). The development of g-glutamyltransferase in a pig renal-epithelial cell line in vitro. *Biochem. J.* **208**: 509-512.
96. Mills, J. W., Macknight, A., Jarrel, J. A., Dayer, J. M., Ausiello, D. A. (1981). Interaction of ouabain with Na^+ pump in intact epithelial cells. *J. Cell Biol.* **88**: 637-643.
97. Viano, I., Eandi, M., and Santiano, M. (1983). Toxic effects of some antibiotics on rabbit kidney cells. *Int. J. Tiss. React.* **2**: 181-186.
98. Williams, P. D., Laska, D. A., Tay, L. K., and Hottendorf, G. H. (1988). Comparative toxicity of cephalosporin antibiotics in a rabbit kidney cell line ($LLC-RK_1$). *Antimicrob. Agents Chemother.* **32**(3): 314-318.
99. Hottendorf, G. H., Laska, D. A., Ford, S. M., and Williams, P. D. (1987). The role of desacetylation in the detoxification of cephalothin in renal cells in culture. *J. Toxicol. Environ. Health* **22**: 101-111.
100. Hori, R., Yamamoto, Saito, H., Kohno, M., and Inui, K. (1984). Effect of aminoglycoside antibiotics on cellular functions of kidney epithelial cell line ($LLC-PK_1$): A model system for aminoglycoside nephrotoxicity. *Pharmacol. Exp. Ther.* **230**: 742-748.
101. Schwertz, D. W., Kreisberg, J. I., and Venkatachalam, M. A. (1986). Gentamicin-induced alterations in pig kidney epithelial ($LLC-PK_1$) cells in culture. *J. Pharmacol. Exp. Ther.* **236**(1): 254-262.
102. Holohan, P. D., Sokol, P. P., Ross, C. R., Coulson, R., Trimble, M. E., Laska, D. A., Kracke, M. J., and Williams, P. D. (1988). Gentamicin-induced increases in cytosolic calcium in pig kidney cells ($LLC-PK_1$). *J. Pharm. Exp. Ther.* **247**: 349-354.
103. Williams, P. D., Laska, D. A., and Hottendorf, G. H. (1986). Comparative toxicity of aminoglycoside antibiotics in cell cultures derived from human and pig kidney. *In Vitro Toxicol.* **1**: 23-32.
104. Fine, L. G., and Sakhrani, L. M. (1986). Proximal tubular cells in primary culture. *Min. Electrolyte Metab.* **12**: 51-57.
105. Grenier, F. C. (1986). Characteristics of renal collecting tubule cells in primary culture. *Min. Electrolyte Metab.* **12**: 58-63.
106. Currie, M. G., Cole, B. R., DeSchryver-Kecskemeti, K., Holmberg, S., and Needleman, P. (1983). Cell culture of renal epithelium derived from rabbit microdissected cortical collecting tubules. *Am. J. Physiol.* **244** (Renal Fluid Electrolyte Physiol. 13), F724-F728.
107. Spielman, W. S., Sonnenburg, W. K., Allen, M. L., Arend, L. J., Gerozissis, K., and Smith, W. L. (1986). Immunodissection and culture of rabbit cortical collecting tubule cells. *Am. J. Physiol.* **251** (Renal Fluid Electrolyte Physiol. 20), F348-F357.

108. Chung, S. D., Alavi, N., Livingston, D., Hiller, S., and Taub, M. (1982). Characterization of primary rabbit kidney cultures that express proximal tubule functions in a hormonally defined medium. *J. Cell Biol.* **95**: 118-126.
109. Goligorsky, M. S., Menton, D. M., and Hruska, K. A. (1986). Parathyroid hormone-induced changes of the brush border topography and cytoskeleton in cultured renal proximal tubular cells. *J. Membr. Biol.* **92**: 151-162.
110. Bellemann, P. (1980). Primary monolayer culture of liver parenchymal cells and kidney cortical tubules as a useful new model for biochemical pharmacology and experimental toxicology. Studies *in vitro* on hepatic membrane transport, induction of liver enzymes, and adaptive changes in renal cortical enzymes. *Arch. Toxicol.* **44**: 63-84.
111. Detrisac, C. J., Sens, M. A., Garvin, A. J., Spicer, S. S., and Sens, D. A. (1984). Tissue culture of human kidney epithelial cells of proximal tubule origin. *Kidney Int.* **25**: 383-390.
112. Wilson, P. D., Dillingham, M. A., Breckon, R., and Anderson, R. J. (1985). Defined human renal tubular epithelia in culture: Growth, characterization, and hormonal response. *Am. J. Physiol.* **248**: F436-F443.
113. Yang, A. H., Gould-Kostka, J., and Oberley, T. D. (1987). *In vitro* growth and differentiation of human kidney tubular cells on a basement membrane substrate. *In Vitro Cell. Devel. Biol.* **23**(1): 34-46.
114. Palmoski, M., Masters, B., and Flint, O. (1989). Characterization of primary rabbit proximal tubule kidney cells grown in filter cultures. Annual Meeting of the Tissue Culture Association, Orlando, Florida.
115. Yang, I. S., Goldinger, J. M., Hong, S. K., and Taub, M. (1988). Preparation of basolateral membranes that transport p-aminohippurate from primary cultures of rabbit kidney proximal tubule cells. *J. Cell. Physiol.* **135**: 481-487.
116. Merot, J., Bidet, M., Gachot, B., Le Maout, S., Tauc, M., and Poujeol, P. (1988). Patch clamp study on primary culture of isolated proximal convoluted tubules. *Pflugers Arch.* **413**: 51-61.
117. Aleo, M. D., Taub, M. L., Olson, J. R., Nickerson, P. A., and Kostyniak, P. J. (1987). Cellular uptake and response of primary cultures of rabbit renal proximal tubule cells exposed to mercuric chloride and methylmercury chloride. In *In Vitro Toxicology.* Vol. 5, A. M. Goldberg (Ed.). Mary Ann Liebert, New York.
118. Ford, S. M., Bennett, D., Laska, D. A., Tay, L. K., and Williams, P. D. (1987). Biochemical comparison of fresh kidney homogenates, rabbit primary proximal tubule cultures (RPT), and a rabbit kidney epithelial cell line (LLC-RK_1). FASEB, April.
119. Inamoto, H., Ino, Y., Inamoto, N., Wada, T., Kihara, H., Watanabe, I., and Asano, S. (1976). Effect of $HgCl_2$ on rat kidney cells primary culture. *Lab. Invest.* **34**: 489-493.
120. McLachlin, J. R., Goyer, R. A., and Cherian, M. G. (1980). Formation of lead-induced inclusion bodies in primary rat kidney epithelial cell cultures: effect of actinomycin D and cycloheximide. *Toxicol. Appl. Pharmacol.* **56**: 418-431.
121. Cherian, M. G. (1982). Studies on toxicity of metallothionein in rat kidney epithelial cell culture. *Dev. Toxicol. Environ. Sci.* **9**: 193-202.

122. Sens, M. A., Hennigar, G. R., Hazen-Martin, D. J., and Sens, D. A. (1988). Cultured human proximal tubule cells as a model for aminoglycoside nephrotoxicity. *Ann. Clin. Lab. Sci.* **18**: 204-214.
123. Chatterjee, S., Trifillis, A., and Regec, A. (1984). Morphological and biochemical effects of gentamicin on cultured human-kidney renal tubular cells. *Human Toxicol.* **3**: 455.
124. Trifillis, A., Regec, A., Hallcraggs, M., and Trump B. (1984) Effects of cyclosporine on cultured human renal tubular cells. *Human Toxicol.* **3**: 454.
125. Kreisberg, J. I., Pitts, A. M., and Pretlow, T. G. (1977). Separation of proximal tubule cells from suspensions of rat kidney cells in density gradients of Ficoll in tissue culture medium. *Am. J. Pathol.* **86**: 591-602.
126. Heidrich, H. G., and Dew, M. E. (1977). Homogeneous cell populations from rabbit kidney cortex. *J. Cell Biol.* **74**: 780-788.
127. Dworzack, D. L., and Grantham, J. J. (1975). Preparation of renal papillary collecting duct cells for study *in vitro*. *Kidney Int.* **8**: 191-194.
128. Eveloff, J., Haase, W., and Kinne, R. (1980). Separation of renal medullary cells: isolation of cells from the thick ascending limb of Henle's loop. *J. Cell Biol.* **87**: 672-681.
129. Endou, H., Koseki, C., Kimura, K., Yokokura, Y., Fukida, S., and Sakai, F. (1982). Use of a flow cytometer for the separation of isolated kidney cells. In *Biochemistry of Kidney Functions*. F. Morel (Ed.) Elsevier Biomedical, Amsterdam, pp. 69-78.
130. Smith, W. L., and Garcia-Perez. A. (1985). Immunodissection: use of monoclonal antibodies to isolate specific types of renal cells. *Am. J. Physiol.* **248**: F1-F7.
131. Williams, P. D., and Hottendorf, G. H. (1985). Effect of cisdichlorodiamineplatinum-II (cisplatin) on organic ion transport in membrane vesicles from rat kidney cortex. *Cancer Treat. Rep.* **69**: 875-880.
132. Williams, P. D., and Hottendorf, G. H. (1986). ^{3}H-Gentamicin uptake in brush border and basolateral membrane vesicles from rat kidney cortex. *Biochem. Pharmacol.* **35**: 2253-2256.
133. Tune, B. M., Sibley, R. K., and Hsu, C.-Y. (1988). The mitochondrial respiratory toxicity of cephalosporin antibiotics. An inhibitory effect on substrate uptake. *J. Pharmacol. Exp. Ther.* **245**: 1054-1059.
134. Tune, B. M., Fravert, D., and Hsu, C.-Y. (1989). Oxidative and mitochondrial toxic effects of cephalosporin antibiotics in the kidney: A comparative study of cephaloridine and cephaloglycine. *Biochem. Pharmacol.* **38**: 795-802.
135. Williams, P. D., Bennett, D. B., Gleason, C. R., and Hottendorf, G. H. (1987). Correlation between renal membrane binding and nephrotoxicity of aminoglycosides. *Antimicrob. Agents Chemother.* **31**(4): 570-574.
136. Kasher, J. S., Holohan, P. D., and Ross, C. R. (1983). Effect of cephaloridine on the transport of organic ions in dog kidney plasma membrane vesicles. *J. Pharmacol. Exp. Ther.* **225**(3): 606-610.
137. Williams, P. D., Hitchcock, M. J. M., and Hottendorf, G. H. (1985). Effect of cephalosporins on organic ion transport in renal membrane vesicles from

rat and rabbit kidney cortex. *Res. Comm. Chem. Pathol. Pharmacol.* **47**(3): 357-371.

138. Williams, P. D., Hottendorf, G. H., and Bennett, D. B. (1986). Inhibition of renal membrane binding and nephrotoxicity of aminoglycosides. *J. Pharmacol. Exp. Ther.* **237**: 919-925.

5

Neurotoxicity

Alan L. Harvey

University of Strathclyde
Glasgow, Scotland

HUMAN NEUROTOXICOLOGICAL EFFECTS

The Nervous System

The nervous system has essentially two main types of cells: neurons and glia. The neurons are organized in an exquisitely complex and integrated manner to provide the functional controls needed for survival, whereas the glia provide nutritive and supportive functions for the neurons. The central nervous system (i.e., the brain and spinal cord) is characterized by the high density of cells that it contains. The peripheral nervous system is unusual in having many cells with extremely long processes; for example, the axons of some motor neurons can be over 1 m long. As a result of these anatomical peculiarities, cells in the nervous system have exceptional metabolic demands, and can, consequently, be prone to damage.

The brain is absolutely dependent on glucose and oxygen for its energy metabolism. These are delivered via the blood circulation. Although the brain is only about 2% of total body weight, in order to maintain its metabolic activity the brain constantly receives about 15% of the cardiac output; i.e., about 750 ml/min. Brain oxygen consumption is about 20% of that of the total body. Hence, the brain is vulnerable to falls in blood flow, and to decreases in oxygen or glucose content of the blood. Loss of brain oxygenation for less than 10 min can cause permanent damage or death.

In general, the brain is protected from xenobiotics in the circulation by a functional barrier known as the blood-brain barrier. This barrier is formed by the tight junctions of endothelial cells in capillaries within the circulation in the brain. Substances must be hydrophobic or have a special transport process in order to pass through the blood-brain barrier and gain access to the neurons and glia.

About half of the brain is comprised of glial cells. These are specialized accessory cells, mainly *astrocytes,* which regulate concentrations of ions in the extracellular space and which play some role in the inactivation of neurotransmitters; and *oligodendrocytes,* which provide myelination of axons. The biology of glial cells is relatively poorly understood, but because of their importance in maintaining a stable metabolic environment for neurons, they should be considered in any assessment of neurotoxicity. Recent advances in electrophysiological recording techniques have enabled demonstrations that glial cells have some ion channels that were previously thought to be restricted to neurons (e.g., Ref. 1). Such sites could easily be targets for neurotoxic agents.

Neurotoxic Effects In Vivo

Because of the complexity of the functional organization of the nervous system, many chemicals can elicit neurotoxic effects. The ability of xenobiotics to affect the nervous system generally depends on whether they have access to neural tissue, the concentration attained and the duration of exposure, and the presence of a specific binding site or the chemical reactivity of the substance. Additionally, there is the possibility of xenobiotics causing neurotoxic effects indirectly as a consequence of ischemic damage.

The spectrum of neurotoxic effects in vivo is wide, ranging from localized loss of sensation due to a restricted peripheral neuropathy to subtle behavioural changes, the origin of which is hard to establish (Table 1). As the examples of drugs and chemicals known to be capable of producing some kind of neurotoxic effect are almost unending, it is difficult to prepare a logical classification of neurotoxic agents. Drug-induced neurotoxic effects are described in detail by Blain and Stewart-Wynne (2) and cellular pathology is summarized by Norton (3). The range and complexity of neurotoxic effects have also made it difficult to develop sensitive and specific in vivo assays for potentially neurotoxic agents; some of the problems involved are discussed by Dewar (4). The particular difficulties associated with neuropsychological toxicology have been explored by Hartman (5). Most of the known examples of neurotoxic effects have been found accidently or after prolonged or excessive exposure to a chemical or drug.

Table 1 Examples of Neurotoxic Effects

Target site	Symptom	Causative agent
Behavioral patterns	Lethargy	Carbon monoxide
	Hallucinations	Ergot alkaloids
	Speech disorders	Aluminium
Special senses	Disturbed vision	Chloroquine
	Disturbed smell	Cadmium
	Numbness	Acrylamide
Motor systems	Parkinson-like	MPTP, phenothiazines
	Muscle weakness	Organophosphate, anticholinesterases
	Tremor	Manganese
	Uncoordination	Lead, seleniuim

IN VITRO NEUROTOXICITY ASSAYS

Tissue Cultures

The nervous system is the most complex human organ, and it is difficult to imagine an in vitro assay system that could adequately mimic its functions. For example, in vitro systems will lack many important functional features; there will be no blood-brain barrier and, indeed, no circulation of blood, little normal metabolism, no long axons, and greatly disturbed cell-cell interactions. Given these disadvantages, it is valid to consider whether in vitro systems have any place in neurotoxicity testing. However, the great value of in vitro preparations may lie in their simplicity. They allow cells to be studied directly and they are well suited for use as model systems for investigating cellular and molecular mechanisms underlying neurotoxic effects.

As with other tissues, the nervous system can be studied in vitro using a number of different approaches. The most promising of these is the use of cells in culture because this allows prolonged exposures to defined concentrations of xenobiotics. Again, there are several technical variations, which can be summarized according to the amount of tissue disaggregation that is used. Fragments of brain tissue (explants) or intact ganglia can be maintained in culture for relatively long periods. Alternatively, the tissue fragments can be dissociated into their constituent cells, which are then usually grown as monolayer cultures. There have been many attempts to isolate selective populations of cells in order to reduce the heterogeneity that is inherent in cell cultures made from nervous tissue. Finally, there are several continuously growing cell lines that have mainly been derived from neuronal or glial tumors.

Explant Cultures

Explant cultures consist of small, thin fragments of neural tissue. They suffer from the disadvantage that cells have to migrate from the explant before they can be easily visualized or individually studied. Within the explant, the organization of cells remains nearly as complex as in the intact nervous system, but nutrition of cells in the interior is likely to be poor. An advantage of explants is that they can be taken from more mature tissue than is usually possible with dissociated cultures, and hence it is easier to study the effects of agents causing demyelination. However, it is difficult to prepare large numbers of identical explant cultures.

Explant cultures of neural tissue have been prepared from slices of spinal cord, fragments of brain, and whole or fragmented peripheral ganglia, for example. An improved system for explant cultures involves growing thin slices of neural tissue in slowly rotating flasks. In such roller cultures, the cells spread out, virtually to a monolayer and synaptic connections are maintained (6,7). Another modification that has been used successfully with neural tissue is the "microexplant" technique (8,9). Microexplants are formed by passing brain tissue through a nylon mesh with pores of about 200 μm diameter. Homogeneous clumps of cells are formed. With mammalian cerebellem, it is claimed that essential cellular relationships are maintained, yet the clumps are small enough for good visibility.

Primary Dissociated Cell Cultures

Cell cultures are prepared from tissue that is dissociated by mechanical or enzymatic procedures to produce cell suspensions. Cell cultures can be prepared more reproducibily than explant cultures, and they may survive for longer. Individual cells can be studied more easily than in explant cultures. The actions of toxic substances on neuronal growth as well as on several biochemical systems can be studied and followed over time. However, it can be difficult to obtain enough tissue for quantitative experiments; normal intercellular relationships are usually lost; some cell types do not grow or differentiate fully in cell culture; and neurons usually have to be taken from immature animals. Nevertheless, dissociated cell cultures have been prepared successfully from whole brain or spinal cord, from particular brain regions, and from peripheral ganglia (see Refs. 10-12, for reviews).

Glial cell cultures can also be established. Purified astroglial primary cultures have been prepared from different brain regions of newborn rats or mice, and from chick embryo brain (for details, see Ref. 13). Astroglial cells can be identified by staining for glial fibrillary acidic protein. Primary oligodendroglial cell cultures can also be prepared (14,15). Schwann cells have also been grown in primary cell cultures prepared from dissociated peripheral nerves (16).

Another form of cell culture involves growing dispersed cells in suspension in rotating culture vessels (17-19). Under these conditions, cells reaggregate into small clumps, and it is claimed that subsequent differentiation is better than in monolayer cultures. Another attempt to increase neuronal differentiation in cell culture is to use cells from embryonic rat midbrains and plate them at very high densities as small islets on culture dishes (20). These micromass cultures result in a high degree of neuronal maturation. Both reaggregate and micromass cultures have been used in toxicological investigations (21-24).

Continuous Cell Lines

Continuous cell lines are formed by subculturing cells of a primary culture (i.e., the repeated passaging of cells into new culture vessels), or by growing cells that have been transformed by carcinogens, radiation, or viruses. After much subculturing, the cells may become stable from generation-to-generation, and more or less permanently adapted to survival in tissue culture conditions. Single transformed cells that have been isolated and allowed to divide to form a culture of a single cell type are called clonal cell lines. The purpose of cloning cells is to provide large quantities of permanently established, functionally and genetically homogeneous populations of specific cell types. However, neural cell lines are not genetically normal or completely stable. A stock of cells needs to be maintained frozen and experiments performed on cultures within a specified range of generations.

Cell lines include central glial cells (e.g., C6 glioma, an astrocytic cell type), peripheral glial cells (Schwann cell tumor lines, RN-2), and many neuronal cell clones (e.g., NE-115E). The shape of these cells varies tremendously depending on the culture conditions. Cells grown in suspension cultures are mostly rounded, with few or no processes. However, when grown in monolayer culture and induced to differentiate, they can develop extensive cell processes and neurites.

A large number of glial cell lines have been established from normal brain tissue, brain tumors, and cells transformed in vitro (e.g., Ref. 25). However, many glial cell lines lose their differentiated phenotype upon continuous passage in culture. Furthermore, tumor cell lines may suffer from inherent deficiencies owing to their neoplastic origin. However, it is possible to immortalize cells and maintain a high degree of differentiation through the use of viral gene sequences. This technique has successfully been applied to neuronal and glial cell types (26,27).

Tumors of the nervous system are obviously able to multiply by cell division and most neural cell lines have been derived from tumor material. The first clonal lines were established in 1969 from the mouse neuroblastoma tumor C-1300 (28,29). The precise origin of the tumor is uncertain, although it was found near the spinal cord. In animals or in suspension cultures, the cells are undifferentiated and spherical, but the cells extend axonlike processes when they are allowed to grow on a compatible surface and in appropriate conditions. Clones derived from C-1300 neuroblastoma contain electrically excitable cells that have functional receptors and enzymes for synthesis of various neurotransmitters. Hence, these neuroblastoma clones provide a suitable model system for the study of many neurotoxicological effects.

Since the successful introduction of clonal lines with neural properties from a mouse neuroblastoma, other lines have been established from a variety of sources, including human and rat neuroblastomas. Another line that has been used in several neurotoxicological studies is PC12, which was derived from a rat adrenal pheochromocytoma (30). These cells synthesise norepinephrine and dopamine, and in response to nerve growth factor can extend long fine processes which are highly branched and have numerous varicosities. PC12 cells, therefore, resemble sympathetic neurons rather than chromaffin cells of the adrenal medulla. However, cells in this line also synthesize and release acetylcholine in addition to norepinephrine.

In order to increase the range of properties available in cloned nerve cells, several groups of workers have made hybrids of neuroblastoma cells and other cell types (see Ref. 31 for review). For example, mouse neuroblastoma cells have been fused with mouse and human fibroblasts, rat glioma cells, rat sympathetic ganglion cells, and Chinese hamster brain cells. The hybrid clones sometimes offer advantages over the parent neuroblastoma cells because neural properties can be expressed more strongly. For example, cells of mouse neuroblastoma clone NG18TG-2 do not form synapses but NG18-TG-2 neuroblastoma X C6BU-1 glioma hybrids (line NG108-15 or 108CC15) form functional neuromuscular junctions when added to cultures of skeletal muscle. In addition, cultures of neuroblastoma hybrids often have a higher proportion of electrically excitable cells than parent cultures (for further details, see Refs. 10,11).

Types of Assays

In vitro assays can be used to detect toxic effects and estimate relative potencies of different compounds, and they can be used for more mechanistic studies.

Detection of Potentially Neurotoxic Compounds

Neuronal cultures may be used to identify substances that may be expected to be neurotoxic in vivo, although this use is not very common. For example, Nardone (32) described a test battery designed to pinpoint acutely neurotoxic compounds. This battery consisted of a number of culture systems, and used several neuronal and nonneuronal endpoints. Consequently, a large number of tests had to be performed before conclusions could be drawn. A similar screening procedure was used by Ericsson and Walum (33) to study neurotoxic effects of acrylamide and cyclophosphamide.

However, rather than have a large number of assays in parallel on different types of homogeneous cultures, it might be more appropriate to mimic some of the structural and functional complexity of the nervous system. More complex in vitro systems that could be used include organotypic cultures, reaggregate cultures (21), and midbrain micromass cultures (34).

One study has used an in vitro neurotoxicity assay as a screening procedure to test drugs that might have protective effects against in vivo neurotoxic stimuli (35).

Mechanistic Studies

Tissue cultures have several advantages for studies on the cellular and molecular mechanisms of action of neurotoxic agents. Most in vitro neurotoxicological work published to date concerns mechanism of action rather than toxicity screening.

Usually in vitro studies are performed on agents that are known to be neurotoxic in vivo. If the in vivo effects are specific to a particular region of the nervous system or to one type of cell, it should be possible to select an appropriate in vitro system to maximize the relevance of the study. However, surprisingly many studies are performed on culture systems chosen solely for experimental convenience. Another important factor is the concentration of the toxicant at the site of action. It is often difficult to obtain accurate values for the levels of xenobiotic in cerebrospinal fluid or in brain tissue. Finally, during in vivo experiments, it is possible to detect concomitant nonspecific toxicity in other tissues, but with in vitro experiments it is necessary to have control assays performed with nonneuronal cells in order to exclude general cellular toxicity.

In vitro assays will be of little use when the neurotoxic agent is acting indirectly via the blood supply or even on normal metabolism. In the latter case, it should be remembered that even monolayer cultures are relatively hypoxic and inactive compared with tissue in vivo.

FUTURE DEVELOPMENTS OF IN VITRO ASSAYS

Current Examples of Neurotoxicological Testing In Vitro

Compared with the vast number of physiological and pharmacological studies using neurons and glia in culture, there are relatively few accounts of neurotoxicological investigations. Some early work focused on mercurials and heavy metals, and more recently there have been several studies on MPTP and on excitatory amino acids. However, there appear to be no wide-ranging, systematic assessments of the value of neurotoxicity tests based on neural cultures. The following section gives some indication of the type of studies that have been performed using two examples, excitotoxins and MPTP. Other specific examples can be found in the reviews by Schrier (36), Dewar (37), Chambers (38), Rowan (39), Vernadakis et al. (40), Harvey (41), Atterwill (42), and Walum et al. (13).

Excitotoxins

Glutamic acid is one of the main excitatory neurotransmitters in the central nervous system (CNS). A number of analogues of glutamic acid can produce selective neurotoxic effects. It is postulated that this is a consequence of overstimulation of receptors for amino acid neurotransmitters, and hence these compounds have been termed excitotoxins (see Refs. 43,44). There is great interest in these compounds, which include kainic acid, ibotenic acid, and quinolinic acid, because some of the symptoms produced by their in vivo administration resemble human neurological disorders, including Huntington's chorea and epilepsy. Kainic acid has been studied most extensively, and a component of the research has been conducted on cultured preparations. More recently, attention has focused on *N*-methyl-D-aspartate (NMDA).

Another area of interest is the neurotoxic actions of the amino acid derivatives β-*N*-oxalylamino-L-alanine (BOAA) and β-*N*-methylamino-L-alanine (BMAA) that have been implicated in human motor disorders (45). Again, neuronal tissue cultures are proving to be useful in studies of the mechanisms of action of these compounds (46-48).

Honegger and Richelson (49) studied the effects of kainic acid on the development of neuronal characteristics in reaggregate cultures of fetal rat brain. Effects were assessed by measuring a range of enzyme activities: Choline acetyltransferase, acetylcholinesterase, glutamic acid decarboxylase, tyrosine hydroxylase, aromatic L-amino acid decarboxylase, and monoamine oxidase. By the use of this range of assays, specific markers for cholinergic, adrenergic, dopaminergic, and GABAergic neurons were available. Also, cultures from different brain regions were used in order to have some enrichment of particular classes of neurons: cultures prepared from telencephalon were relatively enriched with cholinergic neurons, whereas those from mesencephalon-diencephalon and rhombencephalon regions were relatively enriched with catecholamine-containing neurons. Kainic acid (5 or 50 μM) was added after 2 days in culture, and assays were performed on day 14 or day 29. Kainic acid (5 μM) caused a significant decrease (~20-30%) in choline acetyltransferase, acetylcholinesterase, and glutamic acid decarboxylase activities, but only between day 14 and day 29. At higher concentrations (50μM), kainic acid produced effects by day 14, and more extensive and pronounced effects on day 29. The loss of acetylcholinesterase and glutamic acid decarboxylase activity was 80-90%. However, there was relatively little change in monoamine oxidase activity and no change in tyrosine hydroxylase activity. The authors postulated that the selective toxicity of kainic acid for cholinergic and GABAergic neurons is because these cells have glutamate receptors, whereas the dopaminergic neurons do not. This hypothesis could be more readily tested using dissociated cultures.

In another study of the toxicity of kainic acid, microexplant cultures from cerebella of 17- to 19-day fetal mice were used (8). In contrast to the developmental study of Honegger and Richelson (49), the cultures were maintained for 4 weeks before kainic acid was added. The cultures consisted of two types of neurons (cell bodies of 8 and 20 μM diameter) growing on a monolayer of flat nonneuronal cells. Kainic acid at a concentration of 75 μM caused degeneration of the larger neurons within 6 h, but had no effect on smaller cells after 24 h. The mechanism of toxicity was not studied, but this type of culture is well suited for electrophysiological experiments that could determine if kainic acid could induce a long-lasting depolarization of the larger (presumed Purkinje) neurons.

More recent studies using hippocampal, cortical, and striatal cell cultures have concentrated on the ionic dependence of the effects of glutamate and its analogs, and on the prevention of neurotoxicity by antagonists that are selective for particular subtypes of glutamate receptor (50-59). A major involvement of *N*-methyl-D-aspartate (NMDA) receptors has been implicated, although other types of glutamate receptors are also involved (60). As dissociated cell cultures allow response of individual neurons to be monitored electrophysiologically and by use of intracellular Ca^{2+}-sensitive dyes (e.g., 61), there is great potential to explore the mechanism underlying the neurotoxicity of glutamate and its analogs. For example, there has been a preliminary report that the survival of neurons in cultures exposed to glutamate may depend on the presence of a calcium-binding protein (62). The recent finding of a cell line that shows cytotoxic responses to glutamate (55) should also be useful in further investigations. Preliminary studies of the possible role of oxidative stress have been published (56,63,64), and the role of cyclic GMP is under investigation (65). The involvement of acidosis in glial cell toxicity has also been studied (66).

Recent work with BMAA and BOAA has been directed at determining the type of receptor that they might act upon. Both explant cultures (47) and dissociated cells cultures (67,68) have been used. On the basis of selective antagonists, it was concluded that BMAA affects NMDA receptors and that BOAA acts at quisqualate receptors. Rather similar results with BOAA have been obtained using brain slice preparations (48) and isolated synaptosomal membranes (69).

MPTP

1-Methyl-4-phenyl-1,2,3,6-tetrahydropyridine (MPTP) is an analog of the synthetic opioid pethidine. It causes Parkinson-like symptoms in vivo because of a specific loss of dopaminergic neurons (for a review, see Ref. 70). Tissue culture preparations may be more useful for testing hypotheses about the mechanism of action of MPTP than animal studies. However, tissue culture studies have primarily been limited to demonstrating that MPTP or its oxidised metabolite 1-methyl-4-phenylpridinium (MPP^+) can affect neurons in culture. The conversion of MPTP to MPP^+ is catalyzed by monoamine oxidase B.

Denton and Howard (71) studied the effects of MPTP on PC12 cells. Fifty percent block of dopamine uptake occurred at 2 μM MPTP, but choline and 2-deoxyglucose transport were unaffected, indicating some selectivity of action. Incubation for 3 days with 100 μM MPTP led to a decrease in stored dopamine but even higher concentrations were needed for cell death: 1.5 mM killed more than 95% of cells in 7 days. Further studies of the susceptibility of PC12 cells to MPP^+ revealed that some subclones were relatively resistant, and that mitochondrial respiration was depressed by the compound only under certain conditions (72). This led the authors to propose that the neuronal selectivity of MPTP in vitro results from subtle differences in the energy metabolism of different classes of neuron. More recently, it has been demonstrated that MPTP and MPP^+ can cause selective depletion of catecholamines from human and monkey chromaffin cells in culture, without causing gross morphological damage (73).

In another study, explant cultures from midbrain regions of 16-day rat embryos were used (74). These were grown for 8 days before MPP^+ or MPTP was added. Effects were monitored by visual assessment of neurite outgrowth, catecholamine fluorescence, and by measurements of the uptake of [^{3}H]dopamine. MPP^+ (10 μM for 7 days) had no obvious effect on morphology, but it abolished catecholamine fluorescence and reduced high-affinity uptake of dopamine. These effects were apparent within 24 h and were not reversible. MPTP had much less effect (demonstrating the nature of the active metabolite) and reduced MPTP had no activity. Similar effects were found with dissociated cultures of embryonic rat midbrain (75). High concentrations of MPTP had the paradoxical effect of reducing toxicity, probably by blocking uptake of MPP^+. More recent work has revealed an apparently contradictory relationship between MAO-B activity and MPTP toxicity (76). As dissociated mesencephalic cultures mature, there is a marked increase in the specific activity of MAO-B and of the dopamine transport system. This would be expected to enhance the toxicity of MPTP, but the reverse was found. Metabolic changes during development in culture may contribute to these effects (77).

In a rather similar study to those of Mytilineou (74-77), the enhanced visibility of individual neurons in dissociated cell cultures was used to improve the resolution of the histochemical assays (78). The cultures were prepared from the ventral tegmentum of the mesencephalon of 15- to 16-day rat embryos. This area includes the substantia nigra. MPTP and MPP^+ were added to 7 day-old cultures, effects being monitored by catecholamine fluorescence and tyrosine hydroxylase histochemistry. Again, MPP^+ was found to be more potent than MPTP. MPTP (10-100 μM) caused a decrease in fluorescence without affecting cell numbers, whereas 0.1-10.0 μM MPP^+ caused a selective loss of tyrosine hydroxylase-containing cells. More general toxic effects were found at concentrations above 100 μM for MPTP and above 30 μM for MPP^+.

Sanchez-Ramos et al. (78) also assessed the effects of some possible MPTP antagonists. The selective blocker of dopamine uptake, mazindol, partially reduced the effects of MPP^+, but desipramine (which blocks norepinephrine uptake) and deprenil (which inhibits MAO-B) had no effect. Deprenil has been shown to reduce the toxicity of MPTP to rat neurons in culture (79,80), which is consistent with the hypothesis that MPTP is converted to the neurotoxic MPP^+ by MAO-B.

More recently, Hyman et al. (93) have used cultures of embryonic rat mesencephalon to examine the effects of growth factors in lessening the neurotoxic actions of MPP^+. Brain-derived neurotrophic factor (BDNF) increased the survival of dopaminergic neurons in control cultures and also greatly reduced the toxicity of MPP^+. Nerve growth factor and basic fibroblast growth factor had no effect on MPP^+ toxicity.

Primary cultures prepared from rat brain have been used to look for regional differences in the susceptibility to MPTP and MPP^+ (81,82), and to investigate the hypothesis that glial cells convert MPTP to the neurotoxic MPP^+ (79,83,84). As shown in Figure 1a, cells from midbrain regions, including the substantia nigra were slightly more sensitive to MPP^+ than cells from striatum or the raphe nucleus. Glial cells were generally less sensitive than the neurons. This is illustrated in Figure 1b, which shows that neurons are more readily affected than glia by both MPTP and MPP. This work does not exclude the possibility that glial cells can convert MPTP to MPP^+ (which is then released to damage neurons) without being injured. However, it does confirm that neurons cultured in the absence of glia are still sensitive to MPTP.

Attempts have been made to find neural cell lines that are suitable for the investigation of the mechanism of action of MPTP and for the testing of potential antagonists. However, the toxicity seems to be seen preferentially on cells in their undifferentiated state, which might lessen the relevance for in vivo comparisons. N_2AB-1 cells are a subclone from an adrenergic line derived from the original C-1300 mouse neuroblastoma. The cells contain tyrosine hydroxylase, which is the rate-limiting enzyme for dopamine synthesis. Such cells are vulnerable to MPP^+, but not MPTP (85). Exposure of differentiated cells to 3.4 μM MPP^+ for 24 h led to a loss of neuritic processes. Ten times higher concentrations were cytotoxic to N_2AB-1 cells, but not to C_6 glioma cells. A human adrenergic cell line (LA-N-1) has also been reported to be sensitive to MPTP (86). The effects were more pronounced on actively dividing cells rather than on differentiated cells. This was also

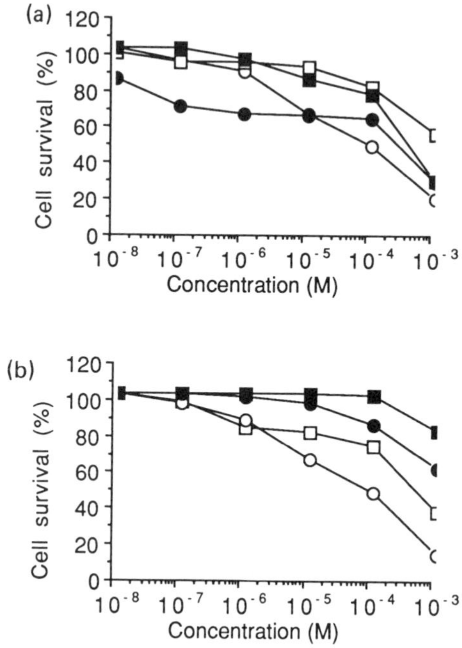

Figure 1 Toxicity of MPP^+ on rat neuronal cell cultures prepared from different brain regions (a). Cultures were exposed to MPP^+ for 24 h and then live and dead cells were stained and counted. ●, frontal cortex; ○, midbrain with substantia nigra; ■, striatum; □, midbrain with raphe nucleus. (Data from Ref. 81.) Relative toxicity of MPTP and MPP^+ on neuronal and glia cell cultures. Midbrain cultures with substantia nigra were used (b). □, MPTP on neuronal cultures; ■, MPTP on glial cultures; ○, MPP^+ on neuronal cultures; ●, MPP^+ on glial cultures. (Data from Ref. 83.)

the case with N_2AB-1 cells (87). In the latter study, a mixture of gangliosides was found to have some protective effect against MPP^+.

These two examples illustrate the valuable role that in vitro systems play in the investigation of basic mechanisms of neurotoxic action.

Possibilities for Developments in Neurotoxicology Testing In Vitro

It should be apparent that in vitro testing for neurotoxic effects has been almost entirely concerned with studies of mechanisms of action. This is a valuable contribution that will continue to develop as techniques become more refined and individual neurotoxicological problems are better defined. However, there has been little progress in establishing in vitro methods that are suited to large-scale screening of potentially neurotoxic chemicals, and hence there is no database to relate in vitro neurotoxic results to human neurotoxic effects.

Certain technical advances are necessary and some, at least, should be achievable. For example, suitable biochemical markers can be identified and used as the basis of routine automated assays. The release of lactic acid dehydrogenase (e.g., Ref. 57) and the staining of metabolically active cells by MTT (88,89) or neutral red (90) can be used to quantify effects of neurotoxic agents, although these assays are not specific to neurons. As they are quantitative assays that can be automated, they have distinct advantages over assays that require manual counting of cells (see, e.g., Ref. 58).

These biochemical techniques may be made more specific if used on cultures containing homogeneous populations of cells. Some progress has been made in preparing relatively pure cultures of different types of glia, but the situation with central neurons is obviously much more complicated and progress has been correspondingly slow. Immortalization of specific types of neurons by viral transformation may offer a way forward.

Two major difficulties remain: the problems associated with in vivo transformation or metabolism of xenobiotics, and the difficulties in studying compounds that may act indirectly by interfering with the blood supply or availability of energy metabolism substrates. These problems are not completely specific to neurotoxicological studies. Some attempts have been made to take into account systemic xenobiotic metabolism by coculturing neuronal cells with liver cells (e.g., Ref. 33), and technical developments along these lines will, no doubt, be possible. It is rather harder to foresee how the problems associated with energy substrate supply and the blood-brain barrier will be overcome.

Despite this, much useful work could be undertaken, simply to improve existing neuronal culture systems, to extend the range of cloned cell lines, and especially to begin a systematic series of validation experiments so that a reliable database for in vitro neurotoxic effects can be established. The studies under the MEIC program may provide a suitable opportunity (91,92).

REFERENCES

1. Tas, P. W. L., Kress, H.-G., and Koschell, K. (1989). Volatile anaesthetics inhibit the ion flux through Ca^{2+}-activated K^+ channels from glioma C6 cells. *Biochim. Biophys. Acta* **983**: 264-268.
2. Blain, P. G., and Stewart-Wynne, E. (1985). Neurological disorders. In *Textbook of Adverse Drug Reactions.* 3rd Ed. D. M. Davies (Ed.). Oxford University Press, Oxford, England, pp. 494-519.
3. Norton, S. (1975). Toxicology of the central nervous system. In *Toxicology. The Basic Science of Poisons.* L. J. Casarett and J. Doull (Eds.). Macmillan, new York, pp. 151-169.

4. Dewar, A. J. (1981). Neurotoxicity testing—with particular reference to biochemical methods. In *Testing for Toxicity*. J. W. Gorrod (Ed.). Taylor & Francis, London, pp. 199-217.
5. Hartman, D. E. (1988). *Neuropsychological Toxicological: Identification and Assessment of Human Neurotoxic Syndromes*. Pergamon Press, New York.
6. Gahwiler, B. H. (1981). Organotypic monolayer cultures of nervous tissue. *J. Neurosci. Meth.* **4**: 329-342.
7. Shahar, A., Frankel, G., David, Y., and Friedmann, A. (1986). *In vitro* cytotoxicity and demyelination induced by Theiler viruses in cultures of spinal cord slices. *J. Neurosci. Res.* **16**: 671-681.
8. Gibbs, W. (1982). Kainic acid sensitivity of mammalian Purkinje cells in monolayer cultures. *Dev. Brain. Res.* **4**: 103-108.
9. Moonen, G., Neale, E. A., MacDonald, R. L., Gibbs, W., and Nelson, P. G. (1982). Cerebellar macroneurons in microexplant cell culture. Methodology, basic electrophysiology and morphology after horseradish peroxidase injection. *Dev. Brain Res.* **5**: 59-73.
10. Nelson, P. G., and Lieberman, M. (1981). *Excitable Cells in Tissue Culture.* Plenum Press, New York.
11. Harvey, A. L. (1984). *The Pharmacology of Nerve and Muscle in Tissue Culture.* Croom Helm, London; Liss, New York.
12. Bottenstein, J. E., and Sato, G. (1985). *Cell Culture and the Neurosciences.* Plenum Press, New York.
13. Walum, E., Hansson, E., and Harvey, A. L. (1989). *In vitro* testing of neurotoxicity. *ATLA* **18**: 153-179.
14. McCarthy, K. D., and de Vellis, J. (1980). Preparation of separate astroglial and oligodendroglial cell cultures from rat cerebral tissue. *J. Cell Biol.* **85**: 890-902.
15. Poduslo, S. E., Curbeam, R., Miller, K., and Reier, P. (1985). Purification and characterization of cultures of oligodendroglia from rat brain. *J. Neurosci. Res.* **14**: 433-447.
16. Brockes, J. P., and Raff, M. C. (1979). Studies in cultured rat Schwann cells. II. Comparison with a rat Schwann cell line. *In Vitro* **15**: 772-778.
17. Honneger, P., and Richelson (1977). Biochemical differentiation of aggregating cell cultures of different fetal rat brain regions. *Brain Res.* **133**: 329-339.
18. Stafstrom, C. E., Johnston, D., Wehner, J. M., and Sheppard, J. R. (1980). Spontaneous neural activity in fetal brain reaggregate cultures. *Neuroscience* **5**: 1681-1689.
19. Kontur, P. J., Hoffmann, P. C., and Heller, A. (1987). Neurotoxic effects of methamphetamine assessed in three-dimensional reaggregate tissue cultures. *Dev. Brain Res.* **31**: 7-14.
20. Flint, O. P. (1983). A micromass culture method for rat embryonic neuronal cells. *J. Cell Sci.* **61**: 247-262.
21. Atterwill, C. K. (1987). Brain reaggregate cultures in neurotoxicological investigations. In *In vitro Methods in Toxicology*. C. K. Atterwill and C. E. Steele (Eds.). Cambridge University Press, Cambridge, England.
22. Flint, O. P. (1987). An *in vitro* test for teratogens using cultures of rat embryo cells. In *In Vitro Methods in Toxicology*. C. K. Atterwill and C. E. Steele, Cam-

bridge University Press, Cambridge, England, pp. 339-2363.
23. Walum, E., and Flint, O. P. (1988). Acrylamide, 2,5-hexanedione and beta-aminopropionitrile toxicity tested in rat embryo mid-brain cell cultures. *ATLA* **15**: 238-244.
24. Clemedson, C., Walum, E., and Flint, O. (1989). Effects of carbon tetrachloride on neuronal differentiation in rat embryo mid!brain micromass cultures. *ATLA* **16**: 287-292.
25. Pfeiffer, S. E., and Wechsler, W. (1972). Biochemically differentiated neoplastic clone of Schwann cells. *Proc. Natl. Acad. Sci. U.S.A.* **69**: 2885-2889.
26. Cepko, C. (1988). Immortalization of neural cells via oncogene transduction. *Trends Neurosci.* **11**: 6-8.
27. Lee, H. J., Hammond, D. N., Lamge, T. H., Roback, J. D., Sim, J. A., Brown, D. A., Otten, U. H., and Wainer, B. H. (1990). Neuronal properties and trophic activities of immortalized hippocampal cells from embryonic and young adult mice. *J. Neurosci.* **10**: 1779-1787.
28. Augusti-Tocco, G., and Sato, G. (1969). Establishment of functional clonal lines of neurons from mouse neuroblastoma. *Proc. Natl. Acad. Sci. U.S.A.* **64**: 311-315.
29. Schubert, D., Humphreys, S., Baroni, C., and Cohn, M. (1969). *In vitro* differentiation of a mouse neuroblastoma. *Proc. Natl. Acad. Sci. U.S.A.* **64**: 316-323.
30. Greene, L. A., and Tischler, A. S. (1976). Establishment of a noradrenergic clonal line of rat adrenal pheochromocytoma cells which respond to nerve growth factor. *Proc. Natl. Acad. Sci. U.S.A.* **73**: 2424-2428.
31. Hamprecht, B. (1977). Structural, electrophysiological, biochemical and pharmacological properties of neuroblastoma-glioma cell hybrids in cell culture. *Int. Rev. Cytol.* **49**: 99-170.
32. Nardone, R. M. (1983). The LD_{50} test and *in vitro* toxicology strategies. *Acta Pharmacol. Toxicol.* **52**: 65-79.
33. Ericsson, A.-C., and Walum, E. (1984). Cytotoxicity of cyclophosphamide in glioma and neuroblastoma cell lines cocultured with liver cell. *Toxicol. Lett.* **20**: 251-256.
34. Flint, O. P., and Orton, T. C. (1984). An *in vitro* assay for teratogens with cultures of rat embryo mid-brain and limb bud cell. *Toxicol. Appl. Pharmacol.* **76**: 383-395.
35. Kenna, J. F. W., McBurney, R. N., Scherz, M. W., Fischer, J. B., Hamilton, P. N., Smith, S. M., Server, A. C., Finkbeiner, S., Stevens, C. F., Jahr, C., and Weber, E. (1989). Synthesis and characterization of a series of diarylguanidines that are noncompetitive *N*-methyl-D-aspartate receptor antagonists with neuroprotective properties. *Proc. Natl. Acad. Sci. U.S.A.* **86**: 5631-5635.
36. Schrier, B. K. (1982). Nervous system cultures as toxicologic test systems. In *Nervous System Toxicology.* C. L. Mitchell (Ed.). Raven Press, New York, pp. 337-348.
37. Dewar, A. J. (1983). Neurotoxicity. In *Animals and Alternatives in Toxicity Testing.* M. Balls, R. J. Riddell, and A. N. Worden (Eds.). Academic Press, London, pp. 230-284.

38. Chambers, P. L. (1984). An overview of in vitro neurotoxicity assays. In *Alternatives to in vivo Bioassays for Risk Assessment.* G. R. Thompson (Ed.). Forum for Scientific Excellence Ltd., Hazlet, New Jersey, pp. 224-240.
39. Rowan, M. J. (1984). Central nervous system toxicity evaluation in vitro: neurophysiological approach. In *Neurotoxicology.* K. Blum and L. Manzo (Eds.). Marcel Dekker, New York, pp. 585-612.
40. Vernadakis, A., and Davies, D. L. (1984). Neural culture: A tool to study cellular neurotoxicity. In *Neurotoxicology.* K. Blum and L. Manzo (Eds.). Marcel Dekker, New York, pp. 559-583.
41. Harvey, A. L. (1988). Possible developments in neurotoxicity testing *in vitro. Xenobiotica* **8**: 625-632.
42. Atterwill, C. K. (1989). Brain reaggregate cultures in neurotoxicological investigations: studies with cholinergic neurotoxins. *ATLA* **16**: 221-230.
43. Collins, R. C. (1987). Neurotoxins and the selective vulnerability of brain. In *Neurotoxins and Their Pharmacological Implications.* P. Jenner (Ed.). Raven Press, New York, pp. 1-17.
44. Choi, D. W. (1990). Cerebral hypoxia: Some new approaches and unanswered questions. *J. Neurosci.* **10**: 2493-2501.
45. Spencer, P. S., Nunn, P. B., Hugon, J., Ludolph, A., and Roy, D. N. (1986). Motor-neurone disease in Guam: Possible role of a food neurotoxin. *Lancet* **1**: 965.
46. Nunn, P. B., Seelig, M., Zagoren, J. C., and Spencer, P. S. (1987). Stereospecific acute neuronotoxicity of 'uncommon' plant amino acids linked to human motor-system diseases. *Brain Res.* **410**: 374-379.
47. Ross, S. M., Seelig, M., and Spencer, P. S. (1987). Specific antagonism of excitotoxic action of 'uncommon' amino acids assayed in organotypic mouse cortical cultures. *Brain. Res.* **425**: 120-127.
48. Bridges, R. J., Stevens, D. R., Kahale, J. S., Nunn, P. B., Kadri, M., and Cotman, C. W. (1989). Structure-function studies on N-oxalyl-diamino-dicarboxylic acids and excitatory amino acid receptors: Evidence that β-L-ODAP is a selective non-NMDA agonist. *J. Neurosci.* **9**: 2073-2079.
49. Honneger, P., and Richelson, E. (1977). Kainic acid alters neurochemical development in fetal rat brain aggregating cell cultures. *Brain Res.* **138**: 580-584.
50. Choi, D. W. (1987). Ionic dependence of glutamate neurotoxicity. *J. Neurosci.* **7**: 369-379.
51. Choi, D. W., Maulucci-Gedde, M., and Kriegstein, A. R. (1987). Glutamate neurotoxicity in cortical cell culture. *J. Neurosci.* **7**: 357-368.
52. Kim, J. P., and Choi, D. W. (1987). Quinolinate neurotoxicity in cortical cell culture. *Neuroscience* **23**: 423-432.
53. Kim, J. P., Koh, J.-Y., and Choi, D. W. (1987). L-Homocysteate is a potent neurotoxin on cultured cortical neurons. *Brain Res.* **437**: 103-110.
54. Rothman, S. M., Thurston, J. H., and Hauhart, R. E. (1987). Delayed neurotoxicity of excitatory amino acids in vitro. *Neuroscience* **22**: 471-480.
55. Murphy, T. H., Maloauf, A. T., Sastre, A., Schnaar, R. L., and Coyle, J. T. (1988). Calcium-dependent glutamate cytotoxicity in a neuronal cell line. *Brain Res.* **444**: 325-332.
56. Murphy, T. H., Miyamoto, M., Sastre, A., Schnaar, R. L., and Coyle, J. T.

(1988). Inhibition of cystine uptake mediates quisqualate type glutamate toxicity in a neuronal cell line. *Neurosci. Abst.* **14**: 420.
57. Choi, D. W., Koh, J.-Y., and Peter, S. (1988). Pharmacology of glutamate neurotoxicity in cortical cell culture: Attenuation by NMDA antagonists. *J. Neurosci.* **8**: 185-196.
58. Finkbeiner, S., and Stevens, C. F. (1988). Applications of quantitative measurements for assessing glutamate neurotoxicity. *Proc. Natl. Acad. Sci. U.S.A.* **85**: 4071-4074.
59. Shalaby, I., Chenard, B., and Prochniak, M. (1989). Glycine reverses 7-Cl kynurenate blockade of glutamate neurotoxicity in cell culture. *Eur. J. Pharmacol.* **160**: 309-311.
60. Frandsen, A., Drejer, J., and Schousboe, A. (1989). Direct evidence that excitotoxicity in cultured neurons is mediated via *N*-methyl-D-aspartate (*N*MDA) as well as non-*N*MDA receptors. *J. Neurochem.* **53**: 297-299.
61. Murphy, S. N., Thayer, S. A., and Miller, R. J. (1987). The effects of excitatory amino acids on intracellular calcium in single mouse striatal neurons *in vitro*. *J. Neurosci.* **7**: 4145-4158.
62. Baimbridge, K. G., and Kao, J. (1988). Neurotoxicity: Studies in culture. Calbindin-D-28K protects against glutamate induced neurotoxicity in rat CA1 pyramidal neuron cultures. *Neurosci. Abst.* **14**: 97.
63. DeLong, M. J., Murphy, T. H., Miyamoto, M., and Coyle, J. T. (1988). NAD (P)H:Quinone reductase protects against glutamate toxicity in a neuronal cell line. *Neurosci. Abst.* **14**: 420.
64. Miyamoto, M., Murphy, T. H., and Coyle, J. T. (1988). Antioxidants protect against glutamate cytotoxicity in a neuronal cell line. *Neurosci. Abst.* **14**: 420.
65. Lysko, P. G., and Henneberry, R. C. (1988). Modulation of glutamate-induced neurotoxicity by the putative neurotoxin β-N-Oxalyamino-L-alanine. *Neurosci. Abst.* **14**: 419.
66. Giffard, R. G., Monyer, H., and Choi, D. W. (1990). Selective vulnerability of cultured glia to injury by extracellular acidosis. *Brain Res.* **530**: 138-141.
67. Allen, C. N., Spencer, P. S., and Carpenter, D. O. (1988). β-N-Oxalylamino-L-alanine (BOAA) and quisqualate activate similar ionic currents. *Neurosci. Abst.* **14**: 97.
68. Weiss, J. H., Koh, J., and Choi, D. W. (1988). Beta-N-Methylamino-L-alanine (BMAA) neurotoxicity on murine cortical neurons. *Neurosci. Abst.* **14**: 417.
69. Ross, S. M., Roy, D. N., and Spencer, P. S. (1989). β-N-Oxalylamino-L-alamine action on glutamate receptors. *J. Neurochem.* **53**: 710-715.
70. Markey, S. P., and Schmuff, N. R. (1986). The pharmacology of the Parkinsonian syndrome producing neurotoxin MPTP (1-methyl-4-phenyl-1,2,3,6-tetrahydropyridine) and structurally related compounds. *Med. Res. Rev.* **6**: 389-429.
71. Denton, T., and Howard, B. D. (1984). Inhibition of dopamine uptake by N-methyl-4-phenyl-1,2,3,6-tetrahydropyridine, a cause of parkinsonism. *Biochem. Biophys. Res. Comm.* **119**: 1186-1190.
72. Denton, T., and Howard, B. D. (1987). A dopaminergic cell line varient resistant to the neurotoxin 1-methyl-4-phenyl-1,2,3,6-tetrahydropyridine. *J. Neurochem.* **49**: 622-630.

73. Kaniucki, M., Hansen, J. T., Fiandaca, M. S., Kordower, J. H., Gash, D. M., Okawara, S., and Notter, M. F. D. (1988). Effect of MPTP on primate adrenal chromaffin cells *in vitro*: An acute and chronic study. *Neurosci. Abst.* **14**: 1265.
74. Mytilineou, C., Cohen, G., and Heikkila, R. E. (1985). 1-Methyl-4-phenylpyridine (MPP^+) is toxic to mesencephalic dopamine neurons in culture. *Neurosci. Lett.* **57**: 19-24.
75. Friedman, L., and Mytilineou, C. (1987). The toxicity of MPTP to dopamine neurons in culture is reduced at high concentrations. *Neurosci. Lett.* **79**: 65-72.
76. Mytilineou, C., and Danias, P. (1988). Dopamine neurons increase their resistance to the neurotoxins MPTP and MPP^+ during development in culture. *Neurosci. Abst.* **14**: 1266.
77. Danias, P., Nicklas, W. J., Ofort, S., Shen, J. O., and Mytilineou, C. (1989). Mesencephalic dopamine neurons become less sensitive to 1-methyl-4-phenyl-1,2,3,6-tetrahydropyridine toxicity during development in vitro. *J. Neurochem.* **53**: 1149-1155.
78. Sanchez-Ramos, J., Barrett, J. N., Goldstein, M., Weiner, W. J., and Hefti, F. (1986). 1-Methyl-4-phenylpyridinium (MPP^+) but not 1-methyl-4-phenyl-1,2,3,6-tetrahydropyridine (MPTP) selectively destroys dopoaminergic neurons in cultures of dissociated rat mesencephalic neurons. *Neurosci. Lett.* **72**: 215-220.
79. Mytilineou, C., and Friedman, L. (1988). Studies on the metabolism and toxicity of 1-methyl-4-phenyl-1,2,3,6-tetrahydropyridine in cultures of embryonic rat mesencephalon. *J. Neurochem.* **51**: 750-755.
80. Barnes, N. M., Cheng, C. H. K., Costall, B., and Naylor, R. J. (1989). The effect of deprenyl on MPTP and MPP^+ neurotoxicity in rat neuronal cell culture. *Br. J. Pharmacol.* **97**: 479P.
81. Barnes, J. M., Cheng, C. H. K., Costall, B., Jenner, P. G., and Naylor, R. J. (1989). The selective toxicity of MPP^+ on rat neuronal cell cultures. *Br. J. Pharmacol.* **96**: 333P.
82. Michel, P. P., Dandapani, B. K., Kneusel, B., Sanchez-Ramos, J., and Hefti, F. (1990). Toxicity of 1-methyl-4-phenylpyridinium for rat dopaminergic neurons in culture: Selectivity and irreversibility. *J. Neurochem.* **54**: 1102-1109.
83. Barnes, J. M., Cheng, C. H. K., Costall, B., Jenner, P. G., and Naylor, R. J. (1989). The toxicity of MPTP and MPP^+ in rat neuronal and glial cell cultures. *Br. J. Pharmacol.* **96**: 332P.
84. Marini, A. M., Schwartz, J. P., and Kopin, I. J. (1989). The neurotoxicity of 1-methyl-4-phenylpyridinium in cultured cerebellar granule cells. *J. Neurochem.* **9**: 3665-3672.
85. Notter, M. F. D., Irwin, I., Langston, J. W., and Gash, D. M. (1988). Neurotoxicity of MPTP and MPP^+ *in vitro*: characterization using specific cell lines. *Brain Res.* **456**: 254-262.
86. Sullivan, S., and Notter, M. F. D. (1988). Affects of MPTP on a human adrenergic cell line, La-N-1. *Neurosci. Abst.* **14**: 1265.
87. Simmons, S. J., and Notter, M. F. D. (1988). Modulation of MPP^+ neurotoxicity in the N_2AB-1 neuroblastoma cell line. *Neurosci. Abst.* **14**: 1265.
88. Manthorpe, M., Fagnani, R., Skaper, S. D., and Varon, S. (1986). An automated colorimetric microassay for neuronotrophic factors. *Dev. Brain. Res.* **25**: 191-198.

89. Lefebvre, P. P., Rogister, B., Delree, P., Leprince, P., Selak, I., and Moonen, G. (1987). Potassium-induced release of neuronotoxic activity by astrocytes. *Brain Res.* **413**: 120-128.
90. Borenfreund, E., BAbich, H., and Martin-Alguacil, N. (1988). Comparisons of two *in vitro* cytotoxicity assays—The neutral red (NR) and tetrazolium MTT tests. *Toxicol. In Vitro* **2**: 1-6.
91. Bernson, V., Bondesson, I., Ekwall, B., Stenberg, K., and Walum, E. (1987). A multicentre evaluation study of in vitro cytotoxicity. *ATLA* **14**: 144-146.
92. Bondesson, I., Ekwall, B., Stenberg, K., Romert, L., and Walum, E. (1988). Instructions for participants in the multicentre evaluation study of in vitro cytotoxicity. *ATLA* **15**: 191-193.
93. Hyman, C., Hofer, M., Barde, Y.-A., Juhasz, M., Yancopoulos, G. D., Squinto, S. P., and Lindsay, R. M. (1991). BDNF is a neurotrophic factor for dopaminergic neurons of the substantia nigra. *Nature* **350**: 230-232.

6

Cardiovascular Toxicity

Kenneth Ramos

Texas A&M University
College Station, Texas

Daniel Acosta

The University of Texas at Austin
Austin, Texas

TOXICOLOGICAL/PATHOLOGICAL CONSEQUENCES OF TOXIC INSULT

Incidence

The cardiovascular system consists of the heart and blood vessels which form a circuit for the transport of oxygen and other blood constituents throughout the body. As a result, cardiovascular cells are repeatedly exposed to drugs and other chemicals delivered via the circulation from their portal of entry to more distant sites. Toxicity may result from the accumulation of toxic chemicals within cardiovascular tissue or from cardiovascular cell-specific bioactivation of protoxicants. Alternatively, toxicity may result from interference with specialized physiological functions unique to cardiovascular cells. In the clinical setting, severe alterations of cardiovascular function are commonly associated with exposure to high drug concentrations during the course of therapy. Under these conditions, toxicity is often related to extensions of autonomic activity. Cardiovascular toxicity has also been associated with exposure to environmental pollutants or toxic chemicals found in the home and workplace. Generalized disturbances of cardiovascular function may also be observed upon exposure to nonspecific toxins such as organic solvents, alcohols, gases, and metals.

Toxic insult to the heart compromises its ability to pump blood through the vasculature, and ultimately results in insufficient delivery of essential substrates and/or inadequate removal of the waste products of metabolism. Angiotoxic insult is often associated with dramatic disturbances of blood pressure and/or blood flow control. However, in general, such alterations are of slow onset and typically exhibit long latency periods. The occurrence of cardiovascular toxicity may also be of significance to other organ systems. Recent studies have suggested that lead-induced neuropathy (1) and cadmium-induced hepatotoxicity (2) are, at least in part, of vascular origin.

Public Health Implications

Acute

Serious complications associated with acute exposure to toxic chemicals are mostly limited to the myocardium, and often represent disturbances in the excitation/contraction coupling process. Because cardiac pumping is essential to support blood flow to vital organs, cardiotoxic insult seldom remains unnoticed. Of particular significance are the life-threatening arrhythmias associated with cocaine intoxication (3); the myocardial dysfunction induced by ethanol (4); the cardiac necrosis induced by isoproterenol and other catecholamines (5); and the dose-related, cumulative cardiotoxicity of anthracycline antibiotics.

Chronic

The health consequences associated with repeated exposure to toxic chemicals represents one of the more significant challenges to modern society. Within this context, more information is needed to define the responses of cardiovascular cells to chronic toxic insult. Although the deleterious cardiovascular effects of tobacco smoke constituents or the "expressway blues" associated with casual carbon monoxide exposure have been recognized for many years, little is known about the mechanisms which mediate the occurrence of toxicity. This concept is further exemplified by the limited amount of information available on the excessive cardiovascular morbidity associated with chronic alcohol consumption (6) or the occupational exposure to several pesticides (7).

In Vivo-In Vitro Correlates

The expression of cardiovascular toxicity ranges from subtle abnormalities of cardiac rhythm to permanent loss of cardiovascular regulation. Because the cardiovascular system is characterized by a large degree of structural and functional heterogeneity, the assessment of toxicity in vivo is often complicated. In this regard, in vitro model systems can be used to define general mechanisms of toxicity or to screen potentially toxic drugs and other chemicals. An essential consideration in attempting to validate in vitro systems is that data obtained in vitro should always be correlated to observations made in vivo.

IN VITRO MODELS—STATE OF THE ART

The application of in vitro model systems to evaluate the toxicity of xenobiotics has significantly enhanced our understanding of drug and chemically induced cardiovascular toxicity. From a scientific perspective, the popularity of in vitro model systems has been justified for several reasons (8). From the public perspective, in vitro model systems enjoy increasing popularity because their application in toxicity testing may allow for a reduction in the number of live animals employed. In vitro models commonly used in cardiovascular toxicity testing include: perfused organ preparations, isolated muscle preparations, single cell suspensions, and tissue culture systems. Because these models are used as predictors of the human response, when applicable, all preparations should be derived from species which respond with fidelity to the toxic challenge.

Perfused Organ Preparations

Methodology

Cardiac Modified Langerdorff preparations (9,10) and the working heart preparation developed by Neely and collegues (11) using hearts from several species have been successfully applied to toxicity testing. Hearts are perfused with a physiological salt solution and equilibrated with a gas mixture of 5% CO_2:95% O_1. High coronary flow rates serve to ensure adequate perfusion of the preparation. In the Langerdorff preparation, the heart is rapidly removed and cooled to induce hypothermic arrest. The aorta is dissected free, tied onto a cannula, and perfused with physiological salt solution at 37 °C. The perfusate flows in a retrograde fashion through the aorta and into the coronary arteries at a rate of 5-12 ml/min/g wet weight. The heart is placed in a water-jacketed chamber and hydrostatic pressure is maintained with a constant head device adjusted from 50-100 cm water. The perfusion fluid flows through the coronary vascular bed to enter the right heart and exit via the pulmonary artery. This preparation constitutes a beating heart which does not perform work, since the left ventricle is empty at all times. The system can be modified to allow recirculation of the perfusion fluid.

In the working heart preparation, the heart is processed as described above. However, perfusion is transferred from the aorta to the left atrium shortly after stabilization to generate a left-heart working preparation. The perfusion fluid passes from the left atrium to the ventricle, where it is ejected via the aorta into a chamber with a hydrostatic pressure of about 100 cm of water to impose a fixed afterload. Coronary arteries are perfused during both ventricular ejection and diastole. The coronary effluent is ejected via the pulmonary artery into the chamber housing the heart. With this type of preparation, myocardial oxygen consumption is within the normal range, while coronary flow (15-25 ml/min/g) is typically higher than that of the Langerdorff preparation. The apparatus can be modified to provide various filling pressures and afterloads. The system also incorporates the capacity for noncirculating perfusion.

Vascular Blood vessel segments from several vascular beds can be isolated and processed for perfusion in vitro. Aortic preparations are most commonly employed to study macrocirculatory function (12). Segments of thoracic aortae (4-5 cm) are excised and nonadventitial tissue is dissected off the wall. A cannula is inserted about 2-3 mm into the proximal end of the vessel and secured in place. The vessel is tied distally to occlude outflow and the length of the vessel is adjusted as needed. Arteries can be perfused and superfused with an oxygenated physiological solution using a pump at constant flow rate conditions (3 ml/min) with pulsatile pressure applied circumferentially to approximate physiological conditions.

Characterization/Validation

The time required for isolation and placement of the tissue under physiological conditions is critical to the preservation of tissue viability. Perfused heart preparations are denervated, beat spontaneously at rates within the physiological range, and can be paced at a constant rate. Potassium-arrested hearts can also be used to examine flow-dependent effects in the absence of myocardial function (13). Since the Langerdorff preparation does not perform work, its oxygen consumption is lower than that of the working heart preparation. In the case of vascular preparations, gentle processing of the vessel serves to preserve the integrity of the endothelial lining. Caution must be exercised to ensure that the length of the vascular segment in vitro approximates that of the vessel in vivo. This variable is particularly important, since contractile function is directly influenced by the length of the vessel (14). Perfused preparations can only be used for short-term studies, since their viability decreases rapidly as a function of time. However, important information can be obtained in preparations which retain the geometry of the intact tissue.

Indices of Toxicity

Parameters commonly applied to the study of xenobiotic-induced toxicity using isolated perfused heart preparations include time to peak tension, maximal rate of tension development, and tension development. In addition, the oxygen concentration of the perfusate entering the aorta and leaving the pulmonary artery can be monitored as an index of myocardial oxygen consumption. Coronary flow can be measured by collecting effluent fractions as a function of time. A left atriotomy can be made to insert a latex balloon connected to a pressure transducer to monitor left ventricular pressure. Pin electrodes connected to the right atrium, apex, and pulmonary vessels can be used to obtain electrocardiographic recordings. In the case of aortic preparations, the cannula employed for vessel perfusion can be equipped with side arms for aortic pressure recording. As with cardiac preparations, measurements of contractility and stress development can also be used to evaluate the effects of drugs and chemicals. The application of perfused preparations to the study of drug-induced or chemically induced cardiovascular toxicity is exemplified by recent reports presented by Pilcher and Langley (9), Hale and Poklis (10), and McFaul and McGrath (13).

Isolated Muscle Preparations

Methodology

Cardiac Strips of atrial, ventricular, or papillary muscles can be placed in a bath and superfused with oxygenated physiological solution as described by Foex (15). Isolated preparations operate under constant conditions of carbon dioxide exchange, ionic gradients, and diffusion of byproducts of cellular metabolism. Although studies using isolated strips have provided valuable information regarding the effects of several cardiotoxic agents on myocardial function (16,17), their application is limited because these preparations do not retain the geometry of the intact heart.

Vascular Segments from several vascular beds can be mounted for isometric tension development. Helical strips are preferred over longitudinal strips to avoid alterations in the geometry of muscle fibers. Segments are fixed at the distal end and attached to a transducer at the proximal end. Transverse ring segments in which two stainless steel wires are inserted through the lumen of the cylinder can also be employed. The lower wire is fixed onto the bath while the upper wire is connected to a transducer. Segments are equilibrated in a physiological solution and subjected to multiple stress/relaxation cycles to define optimal length as described previously (14). Optimal length is defined as the length at which maximal contractility occurs in response to a contractile agonist. Under these conditions, the final load placed on the strips represents about 10% of the total active tension development. Naive and treated preparations must be compared at optimal length to eliminate potential misinterpretation of experimental results (18). Preparations devoid of plasma membrane restrictions in permeability can be obtained by stripping off the plasmalemma using detergents or mechanical disruption (14,19). Contractions can be elicited using standard solutions of free ionized calcium within the physiological range as described by Fabiato and Fablato (19). (20).

Characterization/Validation

As with other in vitro models, exogenous influences of neural and humoral origin are excluded. The initial fiber length (preload) and the force which must be overcome for muscle shortening (afterload) can be controlled accurately. Experiments can be divided into three categories including: (1) isometric force development, which precludes muscle shortening; (2) isotonic force development, where the afterload is predetermined and the muscle is able to shorten, and (3) quick-release contractions in which the afterload is varied during contraction (15). Oxygenation of the tissue is due to diffusion and, thus, the thickness of the strips and the concentration of oxygen in the bath must be carefully monitored. Isolated preparations can be controlled with precision, but their stability is limited to brief periods of time.

Indices of Toxicity

Attachment of force and length transducers make it possible to measure force, length, and velocity of contraction under controlled conditions. The study of these variables provide insights into the state of the muscle before and after chemical exposure. Pertinent reports describing the application of isolated muscle preparations in toxicity testing include Gibbs et al. (16), Togna et al. (21), and Robinson et al. (22).

Organ Culture

Methodology

Cardiac Ingwall and her colleagues (23) have described the use of fetal hearts in culture to study processes associated with myocardial cell injury. Whole fetal hearts are obtained aseptically and placed on stainless steel grids in culture dishes to allow gas exchange. The culture medium consists of a phosphate/bicarbonate buffer solution containing essential salts, glucose, amino acids, and vitamins. A variation of this method using the right atria has been reported by several investigators, including Speralakis and Shigenoubu (24) and Tanaka (25).

Vascular Gotlieb and Boden (26) have described the preparation of organ cultures of aortic tissue. Fat and adventitia are removed and the unopened aorta is cut along its long axis. The surface is kept moist at all times to ensure the viability of endothelial cells. The vessel is pinned with the endothelial side up and rectangular pieces of full thickness wall (3×10 mm) are cut out.

Segments are washed in a buffered salt solution and incubated in plastic dishes with culture medium containing serum for up to 7 days.

Characterization/Validation

Organ culture preparations offer long-term stability relative to other in vitro preparations. Hearts in organ culture beat for 4-8 days and, thus, can be used to evaluate repeated toxicant exposures. As with other in vitro preparations, toxicity can be evaluated in the absence of flow regulation. Evidence of persistent tissue edema, primarily in the first layers of aortic tissue, has been documented (26). However, the extent of swelling is less than that observed in response to endothelial denudation. Nonwounded endothelial cells undergo a change from elongated to polygonal shape within 24 h in vitro. This change may be related to the absence of blood flow in culture. Cell proliferation is observed beneath the nondenuded endothelium. Organ culture systems have been developed to facilitate the study of cellular interactions. For example, the rat endothelium in vivo regenerates at a nonlinear rate peaking at 0.4 mm/day to 0.7 mm/day by the second or third day. In contrast, bovine endothelial cell monolayers show a steady regeneration rate of 1 mm/day, whereas rat aortic explants show qualitatively similar rates to rat arteries in vivo (26).

Indices of Toxicity

Toxicant-induced cell injury can be evaluated at the morphological, ultrastructural, and biochemical levels as described by Ingwall et al. (23) and Kloner and Ingwall (28).

Single Cell Suspensions

Methodology

Cardiac Various combinations of physical, enzymatic, and chelating agents have been successfully employed to isolate cardiac cells. No standarized method is universally accepted for the preparation of single cell suspensions. Generally, suspensions of embryonic or neonatal cells derived from ventricular, atrial, or whole heart tissue can be prepared by enzymatic and/or mechchanical dissociation. Typically, minced tissue is incubated for 1-12 h with stipulated concentrations of single or multiple proteolytic enzymes at 4-37 °C. Physical stirring or agitation are commonly used to enhance tissue disruption. Cell isolation is normally carried out in calcium-free medium in order to weaken the connective matrix which holds the tissue together.

The isolation of adult myocytes which exhibit tolerance to physiological calcium concentrations requires the use of more sophisticated techniques. Jacobson (29) has described the use of a dissociation apparatus consisting of fingerlike projections (bristles) which provide abrasive action for the isolation of adult heart cells. Using this procedure, the apical portion of the ventricle is dissected and a series of staggered cuts are made before the tissue is wrapped around the bristles and incubated with collagenase. However, Bkailey et al. (30) have argued that these cells lose their fast sodium channels after several days in culture, and have suggested that replacement of calcium with stronium or barium prevents this change.

Hearts of adult male rats can also be dissociated by a recirculating Langerdorff perfusion (31). Intact hearts are perfused for 30 min with a calcium-containing collagenase solution to which 0.1% albumin is added. The tissue is then chopped and incubated in medium containing a higher albumin content (1%). Gentle pipeting can be used to enhance the release of myocytes. This preparation contains a high proportion of cells which remain in rod shape and are quiescent in medium containing physiological calcium levels.

Vascular A similar approach can be used to prepare a single cell suspensions of vascular cells. The anatomical distribution of cells within the vessel wall facilitates the isolation of relatively pure suspensions of fibroblastic, endothelial, or smooth muscle cells. In contrast to cardiac preparations, however, vascular cells from embryonic, neonatal, and adult vessels can be efficiently isolated in calcium- and magnesium-containing solutions. Endothelial cells are typically isolated by collagenase perfusion of intact cylinders, whereas collagenase/elastase mixtures or trypsin are employed to isolate medial smooth muscle cells. Recent studies in our laboratory have shown that elastase is not essential for the isolation of viable smooth muscle cells (32).

Characterization/Validation

Enzymes, temperature, osmolarity/pH, and time of incubation are important determinants of cell viability immediately after isolation. Purified collagenase alone cannot be used in the isolation of myocytes. This suggests that other constituents, such as proteinases, are essential to the cell isolation process. Caution must be exercised when purchasing commercially available enzyme preparations, since different lots and suppliers may exhibit different enzymatic activities. Other proteolytic enzymes such as trypsin have been successfully used to isolate neonatal cardiac myocytes and adult vascular myocytes. However, because of its ability to hydrolyze lysine and arginine peptide bonds on the carboxyl side of amino acid residues, trypsin may cause extensive damage to cellular membranes. Other deleterious effects of trypsin include increased aggregation and/or removal of surface enzymes, reduction in receptor binding sites and chromosomal damage. Cell damage during the isolation procedure can be minimized by carrying out the enzymatic digestion at an optimal low temperature and by limiting the time during which the cells are exposed to low external calcium concentrations.

The processing of myocardial tissue yields a heterogeneous population of muscle and nonmuscle cells. Neonatal myocytes are remarkably resistant to injury and exhibit variable degrees of beating shortly after isolation. In contrast, beating of adult cardiac myocytes is thought to be due to the uncontrolled leakage of calcium through a permeable plasma membrane. This phenomenom is thought to represent a calcium-paradox phenomenom similar to that originally described by Zimmerman (33). Under these conditions, cellular injury is characterized by release of intracellular protein, accumulation of calcium and sodium within the cell and loss of intracellular potassium. These cells are said to be calcium intolerant and often can be identified by their rounded appearance. However, assessment of cell shape alone may be misleading, since rod-shaped myocytes may display abnormal resting membrane potentials (30). Viable adult myocytes should exhibit normal sarcomere length and remain quiescent at low external calcium concentrations and contract in response to increasing calcium concentrations. The fact that adult cardiac myocytes are mechanically at rest when isolated properly suggests that fundamental differences exist between adult and neonatal cells.

Indices of Toxicity

Isolated cardiac myocytes can be microinjected with fluorescent dyes for ionic measurements. Cells in suspension can also be voltage clamped to evaluate spontaneous and chemically induced electrophysiological changes. Disruption of the structural integrity of the cells is associated with loss of permeability restrictions, leakage of intracellular constituents, and intracellular accumulation of macromolecules. In general, toxic responses may be of slower onset or differing magnitude relative to those observed in vivo. Recent studies by Allshire and his colleagues (34) serve to exemplify the application of single cell suspensions to evaluate myocardial cell injury.

Cultured Cell Systems

Methodology

Cells in suspension exhibit short-term stability and must be used within 4-8 h after isolation. As a result, cultured systems are preferred when toxicity must be evaluated for long time periods. Although, in the past, embryonic or neonatal cultures have been commonly employed, the use of adult cultures is now more prevalent. Primary cultures can be established from cell suspensions of cardiac and vascular tissues. Vascular cell cultures can also be established by explant methods. Myocardial cells are usually obtained from rats or rabbits, whereas vascular cells are often derived from porcine or bovine sources.

Since the preparation of primary cultures is as much art as science, standarization of the conditions employed during cell isolation and growth is essential to ensure the uniformity of each batch of cells placed in culture. Cells in suspension are innoculated and allowed to settle at the bottom of the culture vessel. Viable cells attach to the surface and flatten out. Neonatal and embryonic cells of cardiovascular origin as well as adult vascular endothelial and smooth muscle cells proliferate readily under appropriate conditions in vitro. The ability of differentiated heart muscle cells from embryonic and neonatal sources (35,36) and vascular endothelial and smooth muscle cells (37) to undergo mitosis allows cultures to reach confluence within relatively short periods.

Cardiac As described previously, the dissociation of cardiac tissue yields a heterogeneous population of cells. Cells can be separated into relatively pure cultures of cardiac muscle and nonmuscle cells by a differential pour-off technique based on the rate of attachment of the cells to the substratum (38). Most of the nonmuscle cells attach to the dishes by 3 h, whereas muscle cells remain in suspension for 16-19 h. Because the percentage of fibroblasts in culture increases logarithmically, if no attempt is made to separate individual cell types fibroblasts will eventually dominate the culture. Pre- or postnatal myoblasts resemble fibroblasts in their physical properties. In contrast, adult cardiac myocytes differ considerably in size from other cellular constituents of heart tissue. A monoclonal antibody to cell surface adhesion factors has been used to enrich preparations of cultured myocardial cells (39). The addition of mitotic inhibitors and the maintenance of cultures in glutamine-free or serum-free media can also be used to enhance culture purity (40). Piper et al. (31) have reported a method for culturing adult cardiac myocytes which preserve normal ultrastructural features in the presence of physiological calcium concentrations for up to 4 days. In these preparations, energy stores can be maintained at normal levels by the addition of exogenous creatine. High seeding densities of adult myocytes may reduce cellular attachment due to excessive overlap of rod-shape cells.

Vascular Vascular cell cultures are often derived from large blood vessels to facilitate manipulation of the tissue. Cautious dissection and processing of the tissue ensures that pure cell suspensions are placed in culture.

Characterization/Validation

The viability of cells in suspension decreases rapidly as a function of time. The density of saturable beta-adrenergic binding sites is significantly reduced in cardiac cell suspensions relative to cardiac myocytes established in primary culture (41). Receptor-mediated calcium exchange is observed in cultured myocytes but not in cell suspensions. In addition to these considerations, cell culture preparations are preferred over cell suspensions for toxicity studies because a larger sample pool can be obtained after several cell divisions in culture. This is particularly important because the yield of cells from cardiovascular tissue under most experimental conditions is considerably low. The use of older animals is typically associated with a reduction in the number of cells which can be successfully established in culture. Although the bases for this phenomenon are not yet clear, alterations in the growth/proliferative programs of cardiovascular cells as a function of age may be involved.

Within 2 days in culture, spontaneous beating of neonatal cardiac myocytes is observed at a rate of 80-150 beats/min. The rate and duration of beating in culture is a function of the plating density (42). Adult myocytes do not contract spontaneously, but exhibit a high degree of electrophysiological and pharmacological integrity (31). The responses of cardiac myocytes in culture to biologically active substances are similar to those of the intact heart (43).

Under most experimental conditions, vascular smooth muscle cells do not exhibit spontaneous contractility. These cells, however, respond to pharmacological stimulation (44). In recent years, more information has become available regarding the physiological functions of cardiac and vascular endothelial cells. Mechanical studies of endothelial morphology show that when cells are subjected to fluid mechanical forces associated with blood flow, cells become elongated and orient themselves in the direction of shear stress (45). Growth of endothelial cells on extracellular matrix components, on layers of smooth muscle cells, and under flow may mimic some aspects of the vascular wall not found when cells are grown on plastic.

The culture of most normal cells requires either serum or plasma for attachment, proliferation, and survival of cells. For example, deprivation of aortic endothelial cell cultures of serum for long time periods can result in extensive cell injury. Sato and his colleagues (46) have demonstrated that the serum or plasma requirement for cell growth of several cell lines can be satisfied by the addition of specific hormones and growth factors to synthetic media. For example, heart muscle cells plated on collagen-coated dishes proliferate actively in serum-free defined media supplemented with endothelial cell growth supplement (47). The influence of this supplement has also been observed in nonmuscle cell preparations.

Factors responsible for the cytological, biochemical, and physiological characteristics of cells in culture must be carefully defined. The growth environment of cells in culture is an important determinant of cellular behavior in vitro. The composition of commercially available media, including the concentrations of glucose, vitamins, and other essential substrates, varies to a significant extent. For instance, different substrates regulate the proliferation and growth of cardiac (47) and vascular (K. Ramos and G. Liau, 1989, unpublished observations) cells to different extents. The presence of serum modulates the antioxidant capabilities of cells in vitro. Variable results due to the composition of enzyme solutions, number of cells plated per culture dish, and composition of the growth medium have been observed in our laboratory. From a toxicological standpoint, this is a potentially significant source of variability.

Barnes (48) has reviewed studies by Koetz and coworkers which show that exposure of heart cell cultures to fibroblast growth factor and insulinlike growth factor gives a noncontracting population of myocytes growth advantage. Removal of the growth factors causes certain markers of differentiation to reappear, including atrial natriuretic factor and titin, a large protein thought to help with the assembly of contractile proteins. Cultured myocardial cells may undergo hypertrophy under certain experimental conditions. Hypertrophy appears to be regulated by the amount of serum in the medium in a manner analogous to serum-dependent cellular proliferation (49). Iron-supplemented bovine calf serum has recently been introduced to enhance cellular growth (50).

The identity of cells established in culture must be carefully evaluated before toxicity studies are initiated. Cultures may be characterized at the morphological, ultrastructural, biochemical, or functional level. Cultured cells exhibit signs of adaptation of life in vitro. This point is exemplified by the reduced surface area of intercalated discs observed in cultured adult cardiac myocytes relative to cells in vivo. Cardiovascular cells in culture lose differentiated features as a function of time. Dedifferentiated myocytes exhibit poorly defined contractile structures (51). At the molecular level, the expression of muscle-specific proteins is often compromised (52). Recent studies have shown that the contractile responsiveness of smooth muscle cells in primary culture is lost if the phenotypic stability of the cells is not preserved (44). The degree of differentiation of myocytes is also influenced by the geometry and age of the culture (53,54).

Indices of Toxicity

Cultured cells may respond to a toxic stimulus with changes in growth rate, culture density, cellular morphology, and/or biochemical expression. The occurrence of gross morphological changes is routinely used to screen chemicals of unknown toxic potential and to assess potentially significant toxic interactions. The advent of flow cytometry and computerized evaluation of cell images has reduced many of the shortcomings inherent to microscopic analysis. In the case of embryonic or neonatal cardiac myocytes, toxicity can also be evaluated based on the arrhythmogenic potential of chemicals (55,56). Arbitrary or computer-assisted grading systems can be implemented to evaluate these responses (57,58). Biochemical approaches can be applied with relative ease to elucidate the molecular basis of toxic insult. Because toxicity is often due to interactions with, or disruption of antioxidant defense systems, measurements of the glutathione status of cells may be particularly useful in the elucidation of mechanisms of toxicity (37,59) Ionic homeostasis can also be used as an index of disturbances in the structural and functional integrity of the plasma membrane (60,61). Additional reports describing the use of cell cultures in toxicity testing include Papa and McCauley (62), and McCall and Ryan (61).

FUTURE PERSPECTIVES

Research and Developmental Needs

The successful application of in vitro model systems to evaluate the cardiovascular toxicity of drugs and chemicals has evolved from many years of coordinated research efforts. Future research should be directed toward the refinement of existing methodology and the development of new alternatives. Of particular interest is the application of coculture systems of muscle and nonmuscle cells from cardiac or vascular tissue to the assessment of cardiovascular toxicity. Cocultures of vascular endothelial and smooth muscle cells have been successfully used to study cell-cell interactions in vitro (63,64). These systems reconstruct the complexities of the cellular environment in vivo but retain the advantages inherent to the cell culture preparation. Additional information is needed to optimize the concomitant growth of multiple cell types in vitro and to define suitable experimental conditions. The complexity of coculture systems is exemplified by studies which show that endothelial cells modulate the extent of binding, internalization, and degration of low-density lipoproteins by arterial smooth muscle cells (65) and produce growth factors for both smooth muscle cells and fibroblasts (63). More widespread application of these systems to evaluate cardiovascular toxicity is desirable.

In cases where multifactorial phenomena in the expression of toxicity must be considered, animals can be exposed in vivo and the tissue of interest isolated and processed in vitro. This approach has been successfully applied to evaluate the effects of subchronic toxicant exposure on the phenotypic expression of vascular smooth muscle cells (44,66). However, caution must always be exercised to ensure the uniformity and consistency of different cell batches derived from multiple experimental groups at different times. An additional consideration is that toxicant exposure may alter the ability of cells to attach and grow in culture. In vitro growth conditions can be manipulated to preserve some differentiated properties in serially passaged smooth muscle cells (67). The availability of stable subcultured systems is essential to the application of cellular and molecular techniques in toxicity testing. Collectively, these approaches will facilitate the study of changes in cellular metabolism, growth regulation, differentiation, and homeostasis associated with toxicant exposure. Additional efforts should be directed toward the optimization of subcultured systems.

Recent evidence suggests that the ability of cardiac myocytes to divide is repressed but not completely lost. This concept is consistent with studies which show that the number of myocytes with multiple nuclei increases as a function of age (48) and that some atrial myocytes synthesize large amounts of deoxyribonucleic acid (DNA) and undergo complete cell division after an infarct to the ventricle (68). Myocardial cell division can also be stimulated by insertion of the large tumor antigen from the SV40 virus into the myocyte genome (69). Field (70) have recently described experiments in which the large tumor antigen gene from the SV40 virus coupled to the promoter for the mouse atrionatruiretic factor gene was injected into fertilized mouse eggs. About 20% of the mouse pups obtained under these conditions carried the transgene and developed right atrial tumors. These tumors divided in an uncontrolled fashion and displayed spontanteous contractility. The enhanced proliferative behavior of these muscle cells may offer the opportunity to establish a permanent cell line of heart muscle cells (48). In the future, these myocytelike cells can be used to better understand the regulation of cardiac-specific genes under a variety of experimental conditions.

As the level of technological sophistication advances, an increasing number of toxic drugs and chemicals will likely be identified. Aggressive strategies must be designed to generate the data base required to successfully manage potential toxicities. Although in vitro model systems are now recognized as powerful tools in toxicity testing, their full potential remains largely unexplored.

REFERENCES

1. Markovac, J., and Goldstein, G. W. (1988). Lead activates protein kinase C in immature rat brain microvessels. *Toxicol. Appl. Pharmacol.* **96**: 14-23.
2. Nolan, C., and Shaikh, Z. A. (1986). The vascular endothelium as a target in acute cadmium toxicity. *Life Sci.* **39**: 1403-1409.
3. Isner, J. M., Estes, N. A. M., Thompson, P. D., Costanzo-Nordin, M. R., Subramanian, R., Miller, G., Kastas, G., Sweeney, K. and Sturner, W. Q. (1986). Acute cardiac events temporally related to cocaine abuse. *New Engl. J. Med.* **315**: 1438-1443.
4. Rubin, J. I., and Rubin, E. (1982). Myocardial toxicity of alcohols, aldehydes and glycols including alcoholic cardiomyopathy. In *Cardiovascular Toxicology.* E. W. Van Stee (Ed.). Raven Press, New York, pp. 353-364.
5. Balazs, T., Johnson, G., Joseph, X., Ehrreich, S., and Bloom, S. (1983). Sensitivity and resistance of the myocardium to the toxicity of isoproterenol in rats. In *Myocardial Injury.* J. Spitzer, (Ed.). Plenum Press, New York, pp. 563-577.

6. Report from the American Medical Society on Alcoholism (1985). Alcohol and cardiovascular disease: Implications for clinical practice and research.
7. Kurppa, K., Hietnamen, E., Klockars, M., Partinen, M., Rantanen, J., Ronnemaa, T., and Viikari, J. (1984). Chemical exposures at work and cardiovascular morbidity. *Scand. J. Environ. Health* **10**: 381-388.
8. Acosta, D., Sorenson, E. M. B., Anuforo, D. C., Mitchell, D. B., Ramos, K., Santone, K. S., and Smith, M. A. (1985). An in vitro approach to the study of target organ toxicity of drugs and chemicals. *In Vitro Cell. Devel. Biol.* **21**: 495-504.
9. Pilcher, G. D., and Langley, A. E. (1986). The effects of perfluoro-n-decanoic acid in the rat heart. *Toxicol. Appl. Pharmacol.* **85**: 389-397.
10. Hale, P. W., and Poklis, A. (1986). Cardiotoxicity of thioridazine and two stereoisomeric forms of thioridazine 5-sulfoxide in the isolated perfused rat heart. *Toxicol. Appl. Pharmacol.* **86**: 44-55.
11. Neely, J. E., Liebermeister, H., Battersby, E. J., and Morgan, H. E. (1967). Effect of pressure development on oxygen consumption in isolated rat hearts. *Am. J. Physiol.* **212**: 804-814.
12. Crass, M. F., Hulsey, S. M., and Bulkley, T. J. (1988). Use of a new pulsatile perfused rat aorta preparation to study the characteristics of the vasodilator effect of parathyroid hormone. *J. Pharmacol. Exp. Ther.* **245**: 723-724.
13. McFaul, S. J., and McGrath, J. J. (1987). Studies on the mechanism of carbon monoxide-induced vasodilation in the isolated perfused rat heart. *Toxicol. Appl. Pharmacol.* **87**: 464-473.
14. Ramos, K. (1986). Sarcolemmal dependence of isosorbide dinitrate-induced relaxation of vascular smooth muscle. *Res. Comm. Chem. Pathol.* **52**: 195-205.
15. Foex, P. (1988). Experimental models of myocardial ischemia, *Br. J. Anaesthesiol.* **61**: 44-55.
16. Gibbs, C. L., Woolley, G., Kotsanas, G., and Gibson, W. R. (1984). Cardiac energetics in daunorubicin-induced cardiomyopathy. *J. Mol. Cell. Cardiol.* **16**: 953-962.
17. Rodgers, R. L., Chou, H-N., Temma, K., Akera, T., and Shimizu, Y. (1984). Positive inotropic and toxic effects of brevitoxin-B on rat and guinea-pig heart. *Toxicol. Appl. Pharmacol.* **76**: 296-305.
18. Herlehy, J. T., and Murphy, R. A. (1973). Length-tension relationships of smooth muscle of the hog carotid artery. *Circ. Res.* **33**: 275-283.
19. Chatterjee, M., and Murphy, R. A. (1983). Calcium-dependent stress maintenance without myosin phophorylation in "skinned" smooth muscle cells. *Science* **221**: 464-466.
20. Fabiato, A., and Fabiato, F. (1979). Calculator programs for computing the composition of the solutions containing multiple metals and ligands used for experiments with skinned muscle cells. *J. Physiol.* **75**: 363-505.
21. Togna, G., Dolci, N., and Caprino, L. (1984). Inhibition of aortic vessel adenosine diphosphate degradation by cadmium and mercury. *Arch. Toxicol.* **7**: 378-381.
22. Robinson, C. P., Baskin, S. I., and Franz, D. R. (1985). The mechanism of action of cyanide on the rabbit aorta. *J. Appl. Toxicol.* **5**: 372-377.

23. Ingwall, J. S., DeLuca, M., Sybers, H. D., and Wildenthal, K. (1975). Fetal mouse hearts: a model for studying ischemia. *Proc. Natl. Acad. Sci.* **72**: 2809-2813.
24. Speralakis, N., and Shigenoubu, R. (1974). Organ cultured chick embryonic heart cells of various ages. Part I. Electrophysiology. *J. Mol. Cell. Cardiol.* **6**: 449-471.
25. Tanaka, H., Kasuya, Y., Saito, H., and Shigenobu, K. (1987). Organ culture of rat heart: maintained high sensitivity of fetal atria before innervation to norepinephrine. *Can. J. Physiol. Pharmacol.* **66**: 901-906.
26. Gotlieb, A. I., and Boden, P. (1984). Porcine aortic organ culture: a model to study the cellular response to vascular injury. *In Vitro* **20**: 535-542.
27. Jackman, R. W., Anderson, S. K., and Sheridan, J. D. (1988). The aortic intima in organ culture. Response to culture conditions and partial endothelial denudation. *Am. J. Pathol.* **133**: 241-251.
28. Kloner, R. A. and Ingwall, J. S. (1980). The cultured fetal mouse heart as a model for studying myocardial ischemic necrosis. *Exp. Mol. Pathol.* **32**: 317-335.
29. Jacobson, S. L. (1977). Culture of spontaneously contracting myocardial cells from adult rats. *Cell. Struct. Funct.* **2**: 1-9.
30. Bkailey, G., Speralakis, N., and Doane, J. (1984). A new method for preparation of isolated single adult myocytes. *Am. J. Physiol.* **247**: H1018-1026.
31. Piper, H. M., Probst, I., Schwartz, P., Hutter, F. J., and Spieckermann, P. G. (1982). Culturing of calcium stable adult cardiac myocytes. *J. Mol. Cell. Cardiol.* **14**: 397-412.
32. Ramos, K., Grossman, S. L., and Cox, L. R. (1988). Allylamine-induced vascular toxicity in vitro: Prevention by semicarbazide-sensitive amine oxidase inhibitors. *Toxicol. Appl. Pharmacol.* **95**: 61-71.
33. Zimmerman,, A. N. E., Hulsmann, W. G. (1966). Paradoxical influence of calcium ions on the permeability of the cell membranes of the isolated rat heart. *Nature* **211**: 646-647.
34. Allshire, A., Piper, H. M., Cuthbertson, K. S. R., and Cobbold, P. H. (1987). Cytosolic free calcium in single rat heart cells during anoxia and reoxygenation. *Biochem. J.* **244**: 381-385.
35. Kasten, F. R. (1972). Rat myocardial cells in vitro: Mitosis and differentiated properties. *In Vitro* **8**: 128-149.
36. Halbert, S. P., Brudere, R., and Thompson, A. (1973). Growth of dissociated beating human heart cells in tissue culture, *Life Sci.* **13**: 969-975.
37. Ramos, K., and Cox, L. R. (1987). Primary cultures of rat aortic endothelial and smooth muscle cells. An in vitro model to study xenobiotic-induced vascular cytotoxicity. *In Vitro Cell. and Devel. Biol.* **23**: 288-296.
38. Ramos, K., and Acosta, D. (1989). The heart. Primary cultures of newborn myocardial cells as a model system to evaluate the cardiotoxicity of drugs and chemicals. In *In Vitro Models in Toxicology*. C. McQueen (Ed.). Telford Press.
39. McDonagh, J. C., Cebrat, E. K., and Nathan, R. D. (1987). Highly enriched preparations of cultured myocardial cells for biochemical and physiological analyses. *J. Mol. Cell. Cardiol.* **19**: 785-793.
40. Wenzel, D. G., and Cosma, G. N. (1984). A model system for measuring comparative toxicities of cardiotoxic drugs with cultured rat heart myocytes, en-

dothelial cells and fibroblasts. I. Emetine, chloroquine and metronidazole. *Toxicology* **33**: 103-115.
41. Welder, A. W., Machu, T., Leslie, S. W., Wilcox, R. E., Bradlaw, J. D., and Acosta, D. (1988). Beta adrenergic receptor characteristics of postanatal rat myocardial cell preparations. *In Vitro Cell. Devel. Biol.* **24**: 771-777.
42. Wenzel, D. G., Wheatley, J. W., and Byrd, G. D. (1970). Effects of nicotine on cultured rat heart cells. *Toxicol. Appl. Pharmacol.* **17**: 774-785.
43. Marsh, J. D., Barry, W. H., and Smith, T. W. (1982). Desensitization to the inotropic effect of isoproterenol in cultured ventricular cells. *J. Pharmacol. Exp. Ther.* **223**: 60-67.
44. Cox, L. R., and Ramos, K. (1989). Allylamine-induced phenotypic modulation of aortic smooth muscle cells. *J. Exp. Pathol.* **71**: 11-18.
45. Ives, C. L., Eskin, S. G., and McIntire, L. V. (1986). Mechanical effects on endothelial cell morphology: In vitro assessment. *In Vitro Cell. Devel. Biol.* **22**:500-507.
46. Sato, G. H. (1979). The growth of cells in serum-free hormone supplemented media. *Meth. Enzymol.* **58**: 94-109.
47. Nag, A. C., Ingland, M., and Cheng, M. (1985). Factors controlling embryonic heart cell proliferation in serum-free synthetic media. *In Vitro Cell. Devel. Biol.* **21**: 553-562.
48. Barnes, D. M. (1988). Joint soviet-U.S. attack on heart muscle dogma. *Science* **242**: 193-195.
49. Simpson, P., McGrath, A., and Savion, S. (1982). Myocyte hypertrophy in neonatal rat heart and its regulation by serum and by catecholamines. *Circ. Res.* **51**: 787-801.
50. Hyclone Laboratories Inc. (1988). Iron-supplemented bovine calf serum: An excellent substitute for fetal bovine serum. *Art to Science* **7**: 1-6.
51. Campbell, J. S., and Campbell, G. R. (1988). Phenotypic modulation of smooth muscle cells in primary culture. In *Vascular Smooth Muscle in Culture.* Vol. I. J. S. Campbell and G. R. Campbell (Eds.). CRC Press, Boca Raton, pp. 39-57.
52. Owens, G. K., and Thompson, M. M. (1986). Developmental changes in isoactin expression in rat aortic smooth muscle cells in vivo. *J. Biol. Chem.* **261**: 13373-13380.
53. Speralakis, N., and McLean, M. (1978). Electrical properties of cultured heart cells. In *Recent Advances in Studies on Cardiac Structure and Metabolism.* Vol. 12. T. Kobayashi, Y. Ito, and G. Rona (Eds.). University Press, Baltimore.
54. Simpson, P., and Savion, S. (1982). Differentiation of rat myocytes in single cell cultures with and without proliferating non-myocardial cells. *Circ. Res.* **50**: 101-116.
55. Wenzel, D. G., and Innis, J. D. (1983). Arrhythmogenec and antiarrhythmic effects of lipolytic factors on cultured heart cells. *Res. Comm. Chem. Pathol. Pharmacol.* **41**: 383-396.
56. Aszalos, A., Bradlaw, J. A., Reynaldo, E. F., Yang, G. C., and El-Hage, A. N. (1984). Studies on the action of nystatin on cultured rat myocardial cells and cell membranes. *Biochem. Pharmacol.* **33**: 3779-3786.
57. Miletich, D. J., Khan, A., Albrecht, R. F., and Jozefiak, A. (1983). Use of heart cell cultures as a tool for the evaluation of halothane arrhythmia. *Toxicol. Appl. Pharmacol.* **70**: 181-187.

58. Yarom, R., Hasin, S., Raz, S., Shimoni, Y., Fixler, R. and Yagen, B. (1986). T-2 toxin effect on cultured myocardial cells. *Toxicol. Lett.* **31**: 1-8.
59. Ramos, K., Combs, A. B., and Acosta, D. (1983). Cytotoxicity of isoproterenol to cultured heart cells: Effects of antioxidants on modifying membrane damage. *Toxicol. Appl. Pharmacol.* **70**: 317-323.
60. Ramos, K., Combs, A. B., and Acosta, D. (1984). Role of calcium in isoproterenol cytotoxicity to cultured myocardial cells. *Biochem. Pharmacol.* **33**: 1989-1992.
61. McCall, D., and Ryan, K. (1987). The effect of ethanol and acetaldehyde on Na pump function in cultured rat heart cells. *J. Mol. Cell. Cardiol.* **19**: 453-463.
62. Papa, L. R., and McCauley, P. T. (1985). Hypochlorite-serum reaction products inhibit porcine vascular endothelial cell growth in culture. *Artery* **13**: 50-60.
63. Davies, P. F., Truskey, G. A., Warren, H. B., O'Connor, S. E., and Eisenhaure, B. H. (1985). Metabolic cooperation between vascular endothelial cells and smooth muscle cells in co-culture: Changes in low density lipoprotein metabolism. *J. Cell Biol.* **101**: 871-879.
64. Weinberg, C. B., and Bell, E. (1986). A blood vessel model constructed from collagen and cultured vascular cells. *Science* **231**: 397-399.
65. Horrigan, S., Campbell, J. H., and Campbell, G. R. (1988). Effect of endothelium on VLDL metabolism by cultured smooth muscle cells of differing phenotype. *Atherosclerosis* **71**: 57-69.
66. Cox, L. R., and Ramos, K. (1987). Morphologic modulation of vascular smooth muscle cells upon subchronic exposure to allylamine: Reversal by dibutyryl cyclic AMP. *In Vitro Toxicol.* **1**: 183-187.
67. Liau, G., and Chang, L. M. (1989). Regulation of extracellular matrix RNA levels in cultured smooth muscle cells: Relationship to cellular quiescence. *J. Biol. Chem.* **264**: 10315-10320.
68. Rumyantsev, P. P. (1977). Interrelations of the proliferation and differentiation processes during cardiac myogenesis and regeneration. *Int. Rev. Cytol.* **51**: 187.
69. Claycomb, W. C., and Lanson, N. A., Jr. (1987). Proto-oncogene expression in proliferating and differentiating cardiac and skeletal muscle. *Biochem. J.* **247**: 701-706.
70. Field, L. J. (1988). Atrial natriuretic factor-SV40T antigen transgenes produce tumors and cardiac arrhythmias in mice. *Science* **239**: 1029-1033.

7

Ocular Irritation

Leon H. Bruner

The Procter & Gamble Company
Cincinnati, Ohio

INTRODUCTION

The eye is the delicate sensory organ that captures visible light energy and converts it into neural impulses. These impulses are processed in the retina and central nervous system, giving rise to vision, our most important sense. Because of its external location and anatomy, the eye is constantly exposed. It can be damaged by drying, natural environmental contaminants, and microorganisms. It also is vulnerable to injury induced by a variety of manmade traumatic insults, including chemical exposure.

Accidental ocular exposure to chemicals or consumer products does occur at home and in the workplace. In order to prevent dangerous products from reaching the market and to correctly advise consumers and workers on the safety of the materials they use, developers of consumer goods and chemicals must perform ocular safety assessments.

Since the 1940s animal assays have been used to make ocular safety assessments. These assays primarily use the albino rabbit as the animal model, and a systematic numerical scoring system for quantifying the irritation (1). These tests are currently the standard for assessing the irritancy potential of new materials.

Although the in vivo eye irritation tests provide important and useful information, they are not without criticism. The in vivo ocular safety tests have been criticized for the subjectivity of the method, for their overprediction of human response, and by animal welfare advocates because they require animals as test subjects. Thus, there is great interest in developing alternative methods that will allow toxicologists to make accurate ocular safety assessments. The goals of programs designed to develop such methods is to find systems that are simple to perform, that give consistent results, and provide the information needed to make appropriate human ocular risk assessments. Accomplishing these goals is a great challenge.

This chapter will focus on this challenge. It will describe the anatomical and physiological features of the anterior eye relevant to ocular safety testing and development of alternative assay systems. Considerable work has been devoted to developing alternatives for ocular safety testing, and many of these assays will be described in detail. The chapter closes with a discussion of how the alternatives may be used in safety assessment today, and the areas where additional research may provide more reliable systems for the future.

HUMAN OCULAR ANATOMY

The eyeball is a fibrovascular spheroid globe suspended in a bony orbit by numerous ligaments and extrinsic muscles (Fig. 1) (2-4). The globe is light-

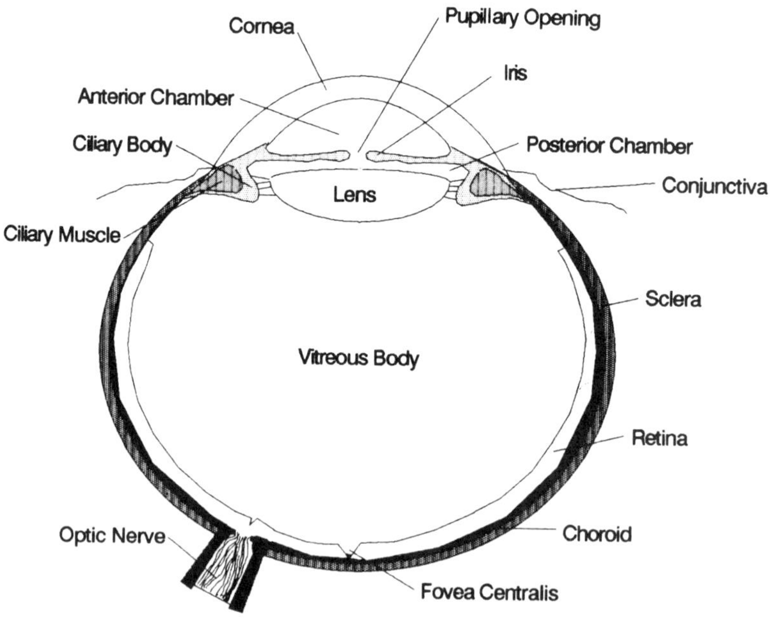

Figure 1 Cross section of the eye.

proof except for the transparent corneal surface. Only the anterior aspect of the eyeball is exposed to the environment. The rest is protected behind the eyelids and bony orbital rim.

The eyeball has three coats that are further divided into subparts. The *outer coat* is the transparent cornea and the gray-white sclera that provides the primary supporting framework of the globe. The *middle coat* is the uvea that contains the choroid, the ciliary body, and the iris. The *inner coat* is the retina, the neural photoreceptive tissue in the eye.

The majority of the nonretinal structures serve secondary functions that aid the photoreception process. These include focusing images on the retina (cornea and lens), regulating the amount of light entering the eye (iris), providing nutrients to ocular tissues (vasculature, aqueous humor, vitreous humor, and lacrimal or tear system), moving the eyes (extrinsic musculature), and protection (somatosensory nerves and eyelids).

Outer Coat

Cornea and Precorneal Tear Film

The cornea is the transparent anterior surface of the eye where light passes to the retina (see Fig. 1). Since the cornea is the main refractive surface of the eye, it also plays a key role in focusing images on the retina. A clear, properly shaped cornea is critical for normal vision. Its exposed location makes it particularly vulnerable to injury, and any scarring that occurs secondary to damage may lead to opacities or shape changes that permanently impair vision.

Percorneal Tear Film The anterior surface of the cornea is covered by a relatively stagnant layer called the precorneal tear film. This outer film is important for proper corneal function. It delays dehydration of the corneal surface and provides a smooth, continuous surface that enhances its optical properties. The tear film has three layers: an anterior lipid layer, a middle aqueous layer, and a thin mucin layer. The lipid layer slows the evaporation of the aqueous layer, and provides a smooth, regular optical surface. The mucin layer wets the microvilli of the corneal epithelial cells and must be intact for the precorneal tear film to form and remain on the corneal surface.

Corneal Structure The cornea has three layers: the epithelium with its basement membrane, the stroma or substantia propria, and the endothelium with its basement membrane (Fig. 2).

Epithelium In humans, the corneal epithelium is approximately 50-90 μm thick and covers the entire stromal surface. It is a stratified, nonkeratinized epithelium, five to six cell layers thick. The outermost layer is two to three cell layers thick. The midzone consists of two to three layers of polyhedral cells, and the bottommost is a single layer of tall, columnar germinal cells. The epithelial cells regenerate in the basal layer, and become progres-

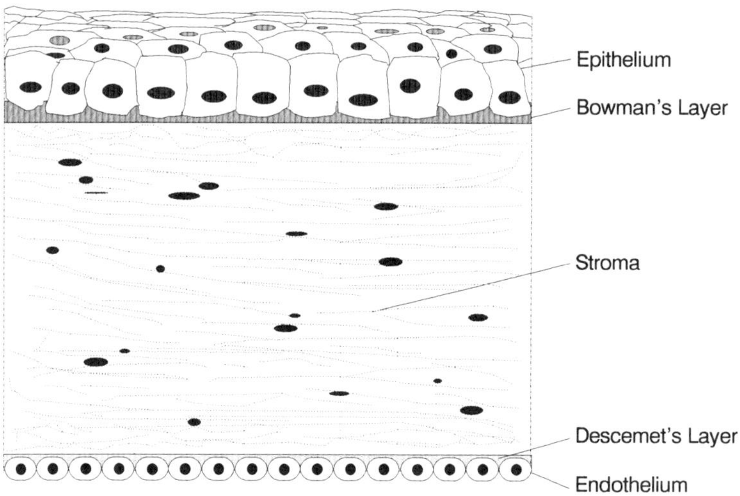

Figure 2 Cross section of the cornea.

sively flatter as they migrate toward the surface. Squamous surface cells are shed from the surface after approximately 7 days. Directly below the basal cell layer is the PAS-positive basement membrane. It is firmly attached to the anterior stroma by irregular filaments.

Corneal Stroma The corneal stroma constitutes approximately 90% of the corneal thickness. Its anterior portion, Bowman's layer, is an acellular region lying just under the epithelial basement membrane. It is more resistant to deformation, trauma, and passage of foreign bodies or infecting organisms than the other layers. Once damaged, its architecture may not be restored, leading to abnormalities in corneal thickness and optical properties that could result in permanent vision deficit.

The remainder of the stroma is composed of layers of type I collagen fibrils gathered together in lamellae that run in parallel with the corneal surface. The fibrils within a lamella are highly organized and are surrounded by a glycosaminoglycan matrix. Corneal glycosaminoglycans are 60% keratin sulfate and 40% chondroitin sulfates. These act as anions and bind cations and water. The posterior surface of the stroma is lined with the loosely attached Descemet's layer that is the basement membrane for the endothelial cells.

Scattered throughout the lamellae are long flat fibroblastlike cells called keratocytes. These cells have long processes that extend to adjacent cells.

There also are a few neutrophils and macrophages that migrate through the stroma.

Corneal Endothelium The endothelium is a single layer of mesothelial cells resting on Descemet's layer. The apical surface is in contact with the aqueous humor of the anterior chamber. The cells are bound tightly to each other with desmosomes. The endothelium serves the important function of maintaining the dehydration (deturgescence) that is also required to maintain corneal clarity (see below).

Sclera

The sclera is a dense, fibrous, collagenous structure that makes up the gray-white part of the globe. Like the cornea, it has three layers. Its major stromal layer lies in the middle and is made up mainly of bundles of irregularly arranged collagen fibrils of varying diameter. The irregular arrangement of these fibrils leads to the white color of the majority of the eyball. The inner surface of the sclera is the choroid. The external scleral surface is covered by the conjunctiva.

The conjunctiva is a transparent mucous membrane that covers the externally exposed scleral surface (bulbar conjunctiva) as well as the inner surface of the eyelids (palpebral conjunctiva). The conjunctival epithelium is continuous with the corneal epithelium and the lacrimal drainage system. The conjunctiva contains many blood vessels, nerves, conjunctival glands, and inflammatory cells. Small blood vessels are present throughout. They are usually not visible, but dilate and become leaky during inflammation. The nerves transmit pain responses and mediate neurogenic vasodilatation and tearing. The conjunctival glands provide moisture and secrete the constituents of the precorneal tear film.

Anterior Chamber, Posterior Chamber, and Aqueous Humor

Between the rear surface of the cornea and the front surface of the lens capsule is a fluid-filled chamber (see Fig. 1). This chamber is divided into anterior and posterior regions by the iris. The two chambers are connected through the pupillary opening. The anterior chamber lies in front of the iris and the posterior chamber lies behind the iris and in front of the lens capsule.

The Middle Coat

The middle coat of the eye is the uvea. It consists of the choroid, the ciliary body, and the iris (see Fig. 1). The choroid is a blood vessel-rich layer that provides blood to the retinal pigmented epithelium and outer half of the adjacent sensory retina. The ciliary body secretes the aqueous humor which fills the anterior and posterior chambers and contains the smooth muscle that alters the lens shape during accommodation. The iris is a diaphragm that lies in front of the lens and ciliary body. Contraction of iridal circular or radial muscles leads to closing or opening of the pupil, which regulates the amount of light entering the eye.

The Inner Coat

The inner coat of the eye is the retina. The two major parts of the retina are the inner sensory layer and the outer pigmented epithelium. The sensory layer lies between the pigmented epithelium on the outside, and the vitreous humor on the inside. It is stratified into several sublayers containing the different photoreceptor and accessory cells involved with sensing and processing the light projected onto the retinal surface. The pigmented epithelium is only one layer thick and lies between the sensory epithelium and choroid.

PATHOPHYSIOLOGY OF OCULAR IRRITATION

Tests used to assess ocular safety focus on three ocular structures: the cornea, iris, and conjunctiva (Table 1) (1). After topical treatment with test substances, the cornea is evaluated for degree of opacity and the area involved. Other changes such as erosions, neovascularization, and scar formation are noted. The iris is evaluated for signs of inflammation that include increased prominence of iridal folds, congestion, swelling, circumcorneal injection, hemorrhage, and gross tissue destruction. The pupillary reflex is assessed. The conjunctiva is evaluated for the degree of redness, swelling (chemosis), and discharge.

Cornea

Damage to the cornea is the most important concern subsequent to chemical exposure. It is therefore important to consider the factors that maintain corneal transparency. The cornea is clear because of three factors: its highly organized microanatomy, the existence of tight junctions between the epithelial and endothelial cells, and an endothelial cell pump mechanism.

Several anatomical features contribute to corneal clarity. These include the lack of blood vessels and pigment, the regular arrangement of the epithelial and endothelial cells, and the presence of only a few nuclei in the stroma. Any injury that leads to proliferation of new cells in the cornea, increased pigmentation, or vascularization will alter corneal transparency.

Another key structural characteristic is the highly organized collagen lamellae that lie in the stroma. The lamellae are arranged in layers from the anterior to the posterior stroma. The collagen fibrils in each layer are perpendicular to the fibrils in the layers directly above and below. The collagen

Table 1 Scale for Scoring Ocular Lesions

(1) CORNEA	
(A) Opacity-degree of density (area most dense taken for reading)	
No Opacity	0
Scattered or diffuse area, details of iris clearly visible	1
Easily discernible translucent area, details of iris slightly obscured	2
Opalescent areas, no details of iris visible, size of pupil barely discernible	3
Opaque, iris invisible	4
(B) Area of cornea involved	
One quarter (or less), but not zero	1
Greater than one quarter, but less than half	2
Greater than half, but less than three quarters	3
Greater than three quarters, up to whole area	4
Score = A × B × 5	Total Maximum = 80
(2) IRIS	
(A) Values	
Normal	0
Folds above normal, congestion, swelling, circumcorneal injection (any or all of these or combination of any thereof) iris still reacting to light (sluggish reaction is positive)	1
No reaction to light, hemorrhage, gross destruction (any or all of these)	2
Score = A × 5	Total Maximum = 10
(3) CONJUNCTIVA	
(A) Redness	
Vessels normal	0
Vessels definitely injected above normal	1
More diffuse, deeper crimson red, individual vessels not easily describable	2
Diffuse beefy red	3
(B) Chemosis	
No swelling	0
Any swelling above normal (includes nictitating membrane)	1
Obvious swelling with partial eversion of lids	2
Swelling with lids about half closed	3
Swelling with lids about half closed to completely closed	4
(C) Discharge	
No discharge	0
Any amount different from normal (does not include small amounts observed in inner canthus of normal animals)	1
Discharge with moistening of the lids and hairs just adjacent to lids	2
Discharge with moistening of the lids and hairs, and considerable area around the eye	3
Score = (A + B + C) × 2	Total maximum = 20

The maximum total score is the sum of all scores obtained for the cornea, iris, and conjunctiva.

fibrils within each lamella are organized in a two-dimensional matrix with approximately equal distance between each fibril. The fibrils have a diameter less than one wavelength of light, so the light passing through is not scattered. The cornea remains transparent as long as the precise configuration of the collagen fibrils is maintained.

Intact epithelial and endothelial cell layers and an endothelial cell pump mechanism also are important for maintenance of corneal clarity. The epithelial and endothelial cell layers form a barrier that slows the movement of water into the corneal stroma from the tears and aqueous humor. The endothelial cell pump mechanism removes water that leaks back into the cornea through the endothelium, epithelium, and periphery of the cornea. This keeps the stroma in a relative state of dehydration required for transparency. Water must be removed from the cornea because the glycosaminoglycan matrix contains only 75% of the water it is capable of holding. If the endothelium or epithelium is damaged, or if the endothelial pump system is poisoned (with ouabain, for example) water will leak into the stroma, causing corneal swelling. This swelling (edema) disrupts the orderly arrangement of the collagen fibrils in the lamellae, resulting in light scattering within the cornea. This light scattering causes the milky, opaque appearance of the edematous cornea.

After the cornea is exposed to foreign materials, the damage occurring will vary depending on the offending agent. The long-term effects resulting from exposure depends largely on the extent of the initial trauma (5,6). If only the outer layers of the corneal epithelium are damaged, the consequences are relatively minor. The changes may include decreased surface luster and slight corneal opacity due to loss of superficial epithelial cells and swelling of the remaining cells (epithelial edema). Fluorescein applied to assess integrity of the corneal epithelium will be retained. As healing begins, the epithelial cells adjacent to the wound flatten and enlarge. They migrate into the denuded area, covering it with a single cell layer. The epithelial cells then undergo mitotic division to replace the multiple layered epithelium which reattaches to the basement membrane by 6 weeks after the injury. There will be no scarring or permanent effects if only the epithelium is involved.

If the Bowman's layer is damaged after a deeper injury, the effects are more serious. Grossly, the cornea may have marked surface lesions (ulcers, deep erosions), and may become edematous. The repair process activated secondary to the deeper injury involves coverage of the lesion by epithelial cells, replication of keratocytes adjacent to the wound, and synthesis of glycosaminoglycan. The reconstruction associated with this repair may not duplicate the original architecture of the cornea and scarring may result. The magnitude of scarring depends on the depth and severity of the initial damage. The consequence of scar formation is that vision may be permanently impaired.

In humans, if the endothelial cells are damaged and lost, they are not replaced. The remaining viable cells spread over a defect. If there are two few remaining cells to completely cover the injured area, then permanent stromal and epithelial edema may occur.

Uvea

Uveitis can occur secondary to severe ocular traumas, including chemical exposure. This inflammation may be due to a direct effect of the chemical that passes through the cornea and sclera to reach the uveal tissues, or may be indirect through extension of significant surface inflammation into the uveal tissues. Since the iris, ciliary body, and anterior choroid share a common blood supply, each structure tends to be involved in the same inflammatory processes. The acute inflammation of the uveal tract is characterized by edema, capillary dilation, and exudation of inflammatory cells and proteinaceous fluids into the anterior chamber. In extensive uveitis, hemorrhage into the anterior chamber may lead to a visible accumulation of blood (hyphema) or leukocytes (hypopyon). The cells may attach to the back of the cornea and form keratitic precipitates. The increased protein concentration in the aqueous humor causes light scattering called aqueous flare. Uveitis also may have associated increased secretion of aqueous humor into the anterior chamber, causing increased intraocular pressure and symptoms of glaucoma.

Uveitis is painful, leading to photophobia and excessive lacrimation, particularly if associated with keratitis. Adhesions between the iris and cornea (posterior synechia) may form. These adhesions can effectively seal the anterior from the posterior chamber. This serious condition, called iris bombé, can lead to increased intraocular pressure because outflow of the aqueous humor is effectively blocked.

Conjunctiva

The conjunctiva is the thin mucous membrane that lines the sclera and inner eyelids. Chemical exposure may cause inflammation of this tissue called conjunctivitis. Conjunctivitis can be due to the direct effects of chemicals on the epithelial cells, or it can be an extension of inflammation from other ocular tissues. The extensive network of blood vessels dilate during the inflammation, leading to a marked increase in redness. Changes in capillary permeability allow fluids to leak into the interstitial spaces, producing edema. If the damage is severe enough, vessels may break, leading to subconjunctival hemorrhage. The numerous conjunctival glands and inflammatory cell secretions as well as lacrimal secretions contribute to the exudate observed. After extensive injury, adhesions between the bulbar and palpebral conjunctiva may form.

CONSEQUENCES OF CHEMICALLY INDUCED OCULAR INJURY

A wide range of effects may occur after ocular tissues are exposed to foreign substances (5,6). Some materials are completely innocuous, causing neither pain nor inflammation. Some produce significant pain without inflammation. Other materials are extremely aggressive, capable of causing massive injury that may never be repaired. Some materials act immediately, and others have significantly delayed effects.

An example of the more serious sequelae of chemical exposure are those occurring on exposure to strongly alkaline substances. The damage may include extensive corneal edema, loss of corneal glycosaminoglycans, corneal vascularization, corneal scarring, permanent corneal opacification, severe conjunctivitis with swelling and hemorrhage, and severe uveitis. Although not observed from the outside, damage to deeper ocular structures such as the lens and retina may occur. In addition to the primary gross damage chemicals may produce, secondary inflammatory processes may cause additional destruction. Repair processes activated after the injury may not restore the architecture of the tissues to their pristine preinjury state. Conjunctival adhesions may require surgical repair, and if the corneal opacification and vascularization are extensive enough, corneal transplantation may be required.

Acids also are capable of producing ocular injury. After exposure to milder, more dilute acids, the corneal epithelium develops slight turbidity or superficial erosion, and the conjunctiva may become swollen and hemorrhaged. The epithelium often will regenerate rapidly and the eye will recover completely with such mild injury. In situations where the exposure involves strong acids, the injury can be severe and irreversible. In the worst case, the ocular tissues can be so severely damaged that massive necrosis results in loss of tissue integrity followed by corneal perforation with extrusion of the intraocular contents.

Surfactants are another class of materials widely used in industry and the home that are a common cause of ocular injury. These materials are used for a variety of purposes in household cleaning products, cosmetics, personal care products, foods, and pharmaceuticals. There are three broad classes of surfactants based on their chemistry. The classes include the cationic surfactants, anionic surfactants, and the nonionic surfactants.

The cationic surfactants are generally quaternary ammonium derivatives and are considered to be the most irritating of the three classes. A common example is benzalkonium chloride (BAC). At low concentrations, BAC is minimally irritating. In fact, it is used as a preservative in some ophthalmic preparations. At higher concentrations, BAC causes severe, extensive corneal damage that may result in permanent injury (5).

Anionic surfactants are usually sodium and potassium salts of straight chain fatty acids (soaps), sulfonic acid salts, sulfuric acid salts, and polyphosphoric acid esters. In general, the anionic surfactants are considered less irritating than the cationic surfactants. The irritant effects of these materials are highly variable depending on the concentration used and the route of application (5).

Nonionic surfactants are generally ester or either combinations of fatty acids or fatty alcohols with polyoxyethylene or sorbitol. They are considered the least irritating surfactants. Several produce no injury when applied undiluted to rabbit eyes. Others have greater irritant potential and some appear to have local anesthetic effects (5).

Investigations on the relationship between the degree of ocular injury and surfactant class suggest that cationic surfactants precipitate cellular proteins, the anionic surfactants cause cell lysis, and the nonionics have neither of these effects (5).

In addition to the alkalis, acids, and surfactants, many other materials can cause ocular injury. These substances mediate their injury through many cellular and biochemical mechanisms, most of which are not well understood. This is because ocular toxicology has been primarily descriptive where relatively little work has been done to define mechanisms of injury.

ASSESSMENT OF IRRITANCY

The need for ocular safety testing became clear early in the 1930s when an untested eyelash product containing p-phenylene diamine was marketed in the United States. Use of this and similar products led to sensitization of the external ocular structures, corneal ulceration, vision loss, and at least one fatality (7). These events resulted in passage of the Food, Drug and Cosmetic Act of 1938, which required that materials sold to consumers be safe.

In response to the need for test methods to assess ocular safety, in vivo assays were developed and put into use. One of the earliest reported experimental animal procedures was devised by Friedenwald to assess the effects of acids and bases on the eye (8). This was the first time the effects of test materials on the cornea, conjunctiva, and iris were separately recorded. Subsequently, Carpenter and Smyth (9) studied many materials and recorded primarily their effects on the cornea. Draize et al. (1) improved the test by standardizing Friedenwald's method and simplifying the scoring system. The Draize procedure and modifications of it have been the standard for assessing the irritancy potential of test materials for decades. Experience with these tests has shown that they provide useful information for making ocular safety assessments.

Draize Eye Irritation Test

In the Draize eye irritation test, 0.1 ml of liquid or weight equivalent of test material is placed into the lower conjunctival cul-de-sac of the albino rabbit eye and the eyelids are held shut for a fixed period. Any ocular response is assessed by an observer at various time points for a period of up to 21 days after treatment. The untreated contralateral eye is used as a control.

The scoring procedure devised by Draize and colleagues evaluates the irritation response of three ocular tissues including the cornea, iris, and conjunctiva (see Table 1). A numerical score is given to different aspects of the irritation observed. The scores are assigned for the degree of corneal opacity and approximate area of corneal involvement, iritis, and conjunctival effects. The contribution of each tissue lesion to the total score is weighted by multiplying each by a factor: five for the cornea and iris and two for the conjunctiva. The maximum possible score is 110 with 80 points possible from the cornea, 10 from the iris and 20 from the conjunctiva. Since damage to the cornea is so critical, its contribution to the scoring is the greatest.

Using the Draize scale as a base, different scoring systems have been devised to classify ocular hazard (10-13). These systems take into account the level of irritation in different tissues of the anterior eye, the relative importance of the tissue damaged, the total number of animals that develop lesions, and the reversibility of the lesions.

Alternatives to the Draize Test

Introduction

Although the Draize eye irritation test has been used as the standard procedure for making ocular risk assessments, it is not without criticism (14). The Draize eye irritation test has been criticized for its lack of repeatability (15), subjective scoring (16,17), different interpretation (10), the high dose of test material used (18,19), its over-predictiveness of human response (16,20), and its use of animals (21,22). Because of the criticisms, significant work has been done to develop alternative methods that address the shortcomings. These alternatives include refining the in vivo procedure as well as attempting to develop in vitro assays with the hope that the in vivo test can ultimately be replaced.

Refinement of the In Vivo Test

Refining the Draize test has been approached in two ways. One has been modification of the test procedures so the assay gives information that is more predictive of the human response and is less stressful to the test animals. The other has been through evaluation of objective measurement procedures.

Modifying the Test Procedure One of the criticisms of the Draize procedure is that its results are biased toward overpredicting the assessment of human risk. The most important factors leading to overprediction of irritancy potential is the amount of test material used and the site of test material application. The Draize procedure requires application of a relatively large volume (100 μl or 100 mg) of test material into the deep conjunctival cul-de-sac of the rabbit eye. Griffith et al. (18) evaluated the relationship between the volume of test materials applied and the resulting irritation level in the rabbit eye. This study demonstrated that 0.01 ml of test substance applied directly to the cornea allows better differentiation between substances of similar irritancy, and produces an irritation response similar in magnitude and duration to the response observed in humans. This study gave rise to a procedure called the Low Volume Eye Test (LVET), which differs from the Draize procedure in three key ways: (1) it uses 0.01 ml of test material instead of 0.1 ml, (2) the test substance is applied directly to the cornea instead of into the conjunctival cul-de-sac, and (3) the eyelids are not held shut following treatment. This method of application and the dose applied much more closely simulates accidental human exposures.

In subsequent studies, Freeberg et al. (23,24) compared the results of animal tests with data collected from actual human exposure and concluded there was good correlation with the LVET results and the human response. Freeberg et al. (25) also directly compared the eye irritation response between humans and animals by measuring responses of human volunteers and rabbits to different doses of four consumer products. The data indicate that the LVET more accurately predicted human ocular response than did the standard Draize protocol. Other studies support the same conclusion (26,27). In addition to being more predictive of the human response, the LVET is less stressful to the test animals because it produces less irritation and more rapid recovery times (18).

Objective Measurement of Injury Another problem with the Draize procedure is the variability in results obtained from the test. Most of this variability is due to the subjective nature of the grading (15). In order to eliminate the subjective components of the test, an effort has been directed toward developing more objective measurements of ocular irritation. Some of the methods evaluated include assessing corneal thickness (28-30), water content (30, 31), permeability (32-34), surface area damaged using fluorescein, wound healing, and exfoliative cytology (35). Objective measurements for conjunctivitis have included assessments of edema (30,31), capillary permeability (30,31), redness, and exfoliative cytology (35). Others have attempted to assess the utility of measuring intraocular pressure (36) and the protein content of the aqueous humor (30,31). None of these methods is in routine use.

IN VITRO ALTERNATIVES TO OCULAR IRRITANCY TESTING

During the last decade, considerable work has been directed toward developing in vitro assays for use in ocular safety assessment. These tests employ a variety of whole tissue and cell cultures, and measure a wide range of endpoints. None of the currently available assays have been shown to be valid replacements for the in vivo ocular safety test. Furthermore, it is unlikely that a single test will ever serve as a replacement. This is because the eye is a complex organ capable of many responses to injury. One in vitro assay alone will not be capable of assessing all the possible effects of test materials on an organ as complex as the eye.

If a replacement is ever developed, it most likely will be composed of a battery containing multiple in vitro tests. If this battery is developed, it is likely to have several characteristics. It will utilize several assays that measure mechanistically diverse endpoints. The endpoints also will have some mechanistic relationship with the in vivo processes being modeled. The endpoints will be easily interpreted so that useful human ocular safety information can be obtained at the end of the testing process. Lastly, the tests will be easy to perform and results will be reproducible between laboratories.

Developing a battery of tests having all these characteristics will be difficult. There is not yet a good understanding of the cellular and molecular mechanisms associated with chemically induced ocular irritation, so it is not possible to design the specific mechanism-based assays desired. Furthermore, there is information obtained from the in vivo tests in addition to inflammation that will be difficult to model with in vitro tests. Examples include models that assess repair after the eyes are chemically injured, tests that accurately assess pain, and methods that assess immune mediated responses (allergic ocular reactions). Development of a test battery that will completely replace the need for in vivo testing is at best years away, if it ever occurs.

Despite these problems there is a developing role for in vitro tests in ocular safety assessment. Recent work suggests that some in vitro assays might be useful as ocular safety screens in a tier testing process. While these tests will not replace the need for in vivo testing, they could serve as adjuncts in the testing process to reduce the number of animals required to make a safety assessment. As research and development proceeds, better cell culture techniques and improved bioanalytical procedures will become available. Our understanding of basic mechanisms will also increase. This information will lead to development of more reliable in vitro methods that will allow additional reduction in our dependence on animal-based methods.

Currently Available In Vitro Tests for Ocular Safety Testing

There are a wide range of in vitro assays that have been proposed as alternatives for ocular safety assessment. Frazier et al. (37) devised a scheme to categorize in vitro alternatives for ocular safety testing. It divides the tests into groups based on the biological components and the endpoints measured. These categories are morphology, cell toxicity, cell and tissue physiology, inflammation and immunity, recovery and repair, and others. The following discussion uses a modification of this framework to review and update the current state of in vitro ocular safety testing alternatives development. One or two key assays within each group will be described in detail.

Morphology-Based Assays

The morphology-based assays use visual changes in the structure of cells or tissue as endpoints. Assays in this group are the highest tolerated dose assay (38-44), the chorioallantoic membrane assays, and the enucleated rabbit eye test (45,46).

Chorioallantoic Membrane Assays The chorioallantoic membrane (CAM) is the vascularized respiratory membrane that surrounds the embryonic bird developing within the egg. It is a complete tissue including arteries, capillaries, and veins. This test was initially developed as a model for the conjunctiva that would respond to test materials with a classic inflammatory reaction after treatment with test materials (47). Since it is not innervated, the embryo developing inside does not sense pain when the membrane is perturbed.

This assay involves isolating an area of the CAM inside the chicken egg. A test material then is applied to the prepared membrane surface. After an incubation period that varies depending on the protocol used, the membrane is inspected visually and the changes in morphology (size of lesion and presence of necrosis or capillary hemorrhage) are scored.

There are two primary variations of this test based on the way the membranes are prepared. One technique uses a modification of a procedure described by Zwilling (48). Fertile eggs are incubated for 3 days at 37 °C, and then the shell is opened in two places. Two milliliters of albumin are drawn from the first opening, a small hole in the pointed end of the egg. A larger rectangular opening is created over the equator of the egg and the CAM is isolated below. The window is sealed with tape, and the egg is incubated until day 14 to allow the CAM to fully develop in the floor of the newly created cavity. The tape is removed, a 10-mm diameter Teflon ring is placed onto the CAM, and test material is dropped onto the CAM inside the ring (47). The window is resealed with tape, the egg incubated for 3 days, and reexamined for the development of test material-induced lesions. The most reliable indices measured are the size of the lesion and necrosis (47,49).

A slightly modified version of the CAM protocol called the CAM vascular assay (CAMVA) has been evaluated (50,51). The eggs are prepared as just described, but the lesions on the CAM are scored at 30 mins after treatment instead of at 3 days. The most significant lesions scored are changes in the CAM vasculature. If hemorrhage occurs or if blood vessels are obstructed after treatment, it is considered a positive test.

Another variation of the CAM assay is the Hen's Egg Test-CAM (HET-CAM) developed by Luepke et al. (52-56). Fresh viable eggs incubated large end up for ten days are used in the assay. The egg shell is opened at the boundary of the air cell and the CAM lying below is exposed. The test substance is dropped onto the membrane and after 20 s the membrane is irrigated with warm water. The membrane is then scored for irritant effects, including hyperemia, hemorrhages, and coagulation.

The HET-CAM assay has also been conducted in combination with an assay that evaluates the effects of test materials on the corneas of excised bovine eyes. This test is called the Bovine Eye-HET CAM (BE-CAM) assay (57). In addition to evaluation in the HET-CAM, test material is placed onto the corneal surface of a freshly excised, undamaged bovine eye for 30 s. The material is washed off and corneal lesions are graded by noting the degree of corneal opacity produced, and whether applied fluorescein is retained in the cornea. A grading scheme has been established for categorizing the irritancy potential of a test material for both the BE and CAM parts of the assay. The final irritancy prediction is made based on the result from either of the two tests that give the most severe score.

Chick Yolk Sac Assay Rosenbruch (58,59) suggested it may be possible to apply test materials to the yolk sac of 2-day-old chicken eggs and evaluate morphological changes after treatment to assess the irritant potential of the substance. Work with this system is preliminary, and more must be done in order to assess its ultimate utility.

Utility of the CAM Assays The CAM assays have been extensively evaluated. Reports on their utility are mixed. There are several reports indicating the test provides information useful for categorizing the ocular irritancy potential of test materials (49,60,61). Others have concluded the CAM has no utility for assessing ocular safety because of high false-positive rates, embryotoxicity, and inaccurate categorization of irritancy potential (52,62-64).

One explanation for the mixed results is that the CAM may not be a good model for conjunctival inflammation. Parish et al. (62) and Lawrence et al. (63) have reported there is little anatomical similarity between the CAM and the conjunctiva. The CAM is a thinner, more primitive structure than the conjunctiva and it lacks goblet cells (62). The CAM also does not respond to test materials by developing a classic inflammatory lesion. Parish et al. (62) compared the histological characteristics of conjunctivitis with responses in the CAM. The conjunctiva from treated rabbit eyes had a classic inflammatory response with infiltration of neutrophils and macrophages. The lesion in the CAM consisted of only necrosis confined just to the area where the test material was applied. Lawrence et al. (63) reported that the primary histological changes in the CAM after treatment were necrosis of varying depth, with little evidence of a classic inflammatory response. This lack of response may, in part, be due to the immaturity of the immune system of the developing embryo and the relative lack of circulating heterophils (chicken neutrophils) in the embryos (63).

Finally, it is also important to note that The British Animals (Scientific Procedures) Act of 1986 defines developing birds as protected animals after half the incubation has elapsed. Thus, a chicken egg-based assay that uses eggs incubated longer than 10.5 days are not considered in vitro tests.

Assays That Measure Adhesion, Proliferation, and Colony-Forming Abilities of Cells

Several assays have been developed to evaluate test material-induced changes in proliferation by measuring the accumulation of cellular protein (65-70), cell growth (71), colony formation (72), and cell adhesion (71). Many of these assays are simple to perform and preliminary results suggest some may be useful as screens in ocular safety assessment.

SIRC Colony-Forming Assay SIRC cells are a fibroblastlike cell derived from rabbit corneas available from the American Type Culture Collection. The SIRC Colony forming assay evaluates the effects of test materials on the ability of the cells to survive an exposure, maintain adherence to the tissue culture plate, and maintain enough viability to proliferate and form colonies after treatment with test materials (73-75).

In the assay, a relatively small number of SIRC cells are seeded into a tissue culture plate. After attachment, different wells are exposed to increasing concentrations of test materials for 1 hr. The cells are washed thoroughly and incubated for 1 week. The colonies with 10 or more cells at the end of the incubation period are counted. The endpoint of this assay is the concentration of test material that decreases the number of colonies formed by 50%. This test has been evaluated with a limited number of surfactants and shampoo formulations. There was good correlation between the in vivo and in vitro data (51,73-75).

Membrane Integrity Tests

These assays measure the effects of test substances on cellular membrane integrity. Large molecular weight dyes or radioactive isotopes normally excluded from, or sequestered within, viable cells are used as markers of the membrane damage. The movement of these markers into or out of the cells can be monitored relatively easily. By following movement of the markers after treatment, the membrane integrity is assessed. Examples include the dye exclusion assays, the ^{51}Cr-release assay (76,77), and the MDCK epithelial barrier integrity assay (78).

Dye Exclusion/Dye Leakage Assays In the dual fluorescent dye staining procedures, cells are treated with two dyes, fluorescein diacetate (FDA) and propidium iodide (PI) or ethidium bromide (EB) (79-82). The lipophillic FDA readily crosses the cell membranes, and once inside is rapidly deacetylated by cytosolic esterases to form impermeable green-fluorescent fluorescein. As long as the cells are viable, the dye remains trapped within the cell and the cells become bright green. Propidium iodide is a large molecular weight dye normally excluded from viable cells. It enters the cell subsequent to membrane injury and stains the nuclear deoxyribonucleic acid (DNA) red.

Cells are exposed to increasing concentrations of test materials in a cocktail containing the FDA and PI. If the membranes are damaged after treatment with test materials, the fluorescein will leak from the cells, causing a decrease in the green fluorescence intensity. At the same time, the PI will enter the cells, causing an increase in the red fluorescence intensity. By monitoring changes in the fluorescence intensity of the two dyes simultaneously, changes in cell viability can be readily assessed.

Metabolism Tests

Measuring test material-induced changes in a wide range of cellular biochemical processes has been evaluated as in vitro alternatives for ocular safety testing. Some of these assays measure changes in active transport processes such as inhibition of uridine uptake (38,43,44,83-85). Neutral red dye retention by viable cells (40,42,44,70,86-89), release of neutral red from preloaded cells (90), and loss of neutral red from cells covered with an agar overlay (91,92) have also been extensively evaluated. Another group measures endpoints related to alterations in cellular energy metabolism. These assays evaluate changes in cellular adenosine triphosphate (ATP) content (93), production of acidic metabolic byproducts (94-97), and alterations in light output from luminescent bacteria (98,99). Lastly, an assay that assesses the release of plasminogen activator from rabbit corneal epithelial cells (100-102) has been evaluated.

Silicon Microphysiometer The silicon microphysiometer is a device that can be used to measure the effects of test materials on cellular metabolic rate. It is based on the light addressable potentiometric sensor (LAPS) (94), a device capable of sensitively measuring pH. This test is useful for assessing cellular metabolism because the principal excreted products of cellular carbohydrate catabolism are carbonic acid (CO_2) and lactic acid, both of which are acidic. Cultured cells tend to depend more on glycolysis than respiration, so lactic acid predominates. Thus, there is a direct connection between cellular metabolic rate and the rate of acidification of a cell's surroundings. Although acidification normally takes days to observe in a standard phenol red-containing indicator system, the silicon microphysiometer provides a nondestructive method of monitoring cellular acidification rates on the time scale of seconds to minutes (94).

The silicon microphysiometer is configured such that the LAPS forms the bottom of a biosensor chamber (Fig. 3). Cells grown on a glass coverslip are placed opposite the LAPS surface. The pH can be determined at each of four ~1 mm^2 sites within the flow chamber. These correspond to regions on the lower surface of the LAPS chip that are illuminated by infrared light conducted via optic fibers from light-emitting diodes. For typical confluent cell densities of ~10^5 cm^{-2}, data are gathered from ~10^3 cells in ~100 nl.

Culture medium is pumped through the chamber by a peristaltic or syringe pump. The rate at which cells produce acidic metabolic products is determined by intermittently stopping the flow of medium. When the flow is on at ~100 μl/min the sensor reads the pH of fresh medium. Stopping the flow results in a buildup of acidic metabolites in the stagnant medium, causing the pH to drop within the chamber. The calculated acidification rate is the slope of a linear least-squares fit to these pH-vs-time data. When the flow is restarted, the pH quickly returns to its previous value as the stagnant medium is flushed out and replaced with fresh medium. This resets the system for subsequent measurements. A personal computer controls most aspects of the instrument.

When evaluating the effects of test materials on cellular acidification rate, an initial baseline rate is determined. Cells, either normal human keratinocytes or mouse fibroblasts, are exposed to dilute test substance. After a short incubation period, the test material is pumped out of the chamber and the acidification rate is remeasured. This cycle is repeated with continually increasing concentrations of test material until the cellular metabolism has ceased. The concentration of test material that decreases the metabolic rate by 50% (MRD_{50}) is the endpoint of the assay.

Parce et al. (95) compared the MRD_{50} values obtained from eight organic materials with the in vivo irritancy potential of the test materials and found good correlation between the data. Bruner et al. (96), in an expanded evaluation using 17 test materials that included both chemicals and consumer products, found the MRD_{50} was correlated with the irritancy potential.

In addition to measuring the MRD_{50}, there is other information available from the test. It can be used to determine if the effects of test materials are reversible. Preliminary data suggest that this may be a very useful endpoint for assessing the irritant potential of test materials. When cells are exposed to the MRD_{50} concentration of mild irritants such as dimethyl sulfoxide or triethanolamine, they recover their baseline metabolic rate within 1-2 h.

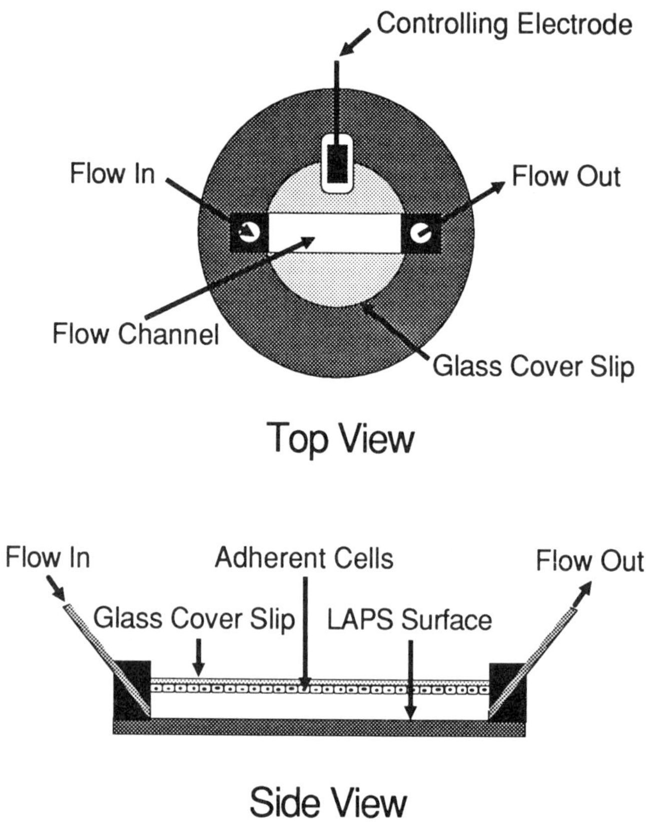

Figure 3 Top view and cross section of the silicon microphysiometer flow chamber.

Conversely, cells exposed to the MRD_{50} concentrations of more significant irritants such as ethanol or a heavy-duty laundry detergent do not recover (95,97).

Another useful alteration observed with some materials is that the metabolic rate increases significantly at subinhibitory concentrations (97). The cause of this increase is unknown at present, but likely represents the cells attempting to return to their baseline state subsequent to perturbation by the test substances. Additional studies designed to determine the cause of the increase may lead to development of other in vitro tests useful for assessing irritant potential.

Another advantage of the silicon microphysiometer is that it will be possible to couple the assay to other technologies, such as image analysis, to assess multiple parameters of cell function simultaneously. The top of the chamber is a transparent glass coverslip that allows visualization of the cells during an assay procedure. There are numerous fluorescent dyes that can be used as indicators of cellular function. Thus, it should be possible to simultaneously measure changes in metabolic rate along with changes in other important functional parameters.

Luminescent Bacteria Toxicity Test The luminescent bacteria toxicity test (LBT) is a test based on a marine organism called *Photobacterium phosphoreum*. This bacterium is one of many species that produces light as a byproduct of cellular metabolism. The bacteria produce light through a biochemical process that requires reduced FMN, a long chain aldehyde, molecular oxygen, and bacterial luciferase (98). The bacterial luciferase catalyzes the bioluminescent oxidation of $FMNH_2$ and a long chain aldehyde by molecular oxygen. The bacterial luciferase is coupled to bacterial respiration via NADH and flavine nucleotide. Thus, measuring the light output from the bacteria is an indirect measure of the respiratory metabolism.

The LBT is distributed commercially under the name Microtox (Microbics Corp., Carlsbad, California), and was developed to provide a rapid, reproducible, and relatively inexpensive toxicity screen. Its greatest use has been in assessing the toxicity of environmental and industrial waste samples. The LBT has also been used in a wide range of other toxicological testing schemes (98). It has been evaluated for its utility in assessing the toxicity of medical devices (103) and for determining ocular irritancy potential of test materials (96).

The test is conducted by exposing suspensions of the bacteria to increasing concentrations of test materials. Light output is measured in a photometric device provided by the vendor. The endpoint of the assay is the concentration of test material that decreases the light output by 50% (EC_{50}).

This test has not yet been extensively evaluated for its utility as an in vitro alternative for ocular safety testing. Bruner et al. (96) reported that there was excellent agreement between the EC_{50} concentration of test material and the in vivo irritancy potential of 17 consumer products and chemicals. Additional work is being done by a nnumber of groups and in the future it will become clearer if this test has utility as a screen for ocular safety testing. Its commercial availability, low cost, ease of use, and fairly extensive experience base in other areas of toxicity testing are other positive features.

Corneal Repair Tests

Since recovery from ocular injury is an important aspect of assessing risk, attempts have been made to develop in vitro assays that predict whether test materials inhibit repair of ocular tissues. One test that approaches this problem has been developed by Jumblatt and coworkers (104-107). A defined area of a rabbit corneal epithelial cell monolayer is damaged using a 6-mm probe frozen in liquid nitrogen. If the damaged monolayer is incubated in the absence of test material, the uninjured epithelial cells at the periphery of the wound migrate over the damaged area, cover the defect, and ultimately the lesion disappears.

During the assay, increasing concentrations of test materials are incubated with a series of wounded monolayers. The concentration of test material that inhibits wound healing rate by 50% compared to nontreated controls is the endpoint. This test has been evaluated with a limited number of materials (106). While the results appear promising, definitive validation has not been completed.

Cell and Tissue Physiology Preparations

A variety of assays that use parts of whole tissues in a variety of bioassays have been evaluated as alternative tests. Models tested include contraction inhibition in isolated ileum strips (108-110), isolated skin models (111), isolated ocular tissues (112,113), and a proposed mouse eye assay (114). Some of these assays are less attractive because they are often technically difficult to perform, their results are difficult to repeat, their relationship to ocular irritation mechanisms is unclear, and they still require animals as a source for tissues.

Assays that Assess Inflammatory Processes

Since ocular irritation is an inflammatory process, it is appropriate to develop in vitro models designed to assess various aspects of inflammation. Research in this area has involved evaluating a wide range of assays that assess release of inflammatory mediators. These assays involve adding test materials to in vitro cultures of inflammatory cells (115,116), epithelial cells (117) or explanted ocular tissues (118,119). After an incubation period, the release of different known mediators of inflammation from the cells or tissues is determined. The mediators evaluated include histamine, serotonin, prostaglandin metabolites, and leukotrienes. From a mechanistic point of view, these assays are well founded. However, because of the large number of mediators involved, and the dynamic interactions that occurs between the mediators during inflammation, it will be very difficult to develop reliably interpretable assays for use as screens in the ocular assessment process.

Other Assays

Two assays that do not easily fit into the categories outlined, the *Tetrahymena thermophila* motility assay and the EYTEX System, have received considerable interest as alternative tests. *Tetrahymena thermophila* is a ciliated protozoan organism. This assay uses test material-induced changes in the motility of *T. thermophila* as an endpoint (120,121). The EYTEX System is based on a jack bean-containing reagent that turns opaque when test materials are added (122). The opacity is measured on a simple spectrophotometer, and the values obtained are converted to eye irritation scores using a standard curve provided with each kit. Reports on the utility of this test are mixed. Good correlation between the in vivo and in vitro data has been reported (122-124). Conversely, Bruner et al. (96) found there was no significant correlation between the in vivo irritancy potential of 17 commercial products and chemicals with the EYTEX System results.

Summary

There are no in vitro assays or a battery of assays that will totally replace the in vivo ocular safety tests today. This does not mean, however, that these tests will not be useful in the ocular safety assessment process in the short term. Several of the currently available in vitro assays appear as though they may be useful as screens prior to confirmation using limited numbers of animals. This has the potential of decreasing the number of animals used for ocular safety assessment.

NEXT STEPS IN OCULAR SAFETY ALTERNATIVES DEVELOPMENT

The goal of in vitro alternatives programs is to develop and validate a series of assays that will provide useful information for assessing the ocular safety of test materials. There are two approaches that can be used to develop such models. One is to develop in vitro tests based on an understanding of the known mechanisms leading to ocular irritation, measure the dose-response relationship for those effects in vitro, and extrapolate the data to provide estimates of irritancy potential. When mechanistic understanding is lacking, a more empirical correlation-based approach must be applied. With this second approach, a series of in vitro tests expected to give useful information on irritancy potential is evaluated with a large set of well-characterized test materials. The in vitro endpoints are evaluated against the in vivo irritant potential of the standard materials, and the degree of correlation between the data sets is calculated. The irritancy potential of new materials is then assessed by comparing the in vitro test results of the new material against the standard curve generated earlier.

Because so little is known about the mechanisms leading to ocular injury, the primary emphasis on developing in vitro alternatives has used the correlation-based approach. Although the information from tests using the correlation-based developmental process may be useful, the approach has a significant disadvantage. Standard curves for a given model will provide data useful for making correct risk assessments only as long as any new materials evaluated are members of the same chemical class and act through similar mechanisms. As soon as new materials of different chemical classes are evaluated in the in vitro assays, the model developed for the first class may no longer fit the new materials. Using the wrong model could result in misclassification of the unknown material. Without a good understanding of the mechanistic basis of a test, determining the proper model to use for making a safety assessment could be very difficult. Thus, with the correlation-based assays, there will always be a possibility that the wrong standard curve will be used, leading to error in risk assessment.

This does not mean the correlation-based tests are useless, but it does impose significant limits on their utility. They likely will be restricted to use as screens in the ocular safety assessment process. In that role, they may be used to classify test materials into broad irritant categories. Then, depending on the degree of certainty required, confirmation using limited numbers of animals may be required to confirm a prediction made with the in vitro screens. All materials will have to be evaluated on a case-by-case basis and judgment will have to be applied in each instance.

If an in vitro test battery is to be developed that will replace the animal tests, the assays in the battery must be based on some mechanistic understanding of the relationship between the in vitro endpoints and events occurring in vivo. If it is possible to obtain such information, it will be far easier to extrapolate risk to humans. Unfortunately, the current state of the art does not provide the basic information on mechanisms needed to establish these kinds of tests. The research required to gain such information will take years to complete.

Moving the Field Forward

What must be done to move the field of in vitro ocular toxicology forward? Significant work has been done to develop in vitro alternatives for ocular safety testing. Some of the tests appear to give information that will be useful as aids for making ocular safety assessments. If toxicologists are to begin using in vitro alternatives in the ocular safety assessment process, evaluation of currently available technology must continue. Effort also should be made to actually begin implementing these tests as screens in ocular safety assessment. The assays will not replace the need for animals in ocular safety testing in the short run, but may provide the means to significantly decrease the number of animals needed to make a safety assessment. Furthermore, pushing in vitro tests into the safety assessment process now will provide much information on where these tests are useful and where the tests fail. In the long term, if a replacement for the animal test is to be found, mechanism-based research must be undertaken.

Development of Screens for Use in the Short Term

There are a wide range of tests available that give different kinds of information on the adverse cellular effects of test materials. Although some tests appear very promising, there is not a clear consensus on whether these tests can be used reliably in the ocular safety assessment process. It is not clear because extensive, well-designed validation studies have not yet been completed. Another reason for the lack of consensus is that the needs of groups doing ocular safety testing are very diverse. The factors important to developers of ocular pharmaceuticals, industrial chemicals, and finished consumer products are all different. Each group is evaluating different tests with different kinds of test materials and it has not yet been possible to codify the data and establish uniform guidelines on using alternatives in these different areas. Finally, there is tremendous pressure being placed on some organizations to stop using animals in ocular safety assessment. This pressure makes it difficult to conduct an unbiased review and discussion of the data necessary to develop useful alternative tests.

How can a community with very diverse needs proceed to accomplish this very difficult problem? The following offers a stepwise program that could be followed to determine if today's technology will meet the needs of individuals needing to conduct ocular safety testing. This process has three steps: preliminary evaluation, parallel testing and expanded test set evaluation, and tier testing (Fig. 4).

Preliminary Evaluation

The purpose of the preliminary evaluation is to identify a limited number of the many currently available in vitro tests that will provide useful information in ocular safety assessment. This evaluation (Fig. 5) is accomplished by assaying a small common set of test materials in a series of in vitro tests that may provide information useful to the developer. When the data are available for all of the assays from the common test set, the utility of infor-

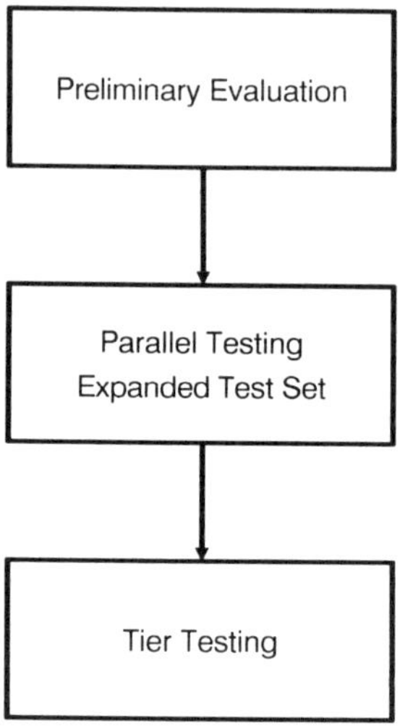

Figure 4 Proposed steps for developing in vitro alternatives for ocular safety testing.

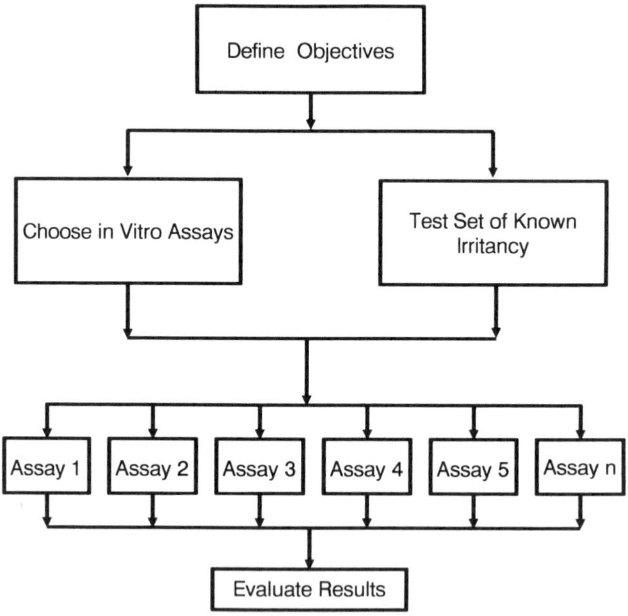

Figure 5 Process useful for assessing the utility of in vitro assays available today.

mation from each test can be evaluated individually and in comparison with the others. At the end of the preliminary evaluation, a small subset of the most useful assays for the testing purpose desired will be identified.

Define Objective In designing a preliminary evaluation program, the first step is to define the objective of the testing. The developer must give consideration to four areas: (1) the types of test materials that must be evaluated in the in vitro tests, (2) the technical problems associated with the test materials, (3) the range and quality of irritant responses expected in routine testing, and (4) the kind of information desired from the in vitro tests.

The kind of information needed will depend on the expected use of the materials needing a safety assessment. Some materials such as industrial chemicals or household products are not intended for use in the eye. Usually, a single accidental splash exposure is the major concern. Other materials, such as ophthalmic drugs, are deliberately instilled into the eyes, often several times per day for long periods. Other materials are developed for use around the eyes, but are not intended to enter the eyes. The safety questions that arise from each situation are different. The in vitro assays needed to assess each of these classes will be quite different. Developers of alternatives must determine their needs and choose the tests that give answers most appropriate for the situation.

In Vitro Assays There are several criteria that should be considered when choosing the in vitro tests for the preliminary evaluation step. These factors include (1) data suggesting the assay provides the kind of information identified in the first step of the process, (2) the mechanistic basis for the test, (3) the ease of test performance, (4) availability of cells, growth factors, and other essential components required to run the test, (5) ease in dealing with technical problems posed by the test materials, (6) cost of performing the assays, and (7) time required to execute a test.

Test Set A set of test materials used to evaluate the assays also must be assembled. There are several criteria that the test set must meet. First, the test set must include both pure chemicals as well as formulations of interest to the developer. Single chemicals are needed in the test set to provide mechanistic information free from additive, subtractive, or synergistic effects that may occur with product formulations. Testing with formulations provides the developer with information on the utility of the tests for products of interest and will give indications where significant interactions may lead to difficulties in the interpretation of results.

Second, the in vivo irritancy potential of the test materials in the set must be well characterized. In the area of ocular irritancy testing, obtaining quality in vivo data is a very significant problem. The ideal data set should be based on human ocular irritancy data, since models are being developed to assess human safety. If sufficient human data are not available, then animal data must be used instead. Ideal animal data should come from tests run in the same laboratory under the same conditions to help minimize the difficulties caused by interlaboratory variation. If in vivo data are not available through testing, then the scientific literature is a source. However, caution should be used with this type of information. Often, the data are reported in subjective rather than objective terms. Significant information about the irritant potential of materials is often lost in the categorization process. Additionally, data may come from tests that are conducted under widely varying conditions perhaps using inconsistent assessment criteria.

Third, the materials within a given test set should be of similar chemical composition and act through a common pathophysiological process. If the developer is interested in assessing multiple classes of materials, then individual sets of materials should be collected and evaluated independently. This will allow standard curves to be constructed for each class of test materials.

Fourth, the materials used in a given test set must cover the range of irritancy potentials encountered in routine testing. This will allow the developer to evaluate whether the tests give information across the range of interest.

Lastly, the quality of the test substances must be assured. Retained samples may decompose with age, meaning that the irritancy potential today may not be the same as was measured previously. If new batches of test materials are manufactured to replace an expired sample, care must be taken to assure that the new test substance is compositionally the same as the old. The materials also should be stable enough or easily replaceable so that they can be used as benchmark internal standards in future assay procedures.

Evaluate Results Once the test materials have been evaluated in the in vitro assays, curves can be constructed that show the relationship between the in vivo and in vitro data for each class of test material. Since a common set of test materials are used in each of the assays, it is not only possible to assess whether there is correlation within an assay, but all of the assays can be evaluated against each other. If the test materials and in vitro tests were chosen well, assays that give the kind of information needed from safety testing should be identified. The best assays of the group can then be further evaluated in the next step of the process.

Parallel Testing and Expanded Test Set

The preliminary evaluation process produces a group of curves that describe the relationship between the in vivo irritant potential of test materials and the in vitro test results. Since the preliminary evaluation was undertaken with a limited number of materials, additional testing must be undertaken to prove the models correct. The additional testing may be accomplished in either of two ways. In situations where the developer has access to an operation that is performing ocular safety tests in vivo, materials can be run in vitro in parallel with the animal-based tests. If access to in vivo testing is not possible, then evaluation of a well-characterized expanded set of new test materials will be required.

In a situation where parallel testing is possible, every time an unknown is submitted for evaluation in vivo, it is assayed in the in vitro test along with internal benchmark standards. When available, the data from the in vivo and in vitro tests can be compared directly to test the correctness of the preliminary evaluation.

Parallel testing accomplishes several goals: (1) it increases the number of materials tested simultaneously in the in vivo and in vitro assays, (2) it allows assessment of the correctness of the conclusions reached in preliminary evaluation, (3) toxicologists have an opportunity to directly compare in vivo and in vitro results and learn how to use in vitro data for making safety assessments, (4) it provides a means to evaluate where the tests predict ocular irritancy correctly, and where the tests fail, and (5) it provides the data necessary for implementing the next step in the process called tier testing.

Tier Testing

Once more practical experience is gained with the in vitro assays in the real-world safety assessment process, and if the tests provide useful information, a tiered testing program should be established (Fig. 6). This tiered process begins with an evaluation of historical eye irritation data and physical/chemical data. If it is possible to make a safety assessment based on this information alone, it would be made without any additional testing. If this initial check does not allow a proper safety assessment, then the materials would be run in the in vitro test battery. Once the data from the in vitro battery are collected, the data would be evaluated along with all other data available for the test material. If the in vitro data provide enough information to complement previously existing historical, physical, chemical, and other information, then it may be possible to make a safety assessment without performing any in vivo testing.

On the other hand, if there are reasons that the in vitro data and other information are not sufficient to make an assessment, it will be necessary to confirm the in vitro prediction with limited in vivo testing. The in vitro data would be used as a guide to determine the type of testing to be done and the numbers of animals used. For materials that appear innocuous based on the in vitro data, confirmatory in vivo assays could be run using limited numbers of animals with reasonable assurance that minimal suffering would result. If the in vitro predictions indicated greater potential irritancy for a test material, judgment on whether testing needs to be done will be made.

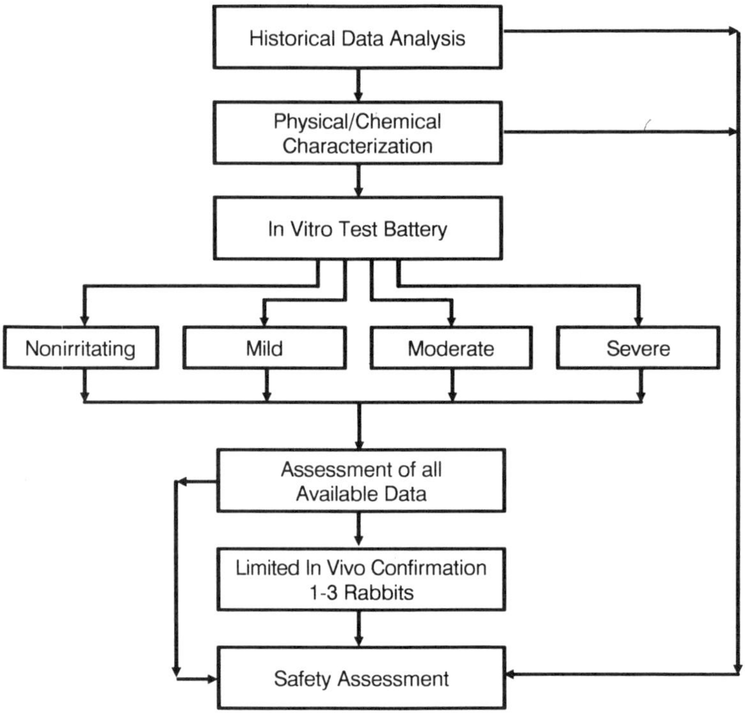

Figure 6 Tier testing process.

By following a protocol similar to that just described, it may be possible to use currently available in vitro alternatives to refine in vivo testing procedures and reduce the numbers of animals required to make a safety decision. As work is done with the in vitro assays, much will be learned about when the tests work best and when they fail. If shared with the scientific and regulatory communities, the new information will be very useful for development of more predictive tests for the future.

Developing Assays Based on an Understanding of Mechanisms for the Long Term

The foregoing discussion outlines a practical approach that can be used in the short term to bring today's state-of-the-art into use in the ocular safety assessment process. Although useful for the short term, it is unlikely this process will provide tests that replace the need for animals in ocular safety assessment. It will only be possible to replace animals completely when we have a much firmer understanding of the mechanistic basis for ocular toxic effects and can design tests based on that understanding.

Most of the currently available in vitro assays are some form of cytolysis test. These assays give little information beyond the concentration of test material that kills a certain number of cells in a tissue culture plate. Although it is important to know how much test material is required to lyse cells in culture, information on the pathophysiological steps that lead to the cells demise will be far more useful. Such information would give a greater understanding of the specific mechanisms by which test materials alter cell function and activate processes leading to inflammation, cytolysis, and tissue destruction. Specific areas where additional research may be beneficial are outlined in the following sections.

Assessment of Direct Cell Injury

Assessing the direct effects of test materials on cellular function will be of great importance in assessing the irritancy potential of test materials in vitro. With modern optical equipment, fluorescent probes, biosensors, and computers, it is possible to probe key cellular physiological processes. These procedures will allow investigators to measure cellular functions that may be altered by test materials. These tests therefore may provide more discriminating information than is offered by the cytolysis assays most commonly considered today.

Modern analytical cytometric techniques such as flow cytometry and image analysis allow simultaneous measurement of multiple parameters of cell function and structure, one cell at a time. Functional assessments possible include measurement of membrane integrity, permeability and microviscosity, cellular energy metabolism, surface and intracellular receptors, cytosolic ion concentrations, transmembrane potential, mitochondrial membrane potential, cytosolic enzyme activity, and intracellular pH. Other characteristics that are relatively easily measurable include cell size and shape, content of DNA, ribonucleic acid (RNA) and other macromolecules, total and basic protein content, intracellular sulfhydryl groups (glutathione content), surface antigens, surface glycoproteins, and cytoskeletal organization. (For review of parameters and probes see Shapiro [125] and Wang and Taylor [126]).

In addition to the cytometric methods, other means can be used to assess the direct effects of test materials on cells. Electron microscopy, histochemistry, and assessment of cellular biochemistry are all viable means to assess cellular injury.

Assessment of Repair Processes

As assays are developed to assess the direct effects of chemicals on cells, another key area is assessment of the consequences of cellular injury at the tissue level. Models need to be developed to answer two questions: (1) after cells are damaged and tissue injury is observed, how long will it take to repair the damage, and (2) what will be the consequences of repair processes initiated after the damage?

Initial work has been done to assess the wound healing processes associated with chemically induced ocular injury. Jumblatt et al. (104-107) have developed a model that uses rabbit corneal epithelial cells in vitro, as discussed above. Uniform lesions are created in corneal epithelial cell monolayers, and healing time is assessed in the presence of increasing concentrations of test materials. This approach is a reasonable start, but the monolayer system lacks many of the microanatomical features that are found in intact ocular tissues. The interactions between migrating epithelial cells, basement membrane components, and a plethora of growth factors released from stromal cells that may be critical for proper repair are not available in this test.

Explanted tissues also could be used to evaluate the extent of damage and as a means to assess repair processes. Several assays using eyes from various sources have been evaluated. These include the superfused enucleated rabbit eye (45,46), a proptosed mouse eye model (114), and enucleated bovine eyes used in conjunction with the CAM assays (57). All three tests as currently used measure the effects of test materials relatively shortly after treatment and the measurements made are relatively gross. It may be possible to refine these tests, making them more predictive of irritancy potential.

An approach that may allow development of consistent and anatomically correct tissue for studying extent of injury and tissue repair are the so-called tissue equivalents (127-129). These are usually composed of a collagen or nylon matrix that contains fibroblasts from the tissue of interest. Once the fibroblasts have fully colonized the matrix, epithelial cells are seeded onto the surface. It may be possible to reconstruct a three-dimensional matrix composed of corneal epithelium, stromal fibroblasts, and endothelial cells that may provide a suitable model for in vitro ocular safety assessment. There are significant technical problems that must be overcome to develop viable corneal tissue equivalent models. If successful, they may be useful for assessing the ability of test materials to alter corneal tissue.

Induction of Inflammation

Test materials can provoke ocular inflammation through a number of mechanisms. Direct injury to ocular cells with changes in cellular function, cytolysis, and tissue destruction will produce inflammation. Besides these gross perturbations, an inflammatory reaction may also be induced by far more subtle effects not associated with overt cellular injury. Since such inflammation can be very damaging, it would be very useful to develop in vitro assays to determine if a test substances is one of these subtle actors.

Developing models that will properly identify noncytolytic inducers of inflammation will be difficult. This is because inflammation is a dynamic, interactive process. The cellular and molecular interactions controlling the induction, maintenance, and resolution of inflammation require multiple cell types and numerous cytokines all acting in a precise, highly regulated manner. Developing an in vitro test battery that assesses these processes is not possible today. The cell types, cell interactions, and mediators involved in the response are just now being unraveled. It will be years before the inflammatory process is understood well enough to develop an in vitro test useful for safety assessment.

Absorption, Distribution, Metabolism, and Excretion from Ocular Tissues

More needs to be learned about the absorption, distribution, metabolism, and excretion of test materials placed in the eye. These factors are important in governing the dose of substances that reach various ocular tissues after treatment. Such information may be useful for more rationally developing realistic dosing schemes for in vitro tests.

Dosing In Vitro Compared to In Vivo

The in vivo ocular saafety tests use a single dose of test substance is placed undiluted into the animal's eye. If the material is a solid, the granules or powders are the dose form. In contrast, cells in most in vitro assays are exposed to test materials after being dissolved or suspended in aqueous tissue culture media. This means there are significant differences in the dosing forms used in vivo compared to the in vitro assays. These differences are necessary because it is difficult to evaluate undiluted test materials in most of the in vitro tests available. In general, cellular monolayers will tolerate undiluted test materials for only a very short period before total cellular destruction occurs.

The consequences of using widely different dosing forms in vivo compared to in vitro may be significant. Diluting mixtures can change the physical characteristics of a test substance making in vitro to in vivo extrapolations very difficult.

One potential solution for this problem is the flow-through system offered by the silicon microphysiometer (94-97). It may be possible to flow neat liquid test substances into a cell-containing chamber for very short times, wash the material away, and measure the effects of the test substance immediately after treatment. It also may be possible to develop other tests that allow brief but well-controlled application of powders to monolayers followed by washing and assessment of injury.

If such tests cannot be developed, then more research is needed to learn how changes in dose form alter the toxic effects in vivo. Such information will be useful for properly interpreting the in vitro test results from diluted or dissolved test materials. Additionally, standard methods on preparing incompatible materials must be developed. The methods used to prepare a suspension of water in-soluble test substance can have profound effects on its biological activity. Colloids prepared must be characterized and standardized in terms of particle number concentration and particle size distribution in order for a proper assessment to be made. An excellent review on this important topic discusses these factors in some detail (130). The interested reader should consult this reference.

CONCLUSIONS

No single test or battery of tests currently available can replace the need for animals in ocular safety testing. Several assays appear promising as screens that may reduce the number of animals required to make a reliable safety assessment. As progress is made, additional tests will be developed that will allow increased reliance on alternative methods. When placed in an appropriate framework that includes analysis of historical data, validation through testing extensive numbers of test materials, parallel testing, and a tier testing program, these tests may play an important role in reducing the need for animal testing.

If complete elimination of animal use in ocular safety assessment is to be achieved, a better understanding of ocular tissue repair, inflammation, and alterations in cellular structure and function is needed. The application of recent progress in tissue culture techniques, cellular and molecular biology, and analytical cytometric techniques will lead us closer to our goal of eliminating the need for animals in ocular safety testing.

REFERENCES

1. Draize, J. H., Woodard, G., and Calvery, H. O. (1944). Methods for the study of irritation and toxicity of substances applied topically to the skin and mucous membranes. *J. Pharmacol. Exp. Ther.* **82**: 377-390.
2. Prince, J. H., Diesem, C. D., Eglitis, I., and Ruskell, G. L. (1960). *Anatomy and Histology of the Eye and Orbit in Domestic Animals.* Charles C Thomas, Springfield, Illinois.
3. Copenhaver, W. M., Kelly, D. E., and Wood, R. L. (1983). The organs of special senses. In *Bailey's Testbook of Histology.* 17th Ed. Williams & Wilkins, Baltimore. pp. 731-765.
4. Newell, F. W. (1986). *Ophthalmology Principles and Concepts.* 6th Ed. Mosby, St. Louis.
5. Grant, W. M. (1986). *Toxicology of the Eye. Effects on the Eyes and Visual System from Chemicals, Drugs, Metals and Minerals, Plants, Toxins and Venoms; Also Systemic Side Effects from Eye Medications.* 3rd Ed. Charles C Thomas, Springfield, Illinois.
6. Potts, A. M. (1991). Toxic responses of the eye. In *Casarett and Doull's Toxicology. The Basic Science of Poisons.* 4th Ed. Amdur, M. O., Doull, J., and Klaassen, C. D. (Eds.). Macmillan, New York, pp. 521-562.

7. McCally, A. W., Farmer, A. G., and Loomis, E. C. (1933). Corneal ulceration following use of lash lure. *J.A.M.A.* **101**: 1560-1561.
8. Friedenwald, J. S., Hughes, W. F., and Herrmann, H. (1944). Acid-base tolerance of the cornea. *Arch. Ophthalmol.* **31**: 279-283.
9. Carpenter, C. P., and Smyth, H. F. (1946). Chemical burns of the rabbit cornea. *Am. J. Ophthalmol.* **29**: 1363-1372.
10. Kay, J. H., and Calandra, J. C. (1962). Interpretation of eye irritation tests. *J. Soc. Cosmet. Chem.* **13**: 281-289.
11. National Academy of Sciences (NAS) (1977). Principles and procedures for evaluating the toxicity of household substances. Vol. 1138. Committee for Revision of NAS Publication Washington, D.C. p. 53.
12. FHSA (Federal Hazardous Substance Act) (1974). Test for eye irritants. In: Code of Federal Regulations, Title 16, paragraph 1500.42, 295. Code of Federal Regulations 295.
13. EEC (European Economic Community) (1983). Commission Directive of 29th July 1983 Adopting to Technical Progress for the Fifth Time Council Directive 61/458/EEC on the Approximation of the Laws, Regulations and Administrative Provisions Relating to the Classification, Packaging and Labeling of Dangerous Substances. Off. J. Eur. Comm. L257/1.
14. Falahee, K. J., Rose, C. S., Olin, S. S., and Seifried, H. E. (1981). Eye irritation testing; an assessment of the methods and guidelines for testing materials for eye irritancy. EPA-560/11-82-001
15. Weil, C. S., and Scala, R. A. (1971). Study of intra- and interlaboratory variability in the results of rabbit eye and skin irritation tests. *Toxicol. Appl. Pharmacol.* **19**: 276-360.
16. Buehler, E. V. (1974). Testing to predict potential ocular hazards of household chemicals. In *Toxicology Annual 1974.* 53rd Ed. by C. L. Winek (Ed.). Marcel Dekker, New York.
17. Heywood, R., and James, R. W. (1978). Towards objectivity in the assessment of eye irritation. *J. Soc. Cosmet. Chem.* **29**: 25.
18. Griffith, J. F., Nixon, G. A., Bruce, R. D., Reer, P. J., and Bannan, E. A. (1980). Dose-response studies with chemical irritants in the albino rabbit eye as a basis for selecting optimum testing conditions for predicting hazard to the human eye. *Toxicol. Appl. Pharmacol.* **55**: 501-513.
19. Swanston, D. W. (1985). Assessment of the validity of animal techniques in eye irritation testing. *Food Chem. Toxicol.* **23**: 169-173.
20. Marzulli, F. N., and Simon, M. E. (1971). Eye irritation from topically applied drugs and cosmetics: Preclinical studies. *Am. J. Ophthalmol.* **48**: 61.
21. Rowan, A. (1983). Shortcomings of alternative techniques for the assessment of acute toxicity. *Acta Pharmacol. Toxicol. (Copenh.)* **52**: 190-200.
22. Rowan, A. N. (1984). The future of animals in research and training. The search for alternatives. *Fund. Appl. Toxicol.* **4**: 508-516.
23. Freeberg, F. E., Griffith, J. F., Bruce, R. D., and Bay, P. H. S. (1984). Correlation of animal test methods with human experience for household products. *J. Toxicol. Cut. Ocular Toxicol* **3**: 53-64.

24. Freeberg, F. E., Hooker, D. T., and Griffith, J. F. (1986). Correlation of animal eye test data with human experience for household products: an update, *J. Toxicol. Cut. Ocular Toxicol.* **5**: 115-123.
25. Freeberg, F. E., Nixon, G. A., Reer, P. J., Weaver, J. E., Bruce, R. D., Griffith, J. F. and Sanders, L. W., III. (1986). Human and rabbit eye responses to chemical insult. *Fundam. Appl. Toxicol.* **7**: 626-634.
26. Johnson, A. W. (1986). CTFA ocular safety testing workshop: In vivo and in vitro approaches, October 6 & 7, 1986, Washington, D. C., Cosmetic, Toiletry and Fragrance Association (unpublished).
27. Williams, S. J. (1985). Changing concepts of ocular irritation evaluation: pitfalls and progress. *Food Chem. Toxicol.* **23**: 189-193.
28. Burton, A. B. G. (1972). A method for the objective assessment of eye irritation. *Food Cosmet. Toxicol.* **10**: 209-217.
29. Kennah, H. E., Hignet, S., Laux, P. E., Dorko, J. D. and Barrow, C. S. (1989). An objective procedure for quantitating eye irritation based upon changes of corneal thickness. *Fundam. Appl. Toxicol.* **12**: 258-268.
30. Conquet, P., Durand, G., Laillier, J., and Plazonnet, B. (1977). Evaluation of ocular irritation in the rabbit: objective versus subjective assessment. *Toxicol. Appl. Pharmacol.* **39**: 129-139.
31. Laillier, J., Plazonnet, B., and LeDourarec, J. C. (1975). Evaluation of ocular irritation in the rabbit: development of an objective method of studying eye irritation. *Proc. Eur. Soc. Toxicol.* **17**: 336-350.
32. Green, K., and Tonjum, A. (1971). Influence of various agents on corneal permeability. *Am. J. Ophthalmol.* **72**: 897-905.
33. Etter, J. C., and Wildhaber, A. (1985). Biopharmaceutical test of ocular irritation in the mouse. *Food Chem. Toxicol.* **23**: 321-323.
34. Maurice, D., and Singh, T. (1986). A permeability test for acute corneal toxicity. *Toxicol. Lett.* **31**: 125-130.
35. Walberg, J. (1983). Exfoliative cytology as a refinement of the Draize eye irritancy test. *Toxicol. Lett.* **18**: 49-55.
36. Walton, R. M., and Heywood, R. (1978). Applanation tonometry in the assessment of eye irritation. *J. Soc. Cosmet. Chem.* **29**: 365-368.
37. Frazier, J. M., Gad, S. C., Goldberg, A. M., and McCulley, J. P. (1987). *A Critical Evaluation of Alternatives to Acute Ocular Irritation Testing. Alternative Methods in Toxicology*. Vol. 4. Mary Ann Liebert, New York.
38. Borenfreund, E., Shopsis, C., Borrero, O., and Sathe, S. (1983). In vitro alternative irritancy assays: Comparison of cytotoxic and membrane transport effects of alcohols. *Ann. N.Y. Acad. Sci.* **407**: 416-419.
39. Borenfreund, E., and Puerner, J. A. (1984). A simple quantitative procedure using monolayer cultures for cytotoxicity assays (HTD/NR-90). *J. Tissue Culture Meth.* **9**: 7-9.
40. Borenfreund, E., and Puerner, J. A. (1986). Cytotoxicity of metals, metal-metal and metal-chelator combinations assayed in vitro. *Toxicology* **39**: 121-134.
41. Borenfreund, E., and Puerner, J. A. (1987). Short-term quantitative in vitro cytotoxicity assay involving an S-9 activating system. *Cancer Lett.* **34**: 243-248.

42. Borenfreund, E., and Puerner, J. A. (1985). Toxicity determined in vitro by morphological alterations and neutral red absorption. *Toxicol. Lett.* **24**: 119-124.
43. Shopsis, C., Borenfreund, E., Walberg, J. and Stark, D. M. (1985). A battery of potential alternatives to the Draize test: Uridine uptake inhibition, morphological cytotoxicity, macrophage chemotaxis and exfoliative cytology. *Food Chem. Toxicol.* **23**: 259-266.
44. Borenfreund, E., and Shopsis, C. (1985). Toxicity monitored with a correlated set of cell-culture assays. *Xenobiotica* **15**: 705-711.
45. Burton, A. B., York, M., and Lawrence, R. S. (1981). The in vitro assessment of severe eye irritants. *Food Cosmet. Toxicol.* **19**: 471-480.
46. Price, J. B., and Andrews, I. J. (1985). The in vitro assessment of eye irritancy using isolated eyes. *Food Chem. Toxicol.* **23**: 313-315.
47. Leighton, J., Nassauer, J., and Tchao, R. (1985). The chick embryo in toxicology: An alternative to the rabbit eye. *Food Chem. Toxicol.* **23**: 293-298.
48. Zwilling, E. (1959). A modified chorioallantoic grafting procedure. *Transplant. Bull.* **6**: 115-116.
49. Kong, B. M., Viau, C. J., Rizvi, P. Y., and DeSalva, S. J. (1987). The development and evaluation of the Chorioallantoic membrane (CAM) assay. In *In Vitro Toxicology. Approaches to Validation. Alternative Methods in Toxicology.* Vol. 5. A. M. Goldberg (Ed.). New York, Mary Ann Liebert, New York, pp. 59-73.
50. Bagley, D. M., Rizvi, B. M., Kong, B. M., and DeSalva, S. J. (1988). An improved CAM assay for predicting ocular irritation potential. In *Progress in in Vitro Toxicology. Alternative Methods in Toxicology.* Vol. 6. A. M. Goldberg (Ed.). Mary Ann Liebert, New York, pp. 131-144.
51. Booman, K. A., De Prospo, J., Demetrulias, J., Driedger, A., Griffith, J. F., Grochoski, G., Kong, B. M., McCormick, W. C., North-Root, H., Rozen, M. G., and Sedlak, R. I. (1989). The SDA alternatives program: Comparison of in vitro data with Draize test data. *J. Toxicol. Cut. Ocular Toxicol.* **8**: 35-49.
52. Luepke, N. P. (1985). Hen's egg chorioallantoic membrane test for irritation potential. *Food Chem. Toxicol.* **23**: 287-291.
53. Luepke, N. P. (1985). HET-Chorionallantois-Test: An alternative to the Draize rabbit eye test. In *Alternative Methods in Toxicology. In Vitro Toxicology.* Vol. 3. A. M. Goldberg (Ed.), Mary Ann Liebert, New York, pp. 593-605.
54. Luepke, N. P., and Wallat, S. (1987). HET-CAM-Reproducibility Studies. In *In Vitro Toxicology. Approaches to Validation. Alternative Methods in Toxicology.* Vol. 5. A. M. Goldberg (Ed.). Mary Ann Liebert, New York, pp. 353-363.
55. Luepke, N. P. (1986). The hen's egg test (HET)-an alternative toxicity test. *Br. J. Dermatol.* **115** (Suppl.): 133-135.
56. Luepke, N. P., and Kemper, F. H. (1986). The HET-CAM test: An alternative to the Draize eye test. *Food Chem. Toxicol.* **24**: 495-496.
57. Weterings, P. J., and Van Erp, Y. H. M. (1987). Validation of the BECAM assay-an eye irritancy screening test. In *In Vitro Toxicology. Approaches to Valida-*

tion. Alternative Methods in Toxicology. Vol. 5. A. M. Goldberg (Ed.). Mary Ann Liebert, New York, pp. 515-521.

58. Rosenbruch, M. (1989). Granulation tissue in the chick embryo yolk sac blood vessel system. *J. Comp. Pathol.* **101**: 363-373.
59. Rosenbruch, M., and Holst, A. (1990). The chick embryo yolk-sac blood vessel system as an experimental model for irritation and inflammation. *Toxicol. In Vitro* **4**: 327-331.
60. Leighton, J., Nassauer, J., Tchao, R., and Verdone, J. (1983). Development of a procedure using the chick egg as an alternative to the Draize rabbit test. In *Product Safety Evaluation. Alternative Methods in Toxicology.* Vol. 1. A. M. Goldberg (Ed.). Mary Ann Liebert, New York, pp. 165-177.
61. Kong, B. M. (1987). The evolution of an alternative to the Draize eye test. *Soap/Cosmetics/Chemical Specialties* **July**: 40-51.
62. Parish, W. E. (1985). Ability of in vitro (corneal injury—eye organ—and chorioallantoic membrane) tests to represent histopathological features of acute eye inflammation. *Food Chem. Toxicol.* **23**: 215-227.
63. Lawrence, R. S., Groom, M. H., Ackroyd, D. M., and Parish, W. E. (1986). The chorioallantoic membrane in irritation testing. *Food Chem. Toxicol.* **24**: 497-502.
64. Price, J. B., Barry, M. P., and Andrews, I. J. (1986). The use of the chick chorioallantoic membrane to predict eye irritants. *Food Chem. Toxicol.* **6/7**: 503-505.
65. Balls, M., and Horner, S. A. (1985). The FRAME interlaboratory programme on in vitro cytotoxicology. *Food Chem. Toxicol.* **23**: 209-213.
66. Horner, S. A., Fry, J. R., Clothier, R. H., and Balls, M. (1985). A comparison of two cytotoxicity assays for the detection of metabolism-mediated toxicity in vitro: A study with cyclophosphamide. *Xenobiotica* **15**: 681-686.
67. Riddell, R. J., Clothier, R. H., and Balls, M. (1986). An evaluation of three in vitro cytotoxicity assays. *Food Chem. Toxicol.* **24**: 469-471.
68. Knox, P., Uphill, P. F., Fry, J. R., Benford, J., and Balls, M. (1986). The FRAME multicentre project on in vitro cytotoxicology. *Food Chem. Toxicol.* **24**: 457-463.
69. Shopsis, C. and Eng, B. (1985). Rapid cytotoxicity testing using a semi-automated protein determination on cultured cells. *Toxicol. Lett.* **26**: 1-8.
70. Shopsis, C. (1989). Validation Study: Ocular irritancy prediction with the total cell protein, uridine uptake and neutral red assays applied to human epidermal keratinocytes and mouse 3T3 cells. *In Vitro Toxicology: New Directions. Alternative Methods in Toxicology.* Vol. 7. A. M. Goldberg (Ed. Mary Ann Liebert, New York, pp. 273-287.
71. Reinhardt, C. A., Pelli, D. A., and Zbinden, G. (1985). Interpretation of cell toxicity data for the estimation of potential irritation. *Food Chem. Toxicol.* **23**: 247-252.
72. Watanabe, M., Watanabe, K., Suzuki, K., Nikaido, O., Sugahara, T., Ishii, I., and Konishi, H. (1988). In vitro cytotoxicity test using primary cells derived from rabbit eye is useful as an alternative for Draize testing. In *Progress in In Vitro Toxicology. Alternative Methods in Toxicology.* Vol. 6. A. M. Goldberg (Ed.). Mary Ann Liebert, New York, pp. 285-289.

73. North-Root, H., Yackovich, F., Demetrulias, J., Gacula, M., Jr., and Heinze, J. E. (1982). Evaluation of an in vitro cell toxicity test using rabbit corneal cells to predict the eye irritation potential of surfactants. *Toxicol. Lett.* **14**: 207-212.
74. North-Root, H., Yackovich, F., Demetrulias, J., Gacula, M., Jr., and Heinze, J. E. (1985). Prediction of the eye irritation potential of shampoos using the in vitro SIRC cell toxicity test. *Food Chem. Toxicol.* **23**: 271-273.
75. Demetrulias, J., and North-Root, H. (1988). Prediction of eye irritation potential for surfactant-based household cleaning products using the SIRC cell toxicity test. In *Progress in In Vitro Toxicology. Alternative Methods in Toxicology.* Vol. 6. A. M. Goldberg (Ed.), Mary Ann Liebert, New York, pp. 145-152.
76. Shadduck, J. A., Render, J., Everitt, J., Meccoli, R. A., and Essex-Sorlie, D. (1987). An approach to validation: Comparison of six materials in three tests. In *In Vitro Toxicology. Approaches to Validation. Alternative Methods in Toxicology.* Vol. 5. A. M. Goldberg (Ed.). Mary Ann Liebert, New York, pp. 75-78.
77. Shadduck, J. A., Everitt, J., and Bay, P. H. S. (1985). Use of in vitro cytotoxicity to rank ocular irritation of six surfactants. In *In Vitro Toxicology. A Progress Report from the Johns Hopkins Center for Alternatives to Animal Testing.* Vol. 3. A. M. Goldberg (Ed.). Mary Ann Liebert, New York, pp. 641-649.
78. Tchao, R. (1988). Trans-epithelial permeability of fluorescein in vitro as an assay to determine eye irritants. In *Progress in In Vitro Toxicology. Alternative Methods in Toxicology.* Vol. 6. A. M. Goldberg (Ed.). Mary Ann Liebert, (Ed.). pp. 271-283.
79. Kemp, R. B., Meredith, R. W., Gamble, S., and Frost, M. (1983). A rapid cell culture technique for assessing the toxicity of detergent-based products in vitro as a possible screen for eye irritancy in vivo. *Cytobios* **36**: 153-159.
80. Aeschbacher, M., Reinhardt, C. A., and Zbinden, G. (1986). A rapid cell membrane permeability test using fluorescent dyes and flow cytometry. *Cell Biol. Toxicol.* **2**: 247-255.
81. Scaife, M. C. (1982). An investigation of detergent action on cells in vitro and possible correlations with in vivo data. *Int. J. Cosmet. Sci.* **4**: 179-193.
82. Scaife, M. C. (1985). An in vitro cytotoxicity test to predict the ocular irritation potential of detergents and detergent products. *Food Chem. Toxicol.* **23**: 253-258.
83. Stark, D. M., Borenfreund, E., Walberg, J., and Shopsis, C. (1985). Comparison of Several Alternative Assays for Measuring Potential Toxicants. In *In Vitro Toxicology. A Progress Report from the Johns Hopkins Center for Alternatives to Animal Testing. Alternative Methods in Toxicology.* Vol. 3. A. M. Goldberg (Ed.). New York, Mary Ann Liebert, New York, pp. 373-390.
84. Shopsis, C. (1984). Inhibition of uridine uptake in cultured cells: A rapid, sublethal cytotoxicity test. *J. Tiss. Cult. Meth.* **9**: 19-22.
85. Shopsis, C., and Sathe, S. (1984). Uridine uptake inhibition as a cytotoxicity test: Correlations with the Draize test. *Toxicology.* **29**: 195-206.
86. Borenfreund, E., Babich, H., and Martin-Alguacil, N. (1988). Comparisons of two in vitro cytotoxicity assays-the neutral red (NR) and tetrazolium MTT tests. *Toxicol. In Vitro* **2**: 1-6.
87. Babich, H., Martin-Alguacil, N., and Borenfreund, E. (1989). Comparisons of the cytotoxicities of dermatotoxicants to human keratinocytes and fibroblasts

in vitro. In *In Vitro Toxicology: New Directions. Alternative Methods in Toxicology.* Vol. 7. A. M. Goldberg (Ed.). Mary Ann Liebert, New York, pp. 153-167.
88. Babich, H., Shopsis, C., and Borenfreund, E. (1986). In vitro cytotoxicity testing of aquatic pollutants (cadmium, copper, zinc, nickel) using established fish cell lines. *Ecotoxicol. Environ. Safety.* **11**: 91-99.
89. Hockley, K., and Baxter, D. (1986). Use of the 3T3 cell-neutral red uptake assay for irritants as an alternative to the rabbit (Draize) test. *Food Chem. Toxicol.* **24**: 473-475.
90. Reader, S. J., Blackwell, V., O'hara, R., Clothier, R. H., Griffin, G., and Balls, M. (1989). A vital dye release method for assessing the short-term cytotoxic effects of chemicals and formulations. *Alternatives Lab. Animals* **17**: 28-37.
91. Wallin, R. F., Hume, R. D., and Jackson, E. M. (1987). The agarose diffusion method for ocular irritancy screening: Cosmetic products, Part I. *J. Toxicol. Cut. Ocular Toxicol.* **6**: 239-250.
92. Jackson, E. M., Hume, R. D., and Wallin, R. F. (1988). The agarose diffusion method for ocular irritancy screening: cosmetic products, part II. *J. Toxicol. Cut. Ocular Toxicol.* **7**: 187-194.
93. Kemp, R. B., Meredith, R. W., and Gamble, S. H. (1985). Toxicity of commercial products on cells in suspension culture: a possible screen for the Draize eye irritation test. *Food Chem. Toxicol.* **23**: 267-270.
94. Hafeman, D. G., Parce, W. J., and McConnell, H. M. (1988). Light-addressable potentiometric sensor for biochemical systems. *Science* **240**: 1182-1185.
95. Parce, J. W., Owicki, J. C., Kercso, K. M., Sigal, G. B., Wada, H. G., Muir, V. C., Bousse, L. J., Ross, K. L., Sikic, B. I., and McConnell, H. M. (1989). Detection of Cell-affecting agents with a silicon biosensor. *Science* **246**: 243-247.
96. Bruner, L. H., Kain, D. J., Roberts, D. A., and Parber, R. D. (1991). Evaluation of seven in vitro alternatives for ocular safety testing. *Fundam. Appl. Toxicol.* **17**: 136-149.
97. Bruner, L. H., Miller, K. M., Owicki, J. C., Parce, J. W., and Muir, V. C. (1991). Testing ocular irritancy with the silicon microphysiometer. *Toxicol. In Vitro.* **5**: 277-284.
98. Bulich, A. A. (1986). Bioluminescence assays. In *Toxicity Testing Using Micro Organisms,* Vol. I. G. Bitton and B. J. Dutka (Eds.). CRC Press, Boca Raton, Florida, pp. 57-74.
99. Bulich, A. A. (1979). Use of liminescent bacteria for determining toxicity in aquatic environments. In *Aquatic Toxicology, ASTM 667.* L. L. Markings and R. A. Kimerle (Ed.), American Society for Testing and Materials, Philadelphia, pp. 98-106.
100. Chan, K. Y. (1985). An in vitro alternative to the Draize test. In *In Vitro Toxicology. A Progress Report from the Johns Hopkins Center for Alternatives to Animal Testing.* Vol. 3. A. M. Goldberg (Ed.). Mary Ann Liebert, New York, pp. 407-422.
101. Chan, K. Y. (1987). Design and correlation of the CEPA test: An in vitro ocular irritation test. *J. Toxicol. Cut. Ocular Toxicol.* **6**: 207-214.

102. Chan, K. Y. (1986). Chemical injury to an in vitro ocular system: Differential release of plasminogen activator. *Curr. Eye Res.* **5**: 357-362.
103. Burton, S. A., Petersen, R. V., Dickman, S. N., and Nelson, J. R. (1986). Comparison of in vitro bacterial bioluminescence and tissue culture bioassays and in vivo tests for evaluating acute toxicity of biomaterials. *J. Biomed. Mater. Res.* **20**: 827-838.
104. Jumblatt, M. M., and Neufeld, A. H. (1985). A tissue culture model of the human corneal epithelium. In *In Vitro Toxicology. A Progress Report from the Johns Hopkins Center for Alternatives to Animal Testing. Alternative Methods in Toxicology.* Vol. 3. A. M. Goldberg (Ed.). Mary Ann Liebert, New York, pp. 393-404.
105. Jumblatt, M. M., and Neufeld, A. H. (1986). A tissue culture assay of corneal epithelial wound closure. *Invest. Ophthalmol. Vis. Sci.* **27**: 8-13.
106. Simmons, S. J., Jumblatt, M. M., and Neufeld, A. H. (1987). Corneal epithelial wound closure in tissue culture: An in vitro model of ocular irritancy. *Toxicol. Appl. Pharmacol.* **88**: 13-23.
107. Jumblatt, M. M., Simmons, S. J., and Neufeld, A. H. (1987). Corneal epithelial wound closure: A tissue culture model of ocular irritancy. In *In Vitro Toxicology. Approaches to Validation. Alternative Methods in Toxicology.* Vol. 5. A. M. Goldberg (Ed.) Mary Ann Liebert, New York, pp. 139-145.
108. Muir, C. K., Flower, C., and Van Abbe, N. J. (1986). The effect of shampoos on rabbit ileum in vitro compared to eye irritancy in vivo. *J. Am. Coll. Toxicol.* **5**: 113-116.
109. Muir, C. K., Flower, C., and Van Abbe, N. J. (1983). A novel approach to the search for in vitro alternatives to in vivo eye irritancy testing. *Toxicol. Lett.* **18**: 1-5.
110. Muir, C. K. (1983). The toxic effect of some industrial chemicals on rabbit ileum in vitro compared with eye irritancy in vivo. *Toxicol. Lett.* **19**: 309-312.
111. Oliver, G. J., and Pemberton, M. A. (1985). An in vitro epidermal slice technique for identifying chemicals with potential for severe cutaneous effects. *Food Chem. Toxicol.* **23**: 229-232.
112. Muir, C. K. (1984). A simple method to assess surfactant-induced bovine corneal opacity in vitro: Preliminary findings. *Toxicol. Lett.* **22**: 199-203.
113. Muir, C. K. (1985). Opacity of bovine cornea in vitro induced by surfactants and industrial chemicals compared with ocular irritancy in vivo. *Toxicol. Lett.* **24**: 157-162.
114. Brooks, D., and Maurice, D. (1987). A simple fluorometer for use with a permeability screen. In: *In Vitro Toxicology. Approaches to Validation. Alternative Methods in Toxicology.* Vol. 5. A. M. Goldberg (Ed.). Mary Ann Liebert, New York, pp. 139-145.
115. Jacaruso, R. B., Bartlett, M. A., Carson, S., and Trombetta, L. D. (1985). Release of histamine from rat peritoneal cells in vitro as an index of irritational potential. *J. Toxicol. Cut. Ocular Toxicol.* **4**: 39-48.
116. Chasin, M., Scott, C., Shaw, C., and Persico, F. (1979). A new assay for the measurement of mediator release from rat peritoneal mast cells. *Int. Arch. Allergy Appl. Immunol.* **58**: 1-10.
117. Dubin, N. H., Wolff, M. C., Thomas, C. L., and DiBlasi, M. C. (1985). Prostaglandin production by rat vaginal tissues, in vitro, in response to ethanol,

a mild mucosal irritant. *Toxicol. Appl. Pharmacol.* **78**: 458-463.
118. Elgebaly, S. A., Herkert, N., O'Rourke, J., and Kreutzer, D. L. (1987). Characterization of neutrophil and monocyte specific chemotactic factors derived from the cornea in response to hydrogen peroxide injury. *Am. J. Pathol.* **126**: 40-50.
119. Elgebaly, S. A., Gillies, C., Forouhar, F., Hashem, M., Baddour, M., O'Rourke, J., and Kreutzer, D. L. (1985). An in vitro model of leukocyte mediated injury to the corneal epithelium. *Curr. Eye Res.* **4**: 31-41.
120. Silverman, J. (1983). Preliminary findings on the use of protozoa (*Tetrahymena thermophila*) as models for ocular irritation testing in rabbits. *Lab. Anim. Sci.* **33**: 56-59.
121. Silverman, J., and Pennisi, S. (1987). Evaluation of *Tetrahymena thermophila* as an in vitro alternative to ocular irritation studies in rabbits. *J. Toxicol. Cut. Ocular Toxicol.* **6**: 33-42.
122. Kelly, C. P. (1989). EYTEX: An in vitro method of predicting ocular safety. *Pharmacopeial Forum* **15**: 4815-4824.
123. Soto, R. J., Servi, M. J. and Gordon, V. C. (1989). Evaluation of an alternative method for ocular irritation. In *In Vitro Toxicology: New Directions. Alternative Methods in Toxicology.* Vol. 7. A. M. Goldberg (Ed.). Mary Ann Liebert, New York, pp. 289-296.
124. Gordon, V. C., Kelly, C P., and Bergman, H. C. (1989). Applications of the EYTEX Method for determination of the ocular irritation of surfactant formulations. In *In Vitro Toxicology: New Directions. Alternative Methods in Toxicology.* Vol. 7. A. M. Goldberg (Ed.). Mary Ann Liebert, New York, pp. 337-345.
125. Shapiro, H. M. (1988). Parameters and probes. In *Practical Flow Cytometry.* 2nd Ed. Liss, New York, pp. 115-198.
126. Wang, Y. L., and Taylor, D. L. (1989). Fluorescence microscopy of living cells in culture. Part A. Fluorescent analogs, labeling cells, and basic microscopy. *Meth. Cell Biol.* **29**: 1-333.
127. Bell, E., Ivarsson, B., and Merrill, C. (1979). Production of a tissue-like structure of contraction of collagen lattices by human fibroblasts of different proliferative potential in vitro. *Proc. Natl. Acad. Sci. U.S.A.* **76**: 1274-1278.
128. Bell, E., Ehrlich, H. P., Buttle, D. J. and Nakatsuji, T. (1981). Living tissue formed in vitro and accepted as skin-equivalent tissue of full thickness. *Science* **221**: 1052-1054.
129. Weinberg, C. B., and Bell, E. (1986). A blood vessel model constructed from collagen and cultured vascular cells. *Science* **231**: 397-400.
130. Frazier, J. M., and Bradlaw, J. A. (1989). *Technical Problems Associated with In Vitro Toxicity Testing Systems. A Report of the Center for Alternatives to Animal Testing Technical Workshop of May 17-18, 1989.* Baltimore, Johns Hopkins University School of Hygiene and Public Health.

8

Cutaneous Irritancy

Vincent A. DeLeo

Columbia University
New York, New York

INTRODUCTION

Human toxicology of manmade and commercially marketed products encompasses damage to the structure and function of literally all bodily tissues. Many of these reactions entail serious health consequences, some with significant mortality. Although such serious consequences rarely occur when the skin is the target organ of toxins, the prevelance of such toxicity makes *cutaneous* primary irritancy of enormous concern in industrialized societies.

Cutaneous primary irritancy is also known as *toxic* contact dermatitis and irritant contact dermatitis and under a myriad of clinical diagnoses, including housewife's eczema, diaper dermatitis, and winter itch. It is one of the most common maladies seen by dermatologists. Importantly, it is the most common cause of industrial dermatitis, which is in turn the most frequently reported occupational disease in the United States (1).

Clinically, cutaneous primary irritancy may appear with diverse morphology. Severe toxins can cause necrosis of the skin with the formation of erythema, bullae, eschar, and ulcerations. Such severe reactions are rare. Usually the cutaneous primary irritant response appears as dermatitis (eczema)—acute, subacute, or chronic. The lesions are confined to the area of toxin contact. Early lesions may consist of erythema and scaling, or macules, papules, and vesicles. These may coalesce to form plaques of erythema with oozing, crusting, and scaling. Long-standing lesions may appear thickened or lichenified and fissured. Histologically, the process involves both epidermis and dermis. The epidermis may show changes of intercellular fluid accumulation (spongiosis) with vesicle formation and/or acanthosis with parakeratosis. Recent studies reveal differences in histological findings depending on the nature and concentration of irritant (2). Toxicologists involved in determining hazard and risk of topical exposure commonly classify primary irritancy into acute primary irritation, cumulative irritation, and corrosion.

The more severe or toxic the irritant, the more rapidly the reaction becomes apparent. Some mild to moderately irritating substances require multiple applications in order to produce a clinical response. Almost any chemical agent has some capacity for producing a cutaneous irritant response. The clinical response in a given situation is dependant on intrinsic and extrinsic factors. While irritant responses tend to be universal, there are vast differences in response among individuals to a given toxin (intrinsic factors) with reactions tending to occur more readily in children and the aged. Extrinsic factors include diffusability of these agents through the skin barrier or percutaneous absorption; concentration and quantity of the toxin; duration and frequency of application and surface area of application; and, of course, the inherent irritation capability of the chemical which includes factors such as stability and purity (3).

By definition irritant contact dermatitis occurs when an agent (toxin or irritant) acts directly to damage the skin, resulting in an inflammatory response. This is in contradistinction to allergic contact dermatitis in which the immune system plays a role, with sensitization a prerequisite to the development of the response. The mechanisms by which agents produce irritancy has unfortunately not received adequate research interest and very little is known about the pathophysiology of the irritant response.

In all likelihood, each chemical affects different combinations of structural components and cells of the cutaneous organ which are characteristic for a specific chemical's structure and reactivity. Some agents affect primarily the stratum corneum, others act as toxins to keratinocytes, while still others penetrate to dermal elements where their targets lie (2). Regardless of the initial target component, mediators are produced and released by toxicant action, resulting in an inflammatory response—vascular dilatation, dermal and epidermal edema, and cellular infiltration. Circulating complement components (4), mast cell-released histamine (5), and membrane-derived arachidonic acid metabolites (6,7) have all been suggested as being important in this mediation process.

SKIN IRRITATION TESTING IN ANIMALS

Materials that cause skin irritation in humans are commonly identified using assays based on the work of Draize et al. (8). However, variations of the

Draize assay include differences in the animal species, inclusion of abraded sites, the volume applied, the number of animals used, and length of exposure time. Regulatory requirements also vary between agencies (9).

The rabbit is the most commonly used species. Fur on the backs of the animals, on both sides, are clipped prior to application of the test materials. Up to four samples can be evaluated per animal. The sites are occluded using tape or plastic. After exposure to the test material for 4 or 24 h (depending on the regulatory requirements), the coverings and test materials are removed and the sites are scored for erythema and eschar formation (maximum score of 4) and edema (maximum score of 4) at various intervals over several days. The primary dermal irritation (PDI) index is calculated from these scores with a maximum value of 8. The interpretation of the scores also varies and is dependent on the regulatory agency, but the value of the PDI index determines irritant classification.

Despite all the variations and modifications of the basic Draize method, it is widely accepted as a predictor of human skin irritation. A major problem with the assay is the subjective nature of the grading which can lead to interlaboratory differences in scoring, although within a laboratory the assay is more reproducible (10). False negative and false positive responses have been reported (11,12).

IN VITRO SYSTEMS FOR EVALUATING CUTANEOUS IRRITANCY

While significant research efforts have yielded a large number of in vitro assay systems for eye irritancy in various stages of validation (13), the development of systems for skin irritancy is not as advanced. Although early in their developmental stages, a number of these test systems appear to hold promise. Below and in Table 1, is a brief description of a number of these systems. This is followed by a discussion in greater detail of a system currently under development.

In many cases, general in vitro cytotoxicity assays have been adapted to cutaneous irritancy prediction by incorporating a relevant cell type (keratinocytes or dermal fibroblasts) as well as by simply evaluating known cutaneous irritants in the standard test system.

One of the earliest and most well-investigated techniques for evaluating toxicity in an in vitro system is the neutral red uptake assay adapted by Borenfreund and her colleagues at Rockefeller University (14-17). This is an easily automated cytotoxicity assay in which cell viability is determined by the ability of lysosomes of intact cells to take up and accumulate neutral red dye. The same culture dishes can then be assayed for total protein as a second measure of cell viability. This combined assay system has been studied extensively with many different toxicants. Most studies compared the observed in vitro toxicity of those agents to their in vivo ocular irritancy. More

Table 1 In Vitro Systems for Assaying Cutaneous Irritancy

In vitro system	Endpoint	References
Human fibroblasts and keratinocytes	Neutral red incorporation Cellular protein	14-18
Human keratinocytes	[^{3}H]Uridine Incorporation Cellular protein	19-23
Skin organ culture (human, guinea pig, rabbit)	[^{14}C]Leucine Incorporation Cellular vacuole formation	24,25
	Cellular vacuole formation	
Cell-free Macromolecular mixture (SKINTEX)	Physical/chemical reaction	30,31
Human keratinocytes	Cell growth inhibition and enzyme and ion leakage	26,27
3T3 fibroblast XB-2 keratinocytes	Neutral red uptake MTT cleavage Hexosaminidase leakage Colony area, cell number Keratin staining	28
Keratome skin in diffusion chamber Fibroblast culture with keratin/agar overlay	Amino acid uptake Enzyme release Histochemistry [^{3}H]Thymidine uptake Chromium release	29

recently, however, the authors have extended their work to human skin fibroblasts and keratinocytes as a method of utilizing their assays as an alternative for cutaneous irritancy as well (18).

A related test system developed by the same group of investigators (14-17) is the [^{3}H]uridine uptake assay. This endpoint appears to depend on toxicant-induced sublethal alterations of cellular metabolism relating to the transport and accumulation of this nucleotide, thereby evaluating cell membrane function and enzyme activity which are important to the overall growth status of cultured cells. This assay has also been extensively studied with the goal of utilizing this system as an alternative to the standard Draize ocular irritancy assay (16-22). These investigators have broadened the scope of this assay by utilizing human keratinocytes as the target cell (23). In their original communication concerning the keratinocyte system, the authors compared the in vitro data with ocular irritancy data from animal studies. It will be interesting to see comparisons between the keratinocyte assay and dermal irritancy data obtained in animals. (These authors also utilize the total protein assays as a second measurement of toxicity.)

Dannenberg and his colleagues used organ rather than cell culture in their studies (24,25). They maintained skin of humans, rabbits, and guinea pigs in short-term culture, and examined the effect of irritants by a variety of techniques. After a 24-h exposure to toxicant, the explants were embedded in glycol-methacrylate and examined histologically for the development of vacuoles in basal epidermal cells. A second assay system with a biochemical endpoint consisted of measuring the incorporation of [^{14}C]leucine from culture medium into the protein extracts of the explants. In the first assay the number of paranuclear vacuoles observed increased with increasing concentration of a variety of irritants, whereas examination of various control treated explants revealed few if any vacuoles. For the second endpoint measurement, increasing concentrations of irritants resulted in decreased [^{14}C] leucine incorporation. There was variability among species for both assays, but within a given species and with a given irritant there was good correlation between the two assay systems.

Van Genderen et al. (26,27) transplanted human skin on to nude mice and reported that this skin could be maintained; and that it responded to toxicants with morphological change (blistering). This group also investigated the inhibition of keratinocyte cell growth to determine the cytotoxicity of irritants in cultures. The same cell cultures were used to assay membrane damage by measuring the content of the enzymes lactate dehydrogenase and B-glucosaminidase and the content of K^+ ions in cells after treatment with known membrane-active agents (26,27).

Duffy and colleagues (28), suggesting that a single parameter in vitro assay would not be appropriate for assessing toxicity in a complex tissue like skin, have proposed a novel approach. They utilized both fibroblasts (3T3) and keratinocytes (XB-2) cell lines in culture and determined the effect of various toxicants on a number of different endpoints testing for *viability* (neutral red uptake), *cellular metabolism* [colorimetric measurement of formazan production from MTT (a tetrazolium salt)], *membrane integrity* (hexosaminidase and lactate dehydrogenase leakage), *keratinization* (keratin staining with Rhodamine B and Nile Blue), and *stratification* (cell number and colony area measurements). Validating the predictability of these assays with 18 compounds with Dermal Draize in vivo data revealed good correlation when using stratification combined with any other parameter as endpoints.

Adopting a similar multifaceted approach, Parish (29) has utilized thin keratome skin slices in diffusion chambers to test the effect of irritants on a number of endpoints, including radiolabeled amino acid utilization, enzyme release, and histological and histochemical alterations. He has also studied human fibroblast cultures alone and with an agar/keratin overlay to test irritant effects on radiolabeled thymidine uptake, and enzyme and radiolabeled chromium release. This latter approach, which attempts to add a "skin permeability" aspect to a monolayer culture system, is an interesting innovation. Parish (29) reported a good correlation of both of these in vitro systems with in vivo irritancy for mild irritants but moderate to poor correlation for more potent irritants using a limited number of test substances. In addition, preliminary studies using isolated neutrophils and mast cells by this author as test systems were not thought to be offer much promise (29).

An interesting system has been developed by Gordon and her colleagues, which they have designated SKINTEX (30). This group previously marketed a similar system for ocular irritancy called EYETEK (31). These system are based on cell-free complex mixtures of various macromolecules with physicochemical charge produced by toxicants, resulting in an observable alteration in light transmission. The authors base the relevance of their system on the in vivo alteration of the stratum cornerum—absorption of the toxic agent onto and alteration of the integrity of the stratum cornerum. A recent unpublished validation study with 200 products revealed an excellent correlation between in vivo irritancy as measured by PDII and SKINTEX/PDII EQUILIVANT.

DEVELOPING NEW TESTS

Believing that mechanistically based assays hold the greatest hope of being accepted by industry and regulatory agencies as alternatives to whole animal studies, we have established a two-phase approach to test development in this laboratory. First, we undertook experiments to define one aspect of the mechanism by which irritants (surfactants) induce inflammation in skin. Since this response in vivo involves arachidonate metabolites (6,7), we concentrated on irritant-induced alterations of membrane phospholipid metabolism of mammalian cells in culture. From those studies we reported that pure surfactants induced release of arachidonic acid from cells (32). The data from related studies suggested that this hydrolysis was due to activation of endogenous phospholipases, specifically phospholipase A_2 (33). The released arachidonic acid (AA) was metabolized via cyclooxygenase and lipoxygenase pathways into biologically significant mediators of inflammation. The release of AA was dose dependent and the magnitude of release was correlated with the irritancy of the surfactants in animal skin.

Once we established a basic and clinically relevant biological endpoint in vitro, i.e., surfactant-induced AA release, we proceeded to the second phase of the project. This phase was the development of a workable assay for irritancy.

We have utilized the release of AA in a minivalidation study with five surfactant-containing finished products (FP). We used two different cell systems in this study, normal human epithelial keratinocytes (NHEK) and murine fibroblasts ($C^3H10T1/2$). The NHEK system is commercially available and is supplied with all media (KGM-growth medium; KBM-basal medium) and reagents necessary for propagation and maintenance of the system (Clonetics Corporation, San Diego, California).

Cells were seeded into dishes at a constant density in growth medium and allowed to attach and grow to 90% confluency. Cells were then labeled with [^{3}H]arachidonic acid (1 μCi/ml). After a 24-hr labeling period, labeling medium was removed and cells were washed three times with assay medium. Assay medium alone (control) or assay medium containing surfactant or finished product was added to triplicate dishes. Cells were incubated at 37 °C. At selected times, medium was removed from dishes; centrifuged (10,000 rpm) to remove detached cells; and an aliquot was assayed for radioactivity by liquid scintillation counting. Results are presented in terms of mean total release of label into media.

The release of label for each of the products at multiple dilutions was determined and calculated as percent control:

$$\text{percent control} = \frac{\text{mean CPM surfactant}}{\text{mean CPM control}} \times 100$$

The release of label for the dilutions from a number of replicate assays were combined and subjected to linear regression analysis to plot a best fit line. The formula for this line was then used to compute the irritant dilution 200% (ID 200%). ID 200% was the dilution calculated to induce release of label at a level of 200% of control. The rank order of the ID 200% for the products was then determined and compared to the rank order irritancy of the product in terms of PDII.

In Figure a and b, the log ID200 for the five products are compared to their PDII values. The best fit regression lines and Pearson correlation were determined for four of the products. Product 5 was excluded from the analysis. The nature of the high sensitivity of the test system to product 5 is unknown and illustrates one of the difficulties encountered in new test development. It should be noted that the ID200 for all five finished products (FPs) is higher in the NHEK cells than in the C3H10T1/2 cells.

The predominant cell types in skin are in fact keratinocytes (epidermis) and the fibroblasts (dermis). Both fibroblasts and keratinocytes have been shown to synthesize arachidonic acid cascade metabolites in vitro (9,10). We were interested in further investigation of the effect of irritants on release of label in these cell types and, therefore, conducted experiments with two fibroblast lines (GM0010 and GM8447) and NM1, an immortal kera-

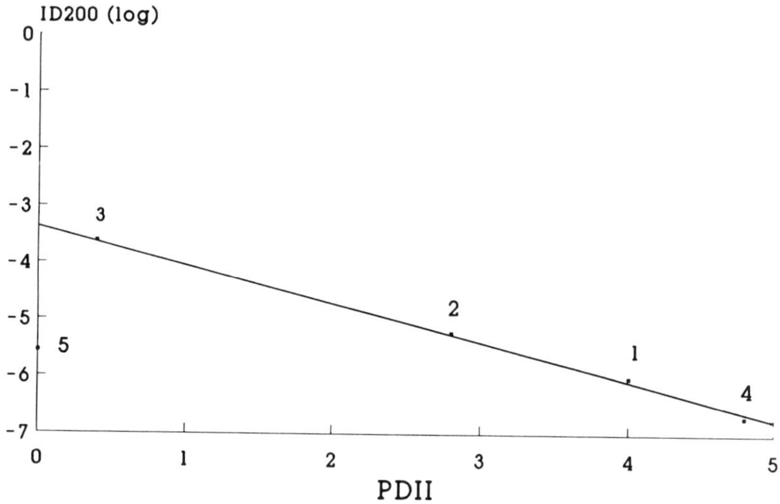

(a)

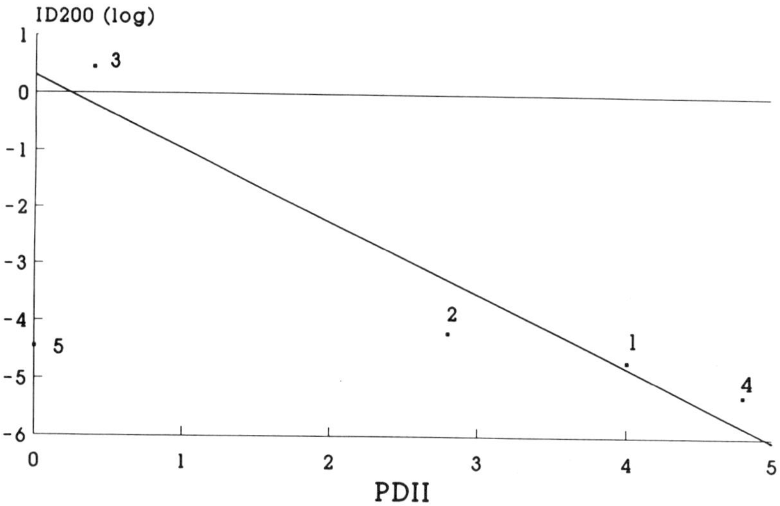

(b)

Figure 1 Comparison of PDII and ID200 for five finished products in (a) 10T1/2 cells and (b) NHEK cells. The best fit regression lines were computed excluding product 5.

tinocyte line obtained from Clonetics Corp. were isolated from either breast or foreskin (34).

For each cell type there was a dose-dependent response to the test materials. The rank order of the response was the same for all cell types, although the magnitude of the response was greater in the fibroblasts than the kerotinocytes. Different cell types have been shown to respond differently in other in vitro systems (18). These results suggest that either cell type may be suitable for an in vitro skin irritation assay.

The role of pH and pKa in vivo skin irritation is unclear. In some situations, it is recommended that all materials with a pH of <2 or >11.5 should be labeled as skin irritants. However, pH alone may not be the sole factor in determining in vivo skin irritation as oxalic acid (pH 1.0) is a mild irritant and aluminum nitrate (pH 0.8) is a nonirritant (35). Similarly at high pH, some materials with pH >10 were shown to be moderately or slightly irritating. The pKa of a chemical may also influence skin irritation. In vivo work of Berner et al. (36) with a homologous series of benzoic acid derivatives has suggested that compounds with pKa <4.1 appear to induce human skin irritation with greater irritation as the pKa decreases. To assess the effect of pH and pKa on keratinocytes in the in vitro radiolabel release assay, we investigated the effect of pH and pKa on radiolabel release.

The pH of the medium was altered by addition of acetic or hydrochloric acid. In experiments with acetic acid the acetate ion concentration was kept constant by addition of sodium acetate. pH effects on radiolabel release were determined in cells alone and also in the presence of test materials known to induce radiolabel release. pKa effects were tested using benzoic acid derivatives, most of which had been tested in humans by Berner et al. (36) in vivo. Each compound was assayed in cell growth medium and also in saline to prevent buffering by KGM. Preliminary experiments indicated that greater radiolabel release occurred after exposure to irritants in saline as compared to KBM.

Decreasing pH in these studies did not induce increased levels of radiolabel release. On the contrary, at low pH, radiolabel release was significantly reduced compared with release from cells at normal pH (Table 2). Furthermore, in the presence of known inducers of radiolabel release, SLS and FPs 2 and 4, the amount of radiolabel released was significantly reduced at lower pH (G. Lamont, personal communication).

There was no trend toward increased radiolabel release with pKa changes in KGM (data not shown) or saline as pKa decreased (Table 3). These results indicate that the response of the monolayer skin model system may not reflect in vivo response with respect to pH and pKa. Since low pH can significantly inhibit an in vitro response, the pH of test materials must be taken into consideration when considering the significance of in vitro responses (G. Lamont, personal communication).

Table 2 Effect of pH on Radiolabel Release

Test material	% Radiolabel release ±SD			
	pH5		pH7	
	HCl	Acetic acid	KGM	Na acetate
Control	1.5 ± 0.1	2.2 ± 0.5	3.7 ± 0.1	3.6 ± 0.8
0.03% FS	5.9 ± 0.4	7.2 ± 0.1	22.2 ± 0.4	21.9 ± 1.0
0.03% PS	1.8 ± 0.2	2.1 ± 0.1	6.6 ± 2.0	6.7 ± 1.0
0.03% BS	2.2 ± 0.3	2.8 ± 0.3	8.8 ± 0.9	9.1 ± 3.5
0.01% SLS	59.5 ± 1.8	62.6 ± 2.5	74.1 + 3.7	77.1 ± 4.4

Table 3 Effect of pKa on Radiolabel Release from NHEK Keratinocytes

		% Radiolabel release ± SD			
		salicylic acid	salicylamide	m-nitrobenzoic acid	m-anisic acid
Conc. (mM)	pKa	2.95	8.1	3.56	4.09
10		2.6 ± 0.1	2.0 ± 0.0	2.0 ± 0.0	1.5 ± 0.2
2		1.7 ± 0.2	2.6 ± 0.5	1.5 ± 0.1	1.6 ± 0.1
0.3		1.9 ± 0.0	2.9 ± 0.5	1.7 ± 0.1	1.6 ± 0.1
0.05		2.1 ± 0.7	2.7 ± 0.3	1.7 ± 0.1	1.6 ± 0.1

Saline control 2.2 ± 0.3.

SUMMARY

The cutaneous reaction patterns in human skin caused by chemical toxicants has long been observed and described at macro- and microscopic levels. Although this irritant reaction is frequently encountered at home and in the workplace, the mechanism of its development is poorly understood. A large body of literature and even more unpublished experience have yielded animal systems that predict with a moderately high level of success the irritancy of chemical products in human skin.

With our society's increased awareness and concern over animal pain and distress in biomedical research, scientists have made a beginning effort to develop alternatives to these standard animal assays. The effort has yielded rewards on two levels. Assays are being developed for prediction of cutaneous irritancy utilizing non-whole animal systems. A second and, in the end, possibly more useful result is the increased understanding of the cutaneous irritant response generated by this experimentation. This understanding, in turn, should yield many benefits, including the development and marketing of less irritating products, the development of new therapeutic agents to ameliorate the response when it occurs, and finally this understanding should lead to the development of mechanistically based non-whole animal test systems. Such systems hold the greatest hope for acceptance as alternatives by industry and regulatory agencies.

We have learned that the primary irritant response is a complex one involving many cell types and noncellular components of the cutaneous organ. These components and cells respond in a variety of ways when they contact different chemical substances. In all likelihood, the future of cutaneous irritancy testing will depend on the development of a battery of assays, some screening, nonspecific, cytotoxicity determinations followed by others more specifically designed to evaluate various classes of toxicants.

The development of alternatives for use in detecting ocular irritancy has laid the framework for those investigators interested in developing skin systems. Many systems are being investigated and the long but necessary validation process is underway.

REFERENCES

1. Fisher, A. *Contact Dermatitis,* 3rd Edition, Lea & Febiger, Philadelphia.
2. Willis, C. M., Stephens, C. J. M., and Wilkinson, J. D. (1989). Epidermal damage induced by irritation in man > a light and electron microscopic study. *J. Invest. Dermatol.* **93**: 695-700.
3. Mathias, C. G. T. (1989). Clinical and experimental aspects of cutaneous irritation. In *Dermatotoxicology.* Marzulli, F. N. and Miabach, H. I. (Eds.). Hemisphere, Washington, D.C., p. 1083.
4. Di Rosa, M., Giroud, J. P., and Willoughby, D. A. (1971). Studies of the mediators of the acute inflammatory response induced in rats in different sites by carrageenan and turpentine. *J. Pathol.* **104**: 15-29.
5. Prottey, C., and Ferguson, T. F. M. (1976). The effect of surfactants upon rat peritoreal mast cells in vitro, *Food Chem. Toxicol.* **14**: 425-530.
6. Sondergaard, J., Greaves, M. W., and Jorgensen, H. P. (1974). Recovery of Prostaglandins in human primary irritant dermatitis. *Arch. Dermatol.* **110**: 556-558.
7. Kassis, V., Mortevsen, J., and Sondergaard, J. (1981). Prostaglandin E, in suction separated human epidermal tissue in primary irritant dermatitis. *Acta Dermatol.* **61**: 424-461.
8. Draize, J. H., Woodward, G., and Calvery, H. O. (1944). Methods from the study of irritation and toxicity of substances applied topically to the skin and mucous membranes. *J. Pharmacol. Exp. Ther.* **82**: 377-390.
9. McGreesh, A. H., and Steinberg, M. (1987). Skin irritation testing in animals. In *Dermatotoxicology.* F. N. 1Marzulli and H. I. Maibach (Eds.). Hemisphere, Washington, D.C., pp. 153-172.

10. Weil, C. S., and Scala, R. A. (1971) Study of intra- and interlaboratory variability in the results of rabbit eye and skin irritation test. *Toxicol. Appl. Pharmacol.* **19**: L276-360.
11. Nixon, G. A., Tyson, C. A., and Wertz, W. C. (1975). Interspecies comparisons of skin irritancy. *Toxicol. Appl. Pharmacol.* **31**: 481-490.
12. Phillips, L., Steinberg, M., Masibach, H. I., and Akers, W. A. (1972). A comparison of rabbit and human skin response to certain irritants. *Toxicol. Appl. Pharmacol.* **21**: 369-382.
13. Frazier, J. M., Gad, S. C., Goldberg, A. M., and McCulley, J. P. (1987). A critical evaluation of alternatives to acute ocular testing. In *Alternative Methods in Toxicology*. Vol. 4. Mary Ann Liebert, New York.
14. Borenfreund, E., and Puerner, J. A. (1984). A simple quantitative procedure using monolayer cultures for cytotoxicity assays (HTD/NR-90). *J. Tiss. Cult. Meth.* **9**: 7-9.
15. Borenfreund, E., and Puerner, J. A. (1985). Toxicity determined *in vitro* by morphological alterations and neutral red absorption. *Toxicol. Lett.* **24**: 119-124.
16. Borenfruend, E., and Puerner, J. A. (1986). Cytotoxicity of metals, metal-metal and metal-chelator combinations assayed *in vitro Toxicology* **39**: 121-134.
17. Borenfreund, E., and Puerner, J. A. (1987). Short-term quantitative *in vitro* cytotoxicity assay involving an @-9 activating system. *Cancer Lett.* **34**: 243-248.
18. Babich, H., Martin-Alguacil, N., and Borenfreund, E. (1989). Comparisons of the cytotoxicities of dermatotoxicants to human keratinocytes and fibroblasts *in vitro*. In *Progress in Toxicology*. Vol. 7. A. M. Goldberg (Ed.). Mary Ann Liebert, New York.
19. Shopsis, C. S. (1984). Inhibition of uridine uptake by cultured cells: A rapid, sub-lethal cytotoxicity test. *J. Tiss. Cult. Meth.* **9**: 19.
20. Shopsis, C. S., and Sathe, S. (1984). Uridine uptake as a cytotoxicity test: correlations with the Draize test. *Toxicology,* **29**: 195.
21. Shopsis, C. S., Borenfreund, E., Walberg, J., and Stark, D. M. (1985). A battery of potential alternatives to the Draize test: Uridine uptake inhibition, morpholgical cytotoxicity, macrophage chemotaxis and exfoliative cytology. *Food Chem. Toxicol.* **23**: 259.
22. Shopsis, C. S., and Eng, B. (1985). Rapid cytotoxicity testing using a semi-automated protein determination on cultured cells. *Toxicol. Lett.* **26**: 1.
23. Shopsis, C. S., and Eng, B. (1988). In vitro occular irritancy prediction: assays in seven free media correlate better with in vivo data. In *Progress in In Vitro Toxicology*. Vol. 6. A. M. Goldberg (Ed.). Mary Ann Liebert, New York.
24. Dannenberg, A. M., Jr., Moore, K. G., Schofield, B. H., Higuchi, K., Kajiki, A., Au, K.-W., Pula, P. J., and Bassett, D. P. (1987). Two new in vitro methods for evaluating toxicity to skin (employing short-term organ culture): I. Paranuclear vacuolization, seen in glycol methacrylate tissue sections; II. Inhibition of ^{14}C-leucine incorporation. *Alternative Meth. Toxicol.* **5**: 115-127, 1987.
25. More, K. G., Schofield, B. H., Higuchi, K., Kajiki, A., Au, K.-W. Pula, P. J., Bassett, D. P., and Dannenberg, A. M., Jr. (1986). Two sensitive *in vitro* monitors of chemical toxicity to human and animal skin (in short-term organ culture): I. Paranuclear vacuolization, in glycol methacrylate tissue sections; II. Interfer-

ence with ^{14}C-leucine incorporation. *J. Toxicol. Cutan. Ocular Toxicol.* **5**: 285-302.
26. Von Genderman, J., Mol, M. A. E., and Wolthus, O. L. (1985). On the development of skin models for toxicity testing. *Fund. Appl. Toxicol.* **5**: S98-S111.
27. Mol, M. A. E., Von Genderen, J., and Wolthus, O. L. Cultured human epidermal cells as tool in skin toxicology. *Food Chem Toxicol.* **24**: 519-520.
28. Duffy, P. A., Flint, O. P., Onton, T. C., and Fursey, M. J., (1986). Initial validation of an *in vitro* test for predicting skin irritancy. *Food Chem Toxicol.* **24**: 517-518.
29. Parish, W. E. (1985). Relevance of in vitro tests to in vivo acute skin inflammation: potential in vitor applications of skin keratome slices, neutrophils, fibroblasts, mast cells and macrophages. *Food Chem. Toxicol.* **23**(2): 275-285.
30. Gordon, V. C., Kelly, C. P., and Bergman, H. C. (1989). SKINTEX$^{(R)}$ an in vitro method for determining dermal irritation. *Oral Commun. Congr. Toxicol.* Brighton, England.
31. Goldberg, A. M. (Ed.). (1987). A critical evaluation of alternatives to acute ocular irritation testing. *Alternative Meth. Toxicol.* **4**: 109-110.
32. Deleo, V. A., Harber, L. C., Kong, B. M., and DeSalva, S. J. (1987). Surfactant-induced alteration of arachidonic acid metabolism of mammalian cells in culture. *Proc. Soc. Exp. Biol. Med.* **184**: 477-482.
33. DeLeo, V. A., Hanson, D., and Scheide, S. (1989). The effect of surfactants on metabolism of choline phospholipids in human epidermal keratinocytes in culture. *J. Toxicol. Cutan. Ocular Toxicol.* **8**(2): 227-240.
34. Baden, H. P., Kubilus, J. C., Kevdar, Steinberg, M. L., and Wolman, S. R. (1987). Isolation and characterization of a spontaneously arising long-lived line of human keratinocytes (NM 1). *In Vitro Cell. Dev. Biol.* **23**: 205-213.
35. Guillot, J. P., Gonnet, J. F., Clement, C., Gaillard, L., and Truhaut, R. (1982). Evaluation of the cutaneous-irritation potential of 56 compounds. *Food Chem. Toxicol.* **20**: 562-572.
36. Berner, B., Wilson, D. R., Guy, R. H., Mazzenga, G. C., Clarde, F. H., and Maibach, H. I. (1988). The relationship of pKa and acute skin irritation in man. *Pharmol. Res.* **5**: 660-663.
37. DeLeo, V. A., Horlick, H., Hanson, D., Eisinger, M., and Harber, L. C. (1984). Ultraviolet radiation induces changes in membrane metabolism of human keratinocytes in culture. *J. Invest. Dermatol.* **83**: 323-326.

9

Teratogenicity

Barbara F. Hales

McGill University
Montreal, Quebec, Canada

THE HUMAN CONSEQUENCES OF EXPOSURE TO A TERATOGEN

It has been estimated that 3-7% of all infants live born in North America will have birth defects. Additional lives are claimed each year through infant death, spontaneous abortion, stillbirth, or miscarriage due to defective fetal development. Some 10 times as many children die of malformations as from contagious diseases! Close to one-half the children in hospital wards are there because of a prenatally acquired malformation. Some of these malformations are due to gene mutations or chromosomal aberrations, others are related to exposure to an identifiable chemical or drug, but the majority are still of unknown cause.

As many as 60,000 chemicals are in use presently and more enter the marketplace each year. Of these chemicals, only about 5% have been tested for teratogenicity in animals. In the range of 40-60% of the chemicals which have been tested may be teratogenic in certain animal species. Despite this, only about 30 chemicals are known or "established" as human teratogens. It is immediately apparent that there are huge gaps in our present information, both with respect to the causes of malformations in man and the effect of chemicals on the developing human being.

One important consideration in attempting to fill these gaps is our ability to accurately assess human teratogenic risk in an experimental system. The measures of adverse effects of chemical or drug exposure on pregnancy outcome in man are varied from embryo or fetal death, malformations, growth and/or mental retardation, to other functional impairments. The usual approach toward evaluating drug teratogenicity is to administer the drug or chemical to pregnant females from two animal test species throughout organogenesis. The females are killed prior to parturition; the uterus and its contents are then examined. Embryo or fetal death and malformations can be detected, but with this experimental protocol, behavioral effects or other functional impairments are not discovered. One rodent and one "nonrodent" species is used; the rodent species is usually the rat or mouse, the non-rodent, the rabbit. Importantly, the next step is then to attempt to extrapolate first from these test species to man, and second from the experimental doses which are studied to those to which humans are exposed.

It is obvious that the assessment of the human hazard represented by chemical and drug exposures during development using pregnant animal testing procedures is a formidable task. There is a great need for alternative approaches which are both scientifically valid and practical. Within the last decade increasing numbers of scientists have begun to explore in vitro alternatives to test for teratogenicity. In vitro technology is being used extensively to study the mechanism(s) by which chemicals and drugs interfere with biological processes in general and in development in particular. As we learn more and more about these mechanisms, we will also be more readily able to evaluate the significance and relevance of the in vitro tests in human risk assessment.

THE CURRENT IN VITRO SYSTEMS AVAILABLE TO TEST TERATOGENICITY

In developing an in vitro teratogenicity test or bank of tests, the first consideration is the biological target. In whole animal teratogenicity testing procedures, the "target" of the teratogen may actually be the embryo or fetus itself, but it may also be the placenta or the mother. For example, if the teratogen influences placental blood flow, the fetus will be deprived of oxygen and nutrients and may be growth retarded and malformed. It is evident that the "capture" of all of the possible mechanisms of drug teratogenicity in vivo in any one in vitro teratogenicity test is a difficult task.

An additional complication is that the susceptibility of the developing embryo/fetus to insult by any one teratogen will vary during gestation, depending upon the developmental events occurring at the time. Some teratogens have very specific effects at one time or stage of development. One example of such a teratogen is thalidomide, a drug which caused limb reduction malformations specifically during the period of limb development. Other teratogens, such as some of the anticancer drugs, affect various stages of development, causing different malformations depending on the period of exposure. It is also difficult to represent the numerous events which take place throughout organogenesis in any one in vitro system.

As the mechanism(s) by which the suspect teratogen is interfering with development becomes clear, we shall have a much sounder basis for our choice of in vitro test system. Until this is possible, most model systems are based on the premise that the insult or target of the chemical or drug is in fact the developing embryo. The in vitro systems then usually consist of a biological component undergoing differentiation. This "component" may vary from cells in culture to organs in culture all the way up to a whole embryo in culture; each of these "levels" has both advantages and disadvantages. Each has different parameters which can be measured to assess the effect of exposure to a chemical or drug on development. In each the basic requirements for any teratogenicity test can be addressed. Examples of some of these approaches are outlined below.

Cell Cultures

The cells that have served as the biological component of in vitro teratogenicity tests have varied from established cell lines to primary cell cultures. Examples of established cell lines that have been studied include mouse ovarian tumor cells (1,2), human embryonic palatal mesenchymal cells (3,4), and neuroblastoma cells (5). Examples of primary cell cultures that have been most extensively investigated include the micromass or high-density limb bud mesenchymal cell and midbrain neural cell culture systems (6,7). For each cell line or primary cell culture system, the "endpoints" measured have varied. Some of these endpoints detect the general cytotoxic effects of the chemicals to be tested, whereas others measure effects on cell proliferation, attachment, communication, or differentiation.

Cell Lines

In the mouse ovarian tumor cell line assay system developed by Braun et al. (1,2), teratogens interfere with attachment of [^{3}H]thymidine prelabeled cells to concanavalin A-coated polyethylene disks; chemically induced inhibition of cell attachment at noncytotoxic concentrations is assessed by counting the radioactivity in the medium. The hypothesis is that the mechanisms involved in embryonic cell-cell interactions are similar to those of lectin-mediated cell attachment in vitro. Any chemical capable of interfering with cell attachment in vitro at noncytotoxic concentrations is considered a potential teratogen. Braun and his coworkers (2) have reported that of over 100 chemicals tested, greater than 90% of the agents inhibiting attachment were teratogens. Interestingly, metabolic-activating systems can be added to assess the effects of chemicals requiring bioactivation. The addition of such an activating system permits the detection in vitro of teratogens requiring metabolic activation. Thalidomide itself did not inhibit cell attachment, but in the presence of liver microsomes and NADPH an active metabolite was formed which did interfere with cell attachment (8).

The human palatal mesenchymal cell line was established at the National Institute of Environmental Health Sciences (NIEHS) in Pratt's laboratory (3,4). These cells were initially obtained from the secondary palatal mesenchyme of a human abortus, close to the time of palatal shelf closure. The cells proliferate rapidly and are karyotypically stable in vitro (9). The endpoint of the teratogenicity assay is growth inhibition; chemicals which inhibit the growth of these cells, as determined by cell counts relative to control, are detected as positive for teratogenicity. It has been suggested that this assay be used in combination with the mouse ovarian tumor cell attachment assay; when these assays are combined the overall predictability is 90%, and the rate of false negatives is only 3%. The human palatal mesenchymal cell line may also be useful in assays which are based on an inhibition of cell-cell communication (10).

In the cultured neuroblastoma cell line system, the cells can differentiate morphologically under certain culture conditions into neurites (5). It is interesting that suspect teratogens may stimulate as well as inhibit this in vitro differentiation. In fact, more than half of the teratogens tested did stimulate differentiation. These investigators have also suggested that this test may be complementary to the mouse ovarian tumor cell attachment assay; teratogens which were incorrectly identified as nonteratogenic by one of these assays could be correctly assigned by the other (5).

Thus, the three cell line assay systems outlined above, i.e., the mouse ovarian tumor cell line, the human palatal mesenchymal cell line, and the neuroblastoma cell line, are based on drug effects on cell attachment/cell communication, cell proliferation/cell communication and cell differentiation, respectively. It is very probable that any chemical which interferes with these three events or processes will have a direct and toxic effect on the conceptus during development. The use of the three test systems as complementary approaches might indeed be expected to positively identify any teratogen targeted at events in the embryo.

Primary Cell Cultures

A large variety of primary cell cultures could also be used to determine the tissue-specific effects of exposure to a chemical. In practice, the two primary cell cultures studied most extensively have been derived from embryonic limb mesenchymal cells and from midbrain neural cells from rat embryos (6,7). Both cell growth or general cytotoxicity and cell differentiation can be used as indicators of teratogenic potential. High-density limb cell cultures differentiate into chondrocytes with cartilage-specific, alcian blue staining proteoglycans (6,7). Differential inhibition of [^{3}H]thymidine incorporation into deoxyribonucleic acid (DNA) relative to [^{35}S]sulfate incorporation into proteoglycans has been used to indicate teratogenic potential. The inhibition of differentiation of micromass cultures of embryonic midbrain into neurons following exposure to a putative teratogen can also be determined both morphologically and biochemically (6). The advantage of such an approach is that the concentrations of the chemical or drug which inhibit differentiation can be compared to the concentrations that are cytotoxic. We might expect that true developmental hazards should affect differentiation at concentrations below those necessary to produce general cytotoxicity. Flint and Orton (6) reported in a blind trial that 93% of the teratogens tested were correctly identified as teratogens, and that 89% of the nonteratogens were identified as nonteratogenic. With several exceptions, most chemicals caused a very similar degree of inhibition of limb and brain differentiation in vitro. As for the mouse ovarian cell line system, it has been possible to add a metabolic-activating system to these assays to permit the detection of teratogens requiring metabolic activation (6).

There are both advantages and disadvantages associated with the use of primary cell culture systems as compared to cell lines in any widespread screening procedure. The primary cultures are closer to an in vivo situation in that the cells are freshly obtained from an embryo. However, reproducibility and variability may be more of a problem with primary cell cultures than with established cell lines, especially when many laboratories are attempting to replicate the same experiments.

Organ Cultures

To go from an in vitro cell culture system to a pregnant animal is obviously a huge step. One of the intermediate stages, the isolated organ culture system, has also been evaluated for its relevancy to teratogenicity testing. In an organ culture system, in addition to growth and cell differentiation, tissue organization occurs. The organ culture system used most extensively to study teratogenicity in vitro is the limb bud culture system (11,12). Rodent limbs, usually mouse, are explanted on day 11 or 12 of gestation and cultured in chemically defined medium (13) or medium supplemented with fetal bovine serum for periods of from 6 to 9 days (11). The limbs can be grown in a static system on a filter paper or other support or submerged in a rotating roller bottle culture system. An example of mouse limbs excised on day 12 of gestation and cultured in roller bottles for 6 days in BGJ medium supplemented with fetal calf serum is shown in Figure 1.

During the culture period, the limbs undergo extensive morphological and biochemical differentiation, both of which can be quantitatively assessed. The morphological criteria of limb organogenesis include size and shape;

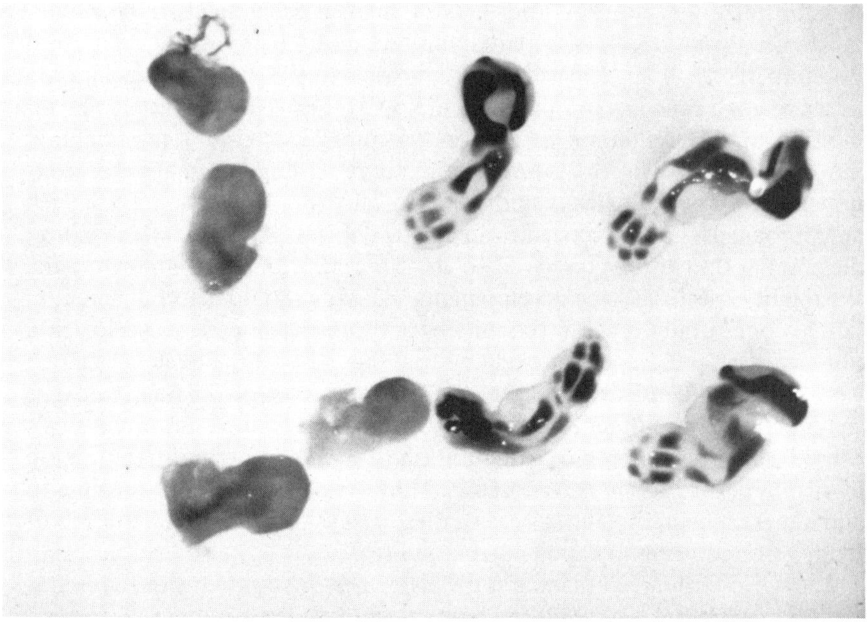

Figure 1 Mouse limb bud culture system. Mouse forelimb buds which were excised on day 12 of gestation are shown on the left. The forelimbs on the right were cultured for 6 days in roller bottles at 37 °C in 75% BGJ medium, 25% fetal calf serum. The limbs were fixed and stained with toluidine blue.

these are frequently evaluated using either a scoring system or image analysis (14,15). The anlagen of the major bones are usually recognizable, but distal anlagen may be missing or greatly distorted, depending on the stage of the embryo from which the buds are explanted. The biochemical criteria of limb development include DNA, ribonucleic acid (RNA), and protein content. Enzymatic activities such as creatine phosphokinase can be measured to assess muscle-specific development, or alkaline phosphatase to assess prebone formation (16,17). The syntheses of tissue-specific collagens and sulfated proteoglycans also serve as biochemical markers of differentiation (18). Some of these "markers" can be measured with easy spectrophotometric assays or localized in the limb histochemically or immunohistochemically.

At this time, limb bud culture procedures have still not been widely standardized. Development of the limb in vitro is still quite variable, depending on the stage of the embryo from which it was explanted and the procedures which are used. However, the endpoints which can be assessed are varied and are becoming more quantitative and less subjective. The general usefulness of the limb bud culture procedure to screen teratogens will depend at least in part on the ability of laboratories to standardize the methodology. Another important consideration will be the ability to culture limbs from embryos at earlier stages of development when effects on long bone anlagen might be more apparent.

Whole Embryo Cultures

The next step is to expose a whole embryo in vitro to a suspect chemical teratogen. We now have fairly extensive experience with both nonmammalian and mammalian embryo culture procedures.

NonMammalian Embryo Cultures

The use of nonvertebrate embryos such as a hydra system (19) as well as nonmammalian embryos such as the chick embryo (20) and fish or frog embryos (21) in teratogenicity testing has received some consideration. The hydra system (19) is attractive because the dose of the test chemical causing toxicity in an adult hydra (A) is compared to that which is toxic to an artificial hydra embryo (D). Adult hydra cells are dissociated and pelleted to form the "artificial" hydra embryo, which will "regenerate" to reform an adult hydra. The ratio of A/D gives an indication of the potential teratogenic hazard of the chemical. A higher ratio would indicate selectively greater toxicity during development.

Chick embryos have also been used to screen for teratogens. In most instances, the suspect teratogen has been injected into the egg and the embryo removed later for evaluation. However, chick embryos can also be explanted during gastrulation and cultured for an additional 3 days in vitro in the presence or absence of chemicals to be screened (20).

A variety of fish embryos, including Japanese medaka and zebra fish, have been used to screen for developmental toxicants. One advantage of a number of fish embryos is the optical clarity of the egg, making observation of any drug effects on the embryo easy without arresting development. Another alternative, the frog embryo has also been studied. A frog embryo teratogenesis assay in *Xenopus* (FETAX) was developed by Dumont and coworkers (21). In this 4-day screening test normally developing *Xenopus* blastulae are exposed to chemicals in vitro and effects are evaluated at 24-h intervals. The numbers of live and dead embryos and of live malformed embryos are ascertained. The head-tail length of each embryo is also measured. Fish and *Xenopus* embryos have limited metabolic activation capabilities, but it has proven possible to add exogenous microsomal metabolizing systems to extend the spectrum of compounds which can be tested using these embryos (22).

Mammalian Embryo Cultures

In the mammalian embryo culture system first developed by New and his colleagues (23), rat or mouse postimplantation embryos are usually excised on day 9 or 10 (rat) or day 8 or 9 (mouse) of gestation, dissected free of decidua, and cultured with the yolk sac intact in a roller bottle system for 48-72 h in a medium containing entirely or largely rat serum. The embryos can be gassed with oxygen concentrations that are appropriate for their stage of development.

During the 2- or 3-day culture period the embryos undergo tremendous growth and differentiation. The embryos at the beginning of the culture period are usually early somite, whereas at the end of the culture they may have 30-45 somites. An example of a rat embryo excised on day 10 of gestation is shown in Figure 2a. The embryo in Figure 2b was cultured for 42 h. During the time in culture, the embryos turn and rotate, the neural tube closes, and the brain, heart, and other organs develop. Examples of a malformed rat embryo (exposed to phosphoramide mustard, an alkylating agent) and a littermate control embryo after culture for 42 h are shown in Figure 3. The major malformations observed in the treated embryo are in brain development, with the most striking being a blunted prosencephalon.

Both all-or-none and quantitative assessments can be made. The all-or-none parameters that are usually measured include the number of dead and live embryos and the number of malformed versus normal embryos. Morphological/quantitative criteria include yolk sac diameter, crown-rump length, head length, and number of somite pairs. A morphological score system developed by Brown and Fabro (24) makes use of 17 morphological features to "stage" embryonic development, aiding in the detection of retardation or dysmorphogenesis of specific organ systems.

The biochemical criteria that have been assessed include DNA, RNA, and protein content. Protein content has been shown to have a close logarithmic relationship with embryonic age (24). Additional criteria that have been determined in the whole embryos in culture include glucose metabolism, hemoglobin content, and ornithine decarboxylase activity (25,26).

It is obviously important to establish whether embryos in vitro respond in a manner similar to their in vivo response. In most respects, both morphological and biochemical development in vitro in these culture systems closely parallels that in vivo during the same time period (27,28). Significantly, when the effects of drug exposure for similar periods of time and in similar concentrations have been studied both in vivo and in vitro, it has been found that the malformations produced in vitro mimic those observed in vivo. Examples of compounds for which this type of comparison has been made include hydroxyurea (28,29), cadmium (29), and vitamin A (30).

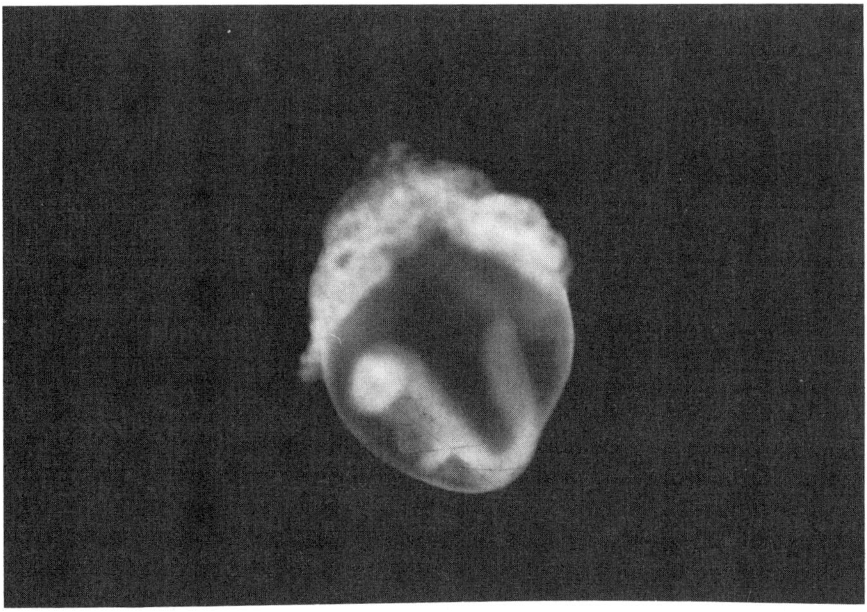

(a)

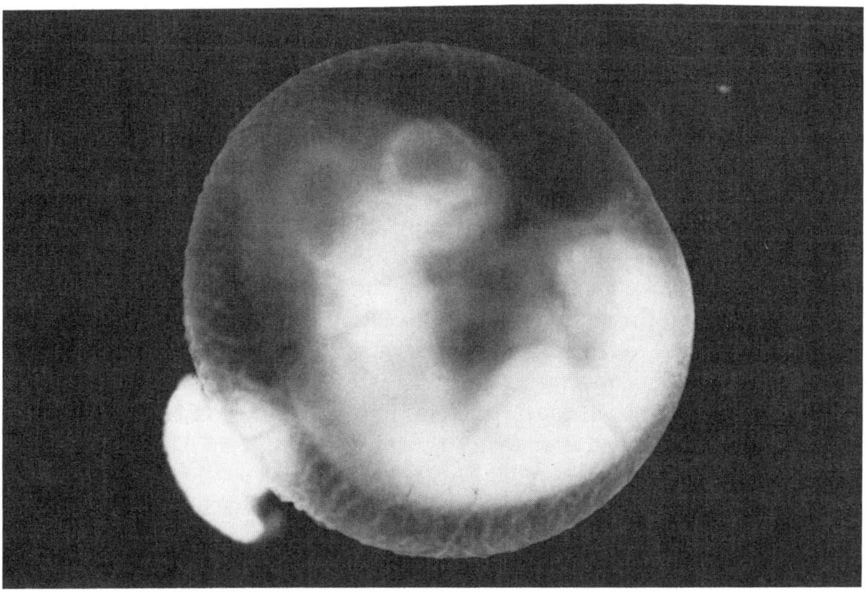

(b)

Figure 2 Rat whole embryo culture system. (a) A rat embryo was excised on day 10 of gestation and dissected free of decidua. Reichert's membrane has been folded back. (b) After excision on day 10 of gestation, this rat embryo was cultured in a roller bottle in 90% rat serum, 10% Tyrode's saline for 42 h at 37°C.

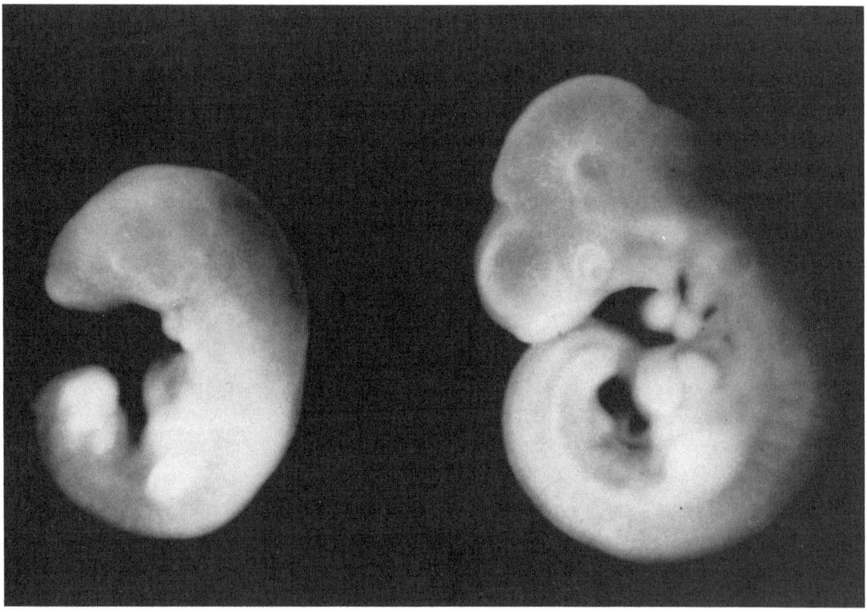

Figure 3 Effect of phosphoramide mustard on a rat embryo in culture. The rat embryo on the left was cultured for 42 h in a roller bottle in the presence of 10 μM phosphoramide mustard. The embryo on the right is a littermate control embryo, cultured in the absence of drug.

Although we now know that the rodent embryo in culture does have some drug-metabolizing capacity, this is relatively limited (31). A number of drugs known to require metabolic activation to be teratogenic are not very effectively activated in the embryo during the culture period. An increase in the ability of the embryos to metabolize chemicals, or the addition of an adult metabolic-activating system, greatly increases the sensitivity and general usefulness of the embryo culture system. Faced with this observation, most investigators have added exogenous sources of drug-metabolizing enzymes, usually from induced male rat liver (32). Alternatively, the embryos have been cocultured with whole hepatocytes (33).

ADVANTAGES/DISADVANTAGES OF THE CURRENT IN VITRO TEST SYSTEMS

Each of the approaches outlined above has some advantages as well as disadvantages. First, in all instances, the effects observed are on a cell or tissue which is either a component of or representative of an embryo, but not of the mother or maternal system. Thus, these in vitro techniques may not be useful in the detection of teratogens targeted at a component of maternal homeostasis. In general, the cell culture systems which make use of established cell lines have the advantage that the biological component of the system is relatively simple and reproducible. It may be feasible to use chemically defined medium and thus limit the confounding factors that are a consequence of using serum from different sources. If necessary, the chemical can be added in a solvent whose effects are minimal or at least have been characterized. In primary cell culture systems, many of these advantages are still maintained, although the biological component may now be more variable. In the cell culture systems the endpoint of chemical or drug exposure which is measured is at the "cellular" level. These endpoints include cell cytotoxicity or effects on cell attachment, cell proliferation, cell communication, or cell differentiation.

The next step in increasing the complexity of the biological component of the test system is to use a whole organ such as in the limb bud culture system. In this system, it has proven possible to use a chemically defined medium, and it is also possible now to add a metabolic-activating system (34). Endpoints of tissue/organ-specific differentiation and organization can be used to attempt to "integrate" the effect of a chemical on the organ. The relationship between any effect of a chemical in vivo and in vitro, e.g., in causing limb reduction malformations, is quite evident. A disadvantage is that not all teratogens will affect one specific organ; e.g., cause any form of limb malformation. In addition, the timing or stage at which the limbs can be cultured and examined is limited to a fairly narrow window.

The most complex system is obviously one where a whole embryo serves as the biological component. To some extent it is possible to take advantage of the complexity of this "biological component" by using littermate control embryos. The endpoints in a whole embryo culture system are much closer to those usually assessed in vivo, i.e., a visible structural malformation. Presumably, all the steps involved in the production of a malformation in vivo also occur during development in vitro, and are thus available to be affected by a teratogenic drug present in the culture system. However, as the size of the embryo increases, the length of time during which normal development can be maintained in vitro becomes shorter. Thus, the events which can be observed in many embryo culture systems are limited to a relatively narrow developmental period. It is also a disadvantage that it has not yet proven possible to grow whole embryos without a substantial amount of serum in the medium.

The scientific basis of any teratogenicity test is of great importance. However, until we have a greater understanding of the basic mechanisms of normal as well as abnormal development, we still do not know what events are critical and must be included. One of the criteria that seems important is that the system be capable of differentiation. Ideally, one should like to have an indication of the toxicity during development or differentiation and be able to compare this to the same system or cells not undergoing differentiation. Such a concept has been developed for the hydra test system (19), but it is more difficult to do this comparison for some of the other systems.

The most practical teratogenicity test system would be rapid, reproducible, inexpensive, and technically easy to perform. Obviously the cell culture approach is more likely to meet most of these criteria than a whole organ or limb approach. On the other hand, the ideal test will also involve all the processes in development which are likely to be susceptible to interference by a teratogen. It may be that this will be more feasible in a whole organ or embryo culture system than in an isolated cell culture system. Thus, it seems unlikely that any one system will be ideal in every context. It is more likely that a battery of tests will be developed, perhaps representing a variety of the different options outlined above.

FUTURE RESEARCH GOALS

A large variety of chemicals and drugs have now been tested in vitro in many of the tests outlined above. In fact, a list of candidate compounds for validation of in vitro teratogenicity test systems was compiled by a 1983 Consensus Workshop on In Vitro Teratogenicity Testing. In a review by Faustman (35) the results of in vitro teratogenicity tests with many of these compounds is tabulated. One of the goals in the future is to standardize a few of the test systems sufficiently to permit multilaboratory validation studies. It is now obvious that such studies should take into consideration the in vivo pharmacokinetics of the chemical and pattern of exposure in vitro. Dose-response relationships in vivo and in vitro will also have to be considered.

An important development in the establishment of useful in vitro teratogenicity tests has been the inclusion of drug-metabolizing enzyme systems. These systems have not yet been well characterized and are not standardized. The systems studied to date have been primarily from the livers of rats pretreated with inducing chemicals. Alternate sources (such as maternal liver) and species (human, primate), perhaps more representative of the human conceptus during periods of susceptibility to chemical insult, need to be considered (36). More information is now available on the individual enzymes and pathways involved in the metabolism of certain drugs and it may be desirable in some circumstances to "tailor" the activating system by using reconstituted or purified enzyme systems for specific chemical or drug families.

Species differences in susceptibility to the action of a teratogen have been an important consideration for in vivo teratogenicity testing. The classic example of a teratogen with species differences in susceptibility to its action is thalidomide (37), but other more recent examples where such differences also exist include 13-cis retinoic acid (38). If such species differences are due to species differences in drug handling and/or metabolism, rather than intrinsic differences in the sensitivity of the embryo, an in vitro test might circumvent these differences. We would then have a sound scientific basis on which to extrapolate from the animal test species to humans; this would be a major breakthrough for human hazard analysis. Preliminary experiments have been done to test this hypothesis using the rat whole embryo culture system and adding an extraembryonic (maternal liver) drug-metabolizing enzyme system from a variety of different species (monkey, rabbit, rat, and hamster (36)). The chemicals which have been tested to date are 2,4,5-trichlorophenoxyacetic acid, acetylsalicylic acid, diazepam, and thalidomide (36,39). The results obtained demonstrate that the in vitro embryolethality and teratogenicity of drugs that are subject to biotransformation can be modified by the addition of the extraembryonic drug-metabolizing enzyme systems, and, importantly, that there are species differences with respect to the effects of these enzyme fractions.

CONCLUSIONS

While there is still no one ideal in vitro teratogenicity test, there are a number of promising alternatives to whole animal screening procedures. It seems likely that the use of a combination or battery of in vitro test procedures, perhaps including one cell culture system, an organ culture system, and one whole embryo culture system, will be necessary at present to encompass all the possible chemical or drug targets during development. The real breakthrough may be that the use of such a battery of test procedures may minimize the "jump" from animal to man, thereby not only replacing whole animal testing, but actually greatly improving on the whole animal teratogenicity tests.

ACKNOWLEDGMENTS

The authors'a laboratory is supported by the Medical Research Council of Canada.

REFERENCES

1. Braun, A. G., Nichinson, B. B., and Horowicz, P. B. (1982). Inhibition of tumor cell attachment to concanavalin A-coated surfaces as an assay for teratogenic agents: Approaches to validation. *Teratogenesis Carcinog. Mutagen* **2**: 343-354.

2. Braun, A. G., Buckner, C. A., Emerson, D. J., and Nichinson, B. B. (1982). Quantitative correspondence between in vivo and in vitro activity of teratogenic agents. *Proc. Natl. Acad. Sci. U.S.A.* **79**: 2056-2060.
3. Pratt, R. M., Grove, R. I., and Willis, W. D. (1982). Prescreening for environmental teratogens using cultured mesenchymal cells from the human embryonic palate. *Teratogenesis Carcinog. Mutagen* **2**: 313-318.
4. Pratt, R. M., Willis, W. D. (1985). An in vitro screening assay for teratogens using growth inhibition of human embryonic cells. *Proc. Natl. Acad. Sci. U.S.A.* **82**: 5791-5794.
5. Mummery, C. L., Van den Brink, C. E., Van der Saag, P. T., and de Laat, S. W. (1984). A short-term screening test for teratogens using differentiating neuroblastoma cells in vitro. *Teratology* **29**: 271-279.
6. Flint, O. P., and Orton, T. C. (1984). An in vitro assay for teratogens with cultures of rat embryo midbrain and limb bud cells. *Toxicol. Appl. Pharmacol.* **76**: 383-395.
7. Paulsen, D. F. and Solursh, M. (1988). Microtiter micromass cultures of limb-bud mesenchymal cells. *In Vitro* **24**: 138-147.
8. Braun, A. G., Harding, F. A. and Weinreb, S. L. (1986). Teratogen metabolism: Thalidomide activation is mediated by cytochrome P-450. *Toxicol. Appl. Pharmacol.* **82**: 175-179.
9. Welsch, F., Stedman, D. B., Willis, W. D., and Pratt, R. M. (1986). Karyotype, growth, and cell cycle analysis of human embryonic palatal mesenchymal cells: relevance to the use of these cells in an in vitro teratogenicity screening assay. *Teratogenesis Carcinog. Mutagen* **6**: 383-392.
10. Welsch, F., and Stedman, D. B. (1984). Inhibition of intercellular communication between normal human embryonal palatal mesenchymal cells by teratogenic glycol ethers. *Environ. Health Perspect.* **57**: 125-133.
11. Kochhar, D. M. (1983). Embryonic organs in culture. In *Handbook of Experimental Pharmacology*. E. M. Johnson and D. M. Kochhar (Eds.). Springer-Verlag, Heidelberg, pp. 301-314.
12. Friedman, L. (1987). Teratological research using in vitro systems. II. Rodent limb bud culture system. *Environ. Health Perspect.* **72**: 211-219.
13. Lessmollmann, U., Hinz, N. and Neubert, D. (1976). In vitro system for toxicological studies on the development of mammalian limb buds in a chemically defined medium. *Arch. Toxicol.* **36**: 169-176.
14. Neubert, D., Hinz, N., Baumann, I., Barrach, H.-J., Schmidt, K. (1978). Attempt upon a quantitative evaluation of the degree of differentiation or the degree of interference with development in organ culture. In *Role of Pharmacokinetics in Prenatal and Perinatal Toxicology*. D. Neubert, H.-J. Merker, H. Nau, and J. Langman (Eds.). Georg Thieme, Stuttgart, pp. 337-349.
15. Kwasigroch, T. E., Skalko, R. G., and Church, J. K. (1984). Mouse limb bud development in submerged culture: quantitative assessment of the effects of in vivo exposure to retinoic acid. *Teratogenesis Carcinog. Mutagen* **4**: 311-326.
16. Hales, B. F., and Jain, R. (1986). Differential effects of 4-hydroperoxycyclophosphamide on limb development in vitro. *Teratology* **34**: 303-311.

17. Hales, B. F. (1989). Effects of phosphoramide mustard and acrolein, cytotoxic metabolites of cyclophosphamide, on mouse limb development in vitro. *Teratology* **40**: 11-20.
18. Barrach, H.-J., Grundmann, K., Hinz, N., and Felies, A. (1981). Comparison of the differentiation of muscle and connective tissue of mouse limb buds in culture and in vivo: A morphological study by indirect immunofluorescence. In *Culture Techniques. Applicability for studies on prenatal differentiation and toxicity*. D. Neubert and H.-J. Merker (Eds.). Walter de Gruyter, Berlin, pp. 135-159.
19. Johnson, E. M., Gorman, R. M., Gabel, B. E. G., and George, M. E. (1982). The Hydra-attenuata system for detection of teratogenic hazards. *Teratogenesis Carcinog. Mutagen* **2**: 263-276.
20. Kucera, P., and Burnand, M.-B. (1987). Routine teratogenicity test that uses chick embryos in vitro. *Teratogenesis Carcinog. Mutagen.* **7**: 427-447.
21. Dumont, J. N., Schultz, T. W., Buchanan, M., and Kao, G. (1983). Frog embryo teratogenesis assay: Xenopus (FETAX)—a short-term assay applicable to complex environmental mixtures. In *Symposium on the Application of Short-term Bioassays in the Analysis of Complex Environmental Mixtures III.* M. D. Waters, S. S. Sandhu, J. Lewtas, L. Claxton, N. Chernoff, and S. Nesnow (Eds.). Plenum Press, New York, pp. 393-405.
22. Fort, D. J., Dawson, D. A., and Bantle, J. A. (1988). Development of a metabolic activation system for the frog embryo teratogenesis assay: Xenopus (FETAX). *Teratogenesis Carcinog. Mutagen* **8**: 251-263.
23. New, D. A. T. (1978). Whole embryo culture and the study of mammalian embryos during organogenesis. *Biol. Rev.* **53**: 81-122.
24. Brown, N. A., and Fabro, S. (1981). Quantitation of rat embryonic development in vitro: a morphological scoring system. *Teratology* **24**: 65-78.
25. Huber, B. E., and Brown, N. A. (1982). Developmental patterns of ornithine decarboxylase activity in organogenesis phase rat embryos in culture and in utero. *In Vitro* **18**: 599-605.
26. Hunter, E. S., III, and Sadler, T. W. (1988). Embryonic metabolism of foetal fuels in whole embryo culture. *Toxicol. In Vitro* **2**: 163-167.
27. Cockroft, D. L. (1976). Comparison of in vitro and in vivo development of rat foetuses. *Dev. Biol.* **48**: 163-172.
28. Warner, C. W., Sadler, T. W., Shockey, J. and Smith, M. K. (1983). A comparison of the in vivo and in vitro response of mammalian embryos to a teratogenic insult. *Toxicology* **28**: 271-282.
29. Sadler, T. W., Shum, L., Warner, C. W., and Smith, M. K. (1988). The role of pharmacokinetics in determining the response of rodent embryos to teratogens in whole-embryo culture. *Toxicol. In Vitro* **2**: 175-180.
30. Steele, C. E., Trasler, D. G., and New, D. A. T. (1983). An in vivo/in vitro evaluation of the teratogenic action of excess vitamin A. *Teratology* **28**: 209-214.
31. Juchau, M. R., Giachelli, C. M., Fantel, A. G., Greenaway, J. C., Shepard, T. H. and Faustman-Watts, E. M. (1985). Effects of 3-methylcholanthrene and phenobarbital on the capacity of embryos to bioactivate teratogens during organogenesis. *Toxicol. Appl. Pharmacol.* **80**: 137-146.

32. Kitchin, K. T., Schmid, B. P. and Sanyal, M. K. (1981). Teratogenicity of cyclophosphamide in a coupled microsomal activating/embryo culture system. *Biochem. Pharmacol.* **30**: 59-64.
33. Oglesby, L. A., Ebron, M. T., Beyer, P. E., Carver, B. D., and Kavlock, R. J. (1986). Co-culture of rat embryos and hepatocytes: In vitro detection of a proteratogen. *Teratogenesis Carcinog. Mutagen.* **6**: 129-138.
34. Kastner, M., Blankenburg, G., Schulz, T., Schack, G., and Neubert, D. (1988). Activation of cyclophosphamide in mouse limb bud cultures using a reconstituted cytochrome P-450 system. *Arch. Toxicol.* **61**: 426-432.
35. Faustman, E. M. (1988). Short-term tests for teratogens. *Mutat. Res.* **205**: 355-384.
36. Hales, B. F. (1987). Incorporation of species differences in metabolism into in vitro teratogenicity testing. In *In Vitro Toxicology. Approaches to Validation.* A. M. Goldberg (Ed.). Mary Ann Liebert, New York, pp. 313-322.
37. Scott, W. J., Fradkin, R., and Wilson, J. G. (1977). Non-confirmation of thalidomide induced teratogenesis in rats and mice. *Teratology* **16**: 333-336.
38. Creech Kraft, J., Kochhar, D. M., Scott, W. J., and Nau, H. (1987). Low teratogenicity of 13-cis retinoic acid (Isotretinoin) in the mouse corresponds to low embryo concentrations during organogenesis: Comparison to the all-trans isomer. *Toxicol. Appl. Pharmacol.* **87**: 474-482.
39. Hales, B. and Jain, R. (1987). Species differences in the effects of drug metabolizing enzymes on the teratogenicity of thalidomide in rat embryo cultures. *Teratology* **35**: 73A.

10

Carcinogenicity: The Use of Animal Models and Short-Term Predictive Tests

David J. Brusick

Hazleton Washington, Inc.
Vienna, Virginia

BACKGROUND

The volatile history of using either animal models or predictive short-term tests to identify potential human carcinogens testifies to the inherent difficulties in accomplishing this goal. There are several characteristics of human carcinogenesis that contribute to the underlying difficulties. These include the fact that human cancers have been described as a collection of related but distinctly different diseases with different etiologies (1). For example, certain adult leukemias have been associated with long-term environmental exposures to cancer-causing agents, whereas the childhood leukemias observed from ages 2-6 would certainly resist such an explanation. Other complicating factors include the lack of definitive mechanisms involved in the initiation of human cancers and the complexities arising from the fact that predisposition for some cancers is inherited (2-4). Classification of chemicals as "known" or "presumed" human carcinogens is based on an assessment system heavily dependent on human epidemiology which is constrained by the difficulties of identifying suitable exposed and control populations. This limits the identification of human carcinogens to only a subset of all agents making up the true prevalence spectrum (5).

However, as difficult as it might be from the practical standpoint, theoretically there are reasons to believe that accurate carcinogen identification of chemical carcinogens using in vivo and in vitro tests should be possible. The types of information leading to this conclusion include the demonstration that many, if not most, human tumors are clonal in origin and result from the expression of a single transformed cell (6). This observation argues for a single step (probably mutation) being common to all cancer processes. Molecular biology studies of normal and tumor cells have demonstrated that proto-oncogenes and tumor-suppressor genes, present in all cells, appear to influence the initiation, expression, and/or expansion of most human tumors following their activation by mutation, chromosome breakage, or gene amplification (7). Such data strongly suggest the existence of a common pathway among neoplasias and detection of these key events may serve as "cancer markers" readily identifiable in experimental animal models or in vitro tests. Consequently, the search continues for the test or group of tests which can reliably detect agents that under the appropriate exposure conditions will produce cancer in humans.

HUMAN CARCINOGENS

Through human use experience or accidental exposure approximately 30 agents (Table 1) have been linked with cancer in humans by the International Agency for Research on Cancer (IARC). For most, a mechanisms has not been defined, but based upon chemical class, molecular structure, and biological reactivity, the majority can be classified as deoxyribonucleic acid (DNA)-reactive, or genotoxic, carcinogens (8). Theoretically then, these chemicals could produce mutations in proto-oncogenes, or other genes affecting the expression of predisposed tumorigenesis, and they should also be detected using a battery of in vivo and/or in vitro tests measuring genotoxicity (8,9). The remaining chemicals classified as human carcinogens are generally not detectable in tests for genotoxicity and appear to act through diverse and not well-understood mechanisms. Some hormones and steroids, such as diethylstilbestrol and progesterone, possibly activate receptor-mediated cell proliferative processes in target organs (10). Other physical agents, such as asbestos, might be active via specific intracellular damage produced by uptake of fiber crystals (11), and carcinogenic metals have been postulated to interfere with the processes of DNA replication, transcription, and/or repair (12,13).

CURRENT STRATEGIES FOR CARCINOGEN IDENTIFICATION

There are four procedures used for the identification of agents that might produce cancer in humans. The first is human epidemiology. This approach, however, is not feasible for evaluating new products (chemicals) prior to release into the environment and has been accomplished for only a few chemicals already present in the environment. The three remaining methods are:

Table 1 Agents Classified by IARC as Human Carcinogens

Agent	Evidence for genotoxicity
1. 4-Amino biphenyl	+
2. Phenacetin	+
3. Azthioprene	+
4. Benzene	+
5. Benzidine	+
6. Bis (chloromethyl) ether	+
7. Chlornaphazine	+
8. Myleran	+
9. MOPP (combined	+
10. chemotherapy)[a]	
11. Chlorambucil	+
12. Mustard gas	+
13. 2-Naphthylamine	+
14. Soots, tars, oils	+
15. Treosulphan[a]	+
16. Vinyl chloride	+
17. Arsenic compounds	+
18. Asbestos	−
19. Chromium 6 compounds	+
20. Methoxalen TUV (PUVA)	+
21. Melphalan	+
22. Diethylstilbestrol	+
23. Conjugated estrogens[a]	−
24. Cyclophosphamide	+

[a]Chemicals for which adequate animal cancer results are unavailable.

Use of animal models
Use of in vitro and in vivo predictive tests
Use of predictive structure activity (SAR) modeling

In the context of this chapter, a distinction is made between models and tests. A model reflects as much as possible all of the characteristics of the actual human disease. Most models for carcinogen assessment would consist of animals in which tumors, with similar histological features to human tumors, occur spontaneously and can be experimentally induced. A test predicts a toxicological phenomenon by monitoring a critical step in the disease process but does not produce responses which reflect clinical manifestations of the disease. A correllary to the definitions is that models should generally be "self-validating," whereas tests must be "validated" before being accepted, usually through correlative performance.

Use of Animal Models

Animal models, because of the characteristics described above, are considered to provide the most definitive carcinogen assessment of a chemical. Typical studies consist of continuous exposure of approximately 400 male and female mice to the test agent for 78 weeks or 104 weeks continuous exposure in male and female rats. Tumorigenicity of the test article is defined on the basis of gross necropsy examination for tumor masses and by extensive histopathological evaluations from a variety (~50) of tissues and organs. Tumor cell foci or lesions are identified, classified, and statistically analyzed against concurrent and historical control data. Several types of statistical analyses are used based upon the number of types of tumors found and the trend of survival over the duration of the study. The results may be presented as a qualitative assessment of carcinogenicity, or a quantitative risk assessment may be made if multiple dose levels are evaluated. Any sex/species combination showing an elevated tumor incidence operationally defines the agent as carcinogenic and is assumed to represent a potential human risk. Human risk estimates based on the animal data are generally derived from a linear extrapolation of the actual animal tumor incidences at the experimental exposure levels to the range of expected human exposures.

The limitations encountered with animal models touch on several critical parameters:

1. For certain types of human carcinogens, the rodents are not relevant models. For example, inhalation studies with two human carcinogens, asbestos or cigarette smoke, will generally not lead to cancer in rodents because of physiological and anatomical differences in the respiratory process between them and humans.
2. Both rodents and humans have genetically controlled predisposition to tumors, but there are significant target organ differences, resulting in some unique susceptibilities (e.g., liver tumors in some mouse strains, mammary tumors in some rat strains). Humans do not have similar high backgrounds for those two tumors. Risk assessments based upon the identification of chemical-induced rodent liver and mammary tumors in mice and rats, respectively, are therefore tenuous, at best.
3. Metabolic, detoxification, compound distribution, and tissue deposition differences between human and nonhuman animal models result in the production of false-positive and false-negative responses. It has been estimated that the false-negative rate in either the mouse or the rat is near 80% for human carcinogens (14), and although it cannot be quantified, there is every reason to suspect a false-positive rate as well (14,15). Phenobarbital, Na saccharin, and DDT are carcinogenic in rodent models, but extensive human exposures have produced no indication of induced cancer.

4. Tumorigenicity appears to be highly correlative with toxicity, which results in study designs with a limited number of dose levels of which all are skewed toward the maximum tolerated dose. Consequently, responses in rodents are obtained at doses which provide very little knowledge of the true induction kinetics expected at the low doses typical of those to which humans might be exposed.

Use of Short-Term Predictive Tests

The development of predictive tests began to receive serious consideration with the maturation of the *Salmonella* reverse mutation assay by Ames and coworkers in 1973 (16). The critical step in this development occurred when it was demonstrated that an in vitro metabolic activation system prepared from rodent hepatic microsomes and required cofactors for oxidative metabolism could be added to the test and would activate aromatic amine and polycyclic hydrocarbon carcinogens to mutagenic intermediates (17,18). The initial correlative performance of 80-95% (Table 2) that the test gave for established animal carcinogens was striking (19), and coupled with its low

Table 2 Changes in the Concordance Between the Ames Test and Rodent Cancer Results from 1973 to 1987

Study	Year	No. clients evaluated	Concordance sens./spec.		Compound selection	Samples coded
McCann et al. (31)	1975	300	90	87	Investigator Selected	No
Sugimura et al. (32)	1976	241	93	77	Investigator Selected	No
Purchase et al. (33)	1978	120	91	93	Investigator Selected	No
Anderson et al. (57)	1979	221	90	100	Investigator Selected	No
Rinkus and Legator (58)	1979	271	77	NA	Literature Search	-
National Cancer Institute (NCI) (59)	1984	59	78	67	Committee Selected	Yes
Environmental Protection Agency (EPA) GeneTox (60)	1986	154	80	67	Literature Search	-
National Toxicology Program (NTP) (20)	1987	73	45	86	Committee Selected	Yes

cost, short duration, and flexibility, the test provided instant appeal to most testing laboratories and to governmental regulatory agencies.

Enthusiastic acceptance of the Ames test in the early 1970s triggered the development and introduction of a large number of other in vitro or submammalian short-term tests assumed to be useful for carcinogen identification (Table 3). During the rapid expansion phase in the mid-1970s, short-term (in vitro) predictive testing eclipsed animal testing in general notoriety. A large in vitro chemical database was very quickly built, and by 1983 or 1984 most chemicals that had been tested in conventional carcinogenicity tests using rodents had a corresponding database in one or more of the short-term tests. Contrary to what had been experienced, based on the early correlation testing (1973-1975), recent comparisons of the responses between the rodent and short-term studies shown in Table 2 failed to continue to find good qualitative agreement across most classes of chemicals (20-22). There have been several attempts to explain the shift (24,30) but some influence certainly resides with the selection process for the chemicals tested and the use of coded samples. The relationship between the results of rodent models and short-term tests suggested that carcinogen/mutagen agreement was highest when electrophic agents predominated in the chemicals selected for validation (i.e., agents capable of forming covalent DNA adducts); however, there was a sizable group of rodent carcinogens that were not readily identified in tests commonly used for genotoxicity (Table 4). This group of agents was considered to represent a composite of the substances acting primarily through nongenotoxic mechanisms. Yet another group of chemicals can be defined which are positive in at least one short-term test but failed to induce tumors when tested in the rodent models (Table 5). These agents are considered false-positive results and have raised the concern that potentially

Table 3 Examples of the Range of Methods Used as Short-Term Tests for Detecting Animal Carcinogens

Test	Type of Event Detected	Organism
Mouse lymphoma assay	Point mutation	CL
Rat hepatocyte DNA repair	Unscheduled DNA synthesis	PC
Balb/c 3T3	Morphological cell cell transformation	CL
Sister chromatid exchange	Reciprocal exchange	0
Alkaline elution	Single/double strand DNA breakage	0
SOS induction	Prophage induction	PR
^{32}P-Post labeling	DNA adduct formation	0
Liver focus	Preneoplastic foci in Rat liver	M

Abbreviations: CL, cell line; PC, primary cell cultures; O, any intact cell from culture or primary tissue; PR, prokaryotic cells; M, intact mammalian species.

Table 4 Examples of Chemicals that Increase Tumors in Rodent Bioassays and Are Not Readily Detected in Short-Term Tests

Arsenic
Chloroform
Ethylene thiourea
Progesterone
PCBs (polychlorinated biphenyls)
Amitrole
Phenobarbital
DEHP (diethylhexylpthalate)
Heptachlor
Dieldrin
Carbon tetrachloride
Asbestos
DDT
2,3,7,8-TCDD
Aldrin
Diethylstilbestrol

Some of these chemicals have been screened in some short-term tests of limited use with reported positive results; however, they are generally negative in the routine short-term tests conducted in most toxicology facilities.

Table 5 Examples of Chemicals that Are Active in Several Short-Term Tests but Which Fail to Produce Cancer in Animal Models

Chemical	Positive in
Sodium ascorbate	Cytogenic assays, in vitro
4-Nitro-o-phenelyene diamine	Ames, SCE, *Drosophila* SLRL
1-Nitronaphtalene	Ames
3-Nitroproprionic acid	Ames
Sodium fluoride	Mouse lymphoma assay
Zearalenone	Cytogenetic assays, in vitro
Caffeine	Cytogenetic assays, in vitro
Methotrexate	Cytogenetic assay, in vitro; UDS
Methoxychlor	Cell transformation

For additional examples, see Ref. 61.

valuable new products might be incorrectly judged as potential human hazards by in vitro testing. The limitations associated with the use of short-term predictive tests can be summarized as:

1. False-positive results for chemicals not carcinogenic in rodents suggest a level of sensitivity which exceeds the animal models which are already believed by more than a few toxicologists to overpredict human susceptibility.
2. Chemicals identified as promotors or tumor enhancers in rodent models are not readily detected with the commonly employed short-term tests measuring genotoxicity.
3. Unlike the rodent models which may be viewed as a battery of two (or four, if one views each sex/species combination as a distinct assay), short-term tests are often used in combinations of four to six tests mixing both in vitro and in vivo techniques. Rodent data are considered positive if any sex/species group show increased numbers of tumors or a reduction in time-to-tumor. While no standard method of interpretation for short-term tests has ever been generally accepted, chemicals are not typically classified as mutagens on the basis of a single positive response among a group of mostly negative test results. This difference in data evaluation between short-term tests and rodent bioassays has resulted in confusion over just how mixed positive and negative results should be interpreted.
4. In vitro predictive tests appear to be particularly susceptible to false responses because the typical metabolic component of the assay (S9 mix) is unable to mimic metabolic transformations and detoxification produced in vivo.

While research activities to refine and strengthen the predictive performance of short-term tests measuring genotoxicity and cell transformation have been emphasized as a result of the correlation problems, additional efforts have been directed to the development and implementation of in vitro short-term tests that detect "key" steps in the secondary nongenotoxic pathways leading to tumor production. For example, an investigation with the phenomenon of cell-to-cell contacts via gap junctions has produced an assay which may be able to identify agents with promoting activity (23). Specific protein receptor molecules, mechanisms of DNA replication, initiation and transcription (gene amplification), peroxisome proliferation, and processes that regulate cell turnover are all being evaluated with the intent of understanding nongenotoxic mechanisms of carcinogenesis (24). At the present time, the number of "routine" assays available in this special area of predictive testing is very small, but continued research into mechanisms of promotion and carcinogenesis is expected to produce valuable technology in the near future.

Structure-Activity Relationship (SAR) Modeling

The identification of agents with carcinogenic activity through an analysis of their molecular structure has been a goal of biochemists for many years. It has been reasonably well documented that strong electrophiles are good candidates as mutagens and/or carcinogens, since they react readily with DNA (nucleophilic center). The initial products of these reactions, DNA adducts, result in DNA bases with alter hydrogen bonding properties or in apurinic sites, either of which might lead to mutation (25). Specific molecular configurations or functional groups are (1) directly associated with electrophilicity or (2) are indicative of susceptibility to oxidative metabolic processes resulting in the production of electrophilic metabolites (26). As more mechanistic knowledge is gained concerning mammalian carcinogenesis, other parameters of molecular structure will be defined and incorporated into SAR predictions. These parameters may be used to predict the ability to induce P448/P450 activity or the ability to stimulate DNA replication (cell proliferative changes). Structural similarities to nongenotoxic hormonal structures such as progesterone or estrogens may also be indicative of carcinogenic potential. Ashby (27) has described a set of "structural alerts" which he considers to be strongly associated with carcinogenic potential in rodents and mutagenic activity in the Ames test. Chemicals with one or more of these alerts are candidates for further evaluation in bioassays. Other SAR investigators rely upon the data-storage capacity of computers. Two excellent sources of sophisticated computer-based SAR information are available from (1) Case Western Reserve University and (2) Health Designs, Inc. Both groups have produced systems that are capable of identifying carcinogenic potential across several well-studied chemical classes (28,29). The basic approaches of the two systems are different. The CASE system relies on computer-derived probabilities of association with cancer generated from an analysis of molecular fragments constructed using sets of known carcinogens and noncarcinogens. A new chemical is broken into fragments and the computer searches to see if the fragments are positive or negative based on the existing data from known carcinogens. A probability is then calculated using the composite of fragment p values. The CASE system does not rely upon a set of traditional structural alerts but generates critical structural elements from the database. This approach should continue to improve in accuracy as the database grows.

The method used by Health Designs relies primarily on traditional key functional groups and complex molecular arrangements known to be associated with model carcinogens. The presence or absence of these key structures and their number determine the probability of carcinogenicity. Both systems use computers which have the capability of on-line direct access to the SAR procedure. The limitations associated with the use of SAR to predict carcinogens include:

1. All information used by the computer software to establish SAR predictions is derived from existing biological test results. Thus, the quality and reliability of the test results and the true accuracy of the tests used to develop the database from which the SAR method is developed will strongly influence the reliability of the SAR prediction. Concern has been expressed by toxicologists that much of the laboratory data supporting the SAR calculations is itself flawed.
2. Experience has shown that extrapolation of biological activity based on similarities in molecular structure, common functional groups, or "structural alerts" cannot be assured. The power and reliability of SAR approaches will improve with greater mechanistic understanding and with larger and more heterogeneous databases supporting the technology and with artificial intelligence programs that can learn from the data input and produce SAR predictions with accuracy exceeding the quality of input test results.

QUALITATIVE PREDICTIVITY OF THE MODELS AND TESTS

Because the human carcinogen database is small and limited only to positive responses, nonhuman animal models have necessarily formed the standard in making regulatory and risk decisions for human populations. The consequences of this approach and the manner in which it has been implemented in toxicological assessments for chemicals has had profound effects on the evaluation and use of short-term predictive tests.

The animal carcinogen database, for all intents, consists of results from two rodent species, the mouse and the rat, and both sexes (Fig. 1). Based on the EPA Genetox work group report on animal carcinogenesis published in 1988, reliable data for approximately 413 chemicals exists (43). Approximately 85% of the chemicals in this database were found to be carcinogens based on tumor findings in at least 1 species/sex subset (Table 6). Results produced by short-term tests from their respective work group reports also showed a relatively high proportion of positive to negative results (Table 6). This situation, especially for data published in the 1970s, resulted from a preference to publish positive findings. The consequence, however, was a database highly biased that in turn produced a high degree of positive correlation between the rodent cancer tests and results of short-term tests. The results could be due to chance just as well as by a true mechanistic association between the phenomena of tumor initiation and mutation.

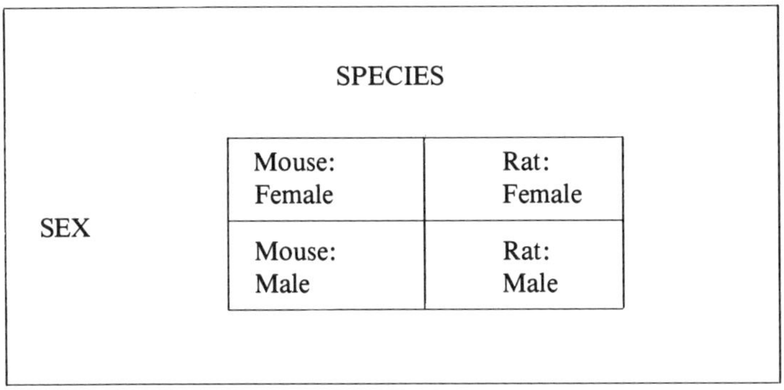

Figure 1 Chemicals may be classified as carcinogens by demonstrating increased tumor incidences in any of the four sex/species quadrants shown. It is generally assumed that the greater the number of quadrants affected, the more likely the agent represents a carcinogen hazard to humans.

Table 6 Relative Distribution of Positive and Negative Agents Among Seven Types of Bioassays Reviewed Under the EPA GeneTox Program

	Chemicals with either sufficient negative or positive responses	Positive agents (%)	Negative agents (%)
Rodent cancer tests	413	351(85)	62(15)
Ames test	1262	820(65)	442(35)
Mouse lymphoma test	138	114(83)	24(17)
In vitro cytogenetics	116	81(70)	35(30)
Micronucleus test	63	60(95)	3(5)
Drosophila (SLRL)	345	238(69)	107(31)

A high degree of association for positive responses for a chemical would be predicted on the basis of random association alone from such biased data sets.

The pattern of effects across the four quadrants of Figure 1 for a given chemical is influenced by the potency and carcinogenic mechanism of the agent and the existence of genetically determined susceptibilities in the target species. The more generalized the response (i.e., number of quadrants affected), the more likely the carcinogenic risks would be extrapolated to other species. It can be seen, then, that the animal cancer results generated for chemicals are derived from four distinct but related species/sex sources. Developing a single short-term predictive test that will accurately reflect the range of animal results possible is not only formidable but probably impossible.

Analyses of several data sets indicate that a test, such as the Ames test, might respond favorably to a single species/sex, either the mouse or the rat, but it will do no better than about 70% in predicting the combined species results for a broad spectrum of chemicals. This probably should not be surprising, since 70% is the approximate level of agreement for chemical carcinogens in mice and rats (30). Early reports by McCann et al. (31), Sugimura et al. (32), and Purchase et al; (33), suggesting correlations exceeding 80%, resulted because the sets of chemicals selected for these studies were probably biased by the inclusion of a high proportion of chemicals where mouse and rat concordance exceeded the 70% level (i.e., positive responses in most of the quadrants of Fig. 1) observed in most recent analyses.

Correlation studies with a broader distribution of chemical classes (see Table 2) produced concordance values in the 60-70% range (20-22). Evaluation of chemicals moved from individual tests to groups of tests (batteries) in the hope that one test might compensate for the deficiency of another.

The use of multiple short-term tests in batteries has thus far failed to improve the correlations because the events detected by these tests involved a single (DNA) target, and thus most commonly used tests proved to be confirming tests rather than complementary (20).

It appears that the requirements for successful prediction of animal carcinogens by short-term tests are:

1. Tests must cover both genotoxic and nongenotoxic mechanisms of carcinogenicity and should be truly complementary.
2. Tests must compensate for genetically determined differences in metabolism, endocrine function, and DNA repair of the rodent species used to detect carcinogens.

Thus, it is clear that one of the most important areas for additional activities in test development is that focused on tests for nongenotoxic cancer mechanisms.

QUANTITATIVE PREDICTIVITY

Even recognizing that at the current state-of-the-art short-term tests are not fully capable of reproducing all of the responses from animal models, several classes of animal carcinogens are predicted quite accurately with short-term tests. This group consists of direct alkylating initiating agents (i.e., nitrosoguanidine, methymethane sulfonate, β-propriolactone, etc.), and some classes of complete carcinogens, including polycyclic aromatic hydrocarbons, aromatic amines, and nitrosamines.

An important question raised relative to the use of short-term tests has been the extent to which short-term tests that accurately identify carcinogen potential can also define the relative potency of the carcinogens for animals. Several attempts to demonstrate that potency of animal carcinogens could be predicted by short-term tests produced results very similar to the results of the qualitative correlation studies:

1. For small structurally biased groups of chemicals, an association between animal carcinogenicity (TD50) and the activity of in vitro test results has been demonstrated (34,35). However, as the composition of the chemical group becomes more representative of the universe of chemicals in the environment, the relationship falls apart (36).
2. While some attempts have been offered by McCann et al. (36) and by Gold et al. (55), it has been difficult to define what is meant by potency, either in the animal cancer studies or the short-term tests. Without a clear and precise understanding of potency, comparisons are not very meaningful.
3. Agreement between animal species and sexes for potency is not very good, making it virtually impossible for a short-term test to be compared generically to "animal cancer" data.

On a broader scale, it has been hypothesized, with some very good supporting evidence, that animal cancer potency is tied very tightly to the acute toxicity of the carcinogen and that potency can be quite accurately predicted from simple acute toxicity (LD_{50}) data (37). This observation may be important in developing and interpreting comparisons between animal carcinogenicity and mutagenicity data, since the association between toxicity and mutagenic potency is also very strong.

Except for some very special exceptions, toxicity alone is probably insufficient to produce either cancer or mutation. These latter two phenomena are initiated by other parameters of the molecules (i.e., electrophilicity, receptor binding, etc.).

There appear, however, to be some special situations where toxicity per se may lead to genotoxicity and to cancer. False-positive responses for cancer and mutagenesis have been observed under treatment conditions of high dose levels of presumed nontoxic chemicals. Sodium saccharin, for example, produces bladder tumors in male rats at 1% in the diet and higher. Sodium saccharin also produces chromosome damage in vitro (aberrations and SCEs) at relativity high concentrations where the osmolality exceeds 400 mOs/kg (38,39). At lower levels, no tumors or genetic damage are observed, suggesting the presence of a common type of toxicity threshold. The link between these two phenomena appears to be the biological activity produced by the associated sodium ions. Sodium ions may be capable of destabilizing DNA in mammalian cells in a manner that leads to chromosomal aberrations, which might then initiate the tumor process. This hypothesis is supported by results from tests using acid saccharin (no sodium ions present) where there is no evidence of genotoxicity with in vitro tests or pretumorigenic activity in male rat bladder tissue (39). The type of toxicity produced by Na^{2+} ions in cells exposed to high concentrations may lead to cancer and genotoxicity experimentally but probably has little relevance to human health.

ROLE OF SHORT-TERM TESTS IN CARCINOGEN TESTING

Short-term methods, particularly in vitro assays, will play a very significant role in a toxicological evaluation of chemicals for cancer induction, primarily because most chemicals released into or found in the environment cannot be assessed by either human epidemiology or with expensive animal models. Thus, nonanimal tests can contribute valuable biological information regarding the genotoxic and carcinogenic potential of agents.

Other roles for short-term tests are those of human monitors and dosimeters. When chemicals known to be animal carcinogens are found in the environment (e.g., formaldehyde, ethylene oxide, EDB), issues of quantitative risk must be considered. Human populations with potential exposure to such agents can be monitored for both qualitative and quantitative DNA damage using techniques such as chromosome breakage determined from cytogenetic analyses of peripheral blood lymphocyte cultures as well as DNA and protein adducts in lymphocytes or hemoglobin (40). The availability of this data is extremely important in (1) defining precisely the exposed populations, (2) calculating the levels of exposure at probable target sites, and (3) identifying hypersusceptible subpopulations. Such data will result in more accurate risk assessments by clarifying the degree of extrapolation of animal test results to human populations over a range of exposure levels (41).

GENERAL STRATEGY FOR TEST DEVELOPMENT

At the present time, there are no fixed guidelines for the selection of short-term tests or the interpretation of their results relative to cancer prediction.

Various federal programs in short-term test "validation" were initiated with the hope of being able to recommend a test battery that would work for all, or at least most, chemical carcinogens that had been detected in rodents. Two of these which have been most visible were established by EPA (Gene-Tox Program) and NTP (Chemical Testing Program). The GeneTox Program consisted of a retrospective analysis of published data from apporoximately 100 different tests (42). The results were compiled and then compared to carcinogenic activity in animals. The NTP program consisted of an assessment of in vitro (and limited in vivo) test performance (conducted with coded samples) on agents previously tested by NTP in mice and rats. The results of these two programs were presented at a conference held in Williamsburg, Virginia, in 1987.

The findings indicated that results from neither program were sufficient to produce a test battery that would satisfy sensitivity, specificity, and predictive requirements for a general test battery (20,43). There were several issues affecting the development of a battery for carcinogens that could not be resolved:

The database composition of the GeneTox Program was largely filled with positive effects. This tended to result in most tests showing high sensitivity and high predictivity but unacceptable specificity. Often the distribution of chemical classes across the various tests evaluated was not good, and the few tests that showed good specificity had significantly underpopulated databases.

The NTP Program selected a more chemically diverse set of chemicals. The results from the four in vitro assays selected (Ames test, Mouse Lymphoma Assay, in vitro SCE, and aberration analyses in cultured CHO cells) failed to demonstrate test complementation or acceptable ratios of sensitivity/specificity. The absence of complementation was totally unexpected. It was also clear from the NTP Program that a significant subset of the chemicals tested were nongenotoxic carcinogens, and that a test battery without provisions to detect this group of chemicals would never achieve the required levels of sensitivity and specificity.

Following the Williamsburg Conference, efforts were initiated or refocused in an attempt to find alternatives to the empirical correlation-based battery development.

CPBS, the Carcinogenicity Prediction and Battery Selection Method, was developed at Case Western Reserve University in 1984 (44). This software uses a statistical approach to take results from the existing databases of short-term tests and construct an optimal battery for a given testing situation and/or chemical class. Using the CPBS, Ennever and Rosenkranz (45) claimed to have generated a test battery that would have provided a better overall prediction for carcinogens and noncarcinogens among the chemicals in the NTP Program than was provided by the four in vitro tests selected.

Ashby and Tennant (46,47) proposed the combined use of structural analysis and minimal genotoxicity testing for assessing rodent carcinogens. Using only structural alerts and results from the Ames test, a high predictivity was obtained for genotoxic carcinogens among 222 chemicals tested in rodents. These results were interpreted as support for the need of a single (Ames) mutagenicity test.

Shelby (8) reported that based on the results from a limited data set the battery of an Ames test combined with in vivo cytogenetic analysis was highly predictive for rodent carcinogens when both short-term tests were positive. Negative results in both tests were associated with noncarcinogenicity. This test battery appeared, therefore, to be not only accurate but also fitted the general testing pattern of regulatory requirements being set up in most developing countries (i.e., one test for gene mutation in bacteria and a test for clastogenicity).

The inclusion of an in vivo test is generally considered essential to raise the correlation coefficient. More recent updates of this test battery, however, have failed to confirm its preliminary level of accuracy (M.D. Shelby, personal communication).

The Reverse Tier approach proposed by Legator (48) is also based upon the assumption that a screening program must include in vivo short-term tests to generate high degrees of predictivity for animal carcinogens. The Reverse Tier screening procedure starts with rodent species and involves the evaluation of multiple genotoxic and nongenotoxic endpoints in the animals exposed to the test agent. In vitro tests are employed subsequent to in vivo tests in an attempt to determine a mechanistic basis for the response of positive chemicals.

In the short term, it is very unlikely that any of these alternatives will provide a satisfactory solution and become generally adopted. Underlying all of the efforts that have gone into the development of in vitro predictive tests for carcinogens are some issues that must be resolved in order to achieve progress in this area of toxicology. For example, most applications of short-term tests utilize multitest batteries. A common battery in genetic toxicology would probably consist of the Ames test, a test for in vitro cytogenetics, a mouse micronucleus assay, and possibly additional tests for either forward mutation in cultured mammalian cells (TK or HGPRT) or a test for unscheduled DNA synthesis (UDS) conducted in primary rat hepatocytes. In the future, at least one assay covering nongenotoxic mechanisms will probably be added. The method of analysis of the composite responses from these assays is a weight-of-evidence approach that will accomodate the occasional outlier response (Fig. 2). The philosophy generally applied in animal carcinogenesis

Chemical: XYZ

Assay	Predictive Test Responses	Assay	Animal Cancer Bioassays
A	–	1	–
B	–	2	+
C	–	3	–
D	+	4	–
E	–	5	–
F	–	6	–
G	–	7	–
H	+	8	–
I	–		
J	–		
K	–		
Responses:	2 positive 9 negative	1 positive 7 negative	
Conclusion:	"Nongenotoxic"	Carcinogenic	

Figure 2 This figure contrasts the fundamental approaches to interpretation of multiple animal cancer studies and data from a battery of short-term predictive tests. A single positive response in any adequate animal test will result in a conclusion that the chemical is an animal carcinogen regardless of the number of negative studies in the same or other species. Interpretation of short-term studies is usually based on a weight-of-the-evidence which accommodates an occasional positive response.

is that evidence of increased tumors in any species/sex group is sufficient to operationally define the chemical as carcinogenic regardless of the number of negative species/sex combinations. The two distinct methods of interpreting multiple assay responses are incompatible and a more unified approach is needed before reasonable agreement can be expected.

FUTURE DIRECTIONS IN CARCINOGEN SCREENING

Except for human epidemiology studies, the other three methods employed to detect carcinogens are technically deficient to some degree and require extensive validation. The degrees of uncertainty for both are great.

The use of animal models, as they are currently configured, to screen all chemicals released into the environment is prohibitively expensive and time-consuming. Reliance entirely on in vitro technology cannot be totally justified today because of (1) technical limitations involved with exogenous in vitro metabolism, (2) the absence of "validated" tests for nongenotoxic carcinogenic mechanisms, and (3) the tendency to generate false-positive results by severe treatment conditions. Dramatic improvements in predicting carcinogenic potential during the past 10 years has been made by SAR modeling, but it still suffers from a dearth of knowledge concerning the steps involved in initiation, promotion, and expansion of tumors in animals.

Advances in technology are beginning to offer some resolution to the multitude of problems encountered in carcinogen screening. Several novel systems have been developed that should result in significant improvements in both animal models and predictive tests.

Animal Models

Activation of proto-oncogenes to oncogenes has been associated with the initiation of tumors in mammals, including humans. In 1988, Leder and Stewart (49) were granted a patent for a transgenic mouse that carries a human oncogene coupled with a mouse promotion region (MMTV). the presence of the oncogene already activated in the specific target cells of the transgenic oncomouse is expected to be more susceptible to chemical carcinogens than conventional mice, enabling studies to be conducted (1) at lower test concentration, (2) with fewer animals, and (3) for shorter periods. This model might well provide more mechanistic information about the molecular steps involved in tumor initiation and could substantially lower testing costs associated with the current animal carcinogen screening models. Transgenic mice engineered with other oncogenes or with DNA target sites for mutation analysis are also currently available for mechanistic studies (50). Some trangenic models for mutation have been shown to respond to a broad range of chemical agents (56).

In Vitro Tests

Shuttle vectors carrying a variety of gene constructs can be introduced into mammalian (including human) cells. These vectors have resulted in an explosive development of cell lines with new and potentially useful genotypes and phenotypes relative to carcinogen screening (51). Table 7 lists examples of the types of gene constructs that have been placed in cells and their proposed use.

Cell transformation assays have been used to detect potential carcinogens for at least 20 years (52). Their use has been most successful with polycyclic aromatic hydrocarbon and a few direct-acting carcinogens. Technical dif-

Table 7 Examples of the Use of Shuttle Vectors in Constructing Mammalian Cell Assays for Carcinogenesis

Type of gene construct	Application
Introduction of recoverable target genes	Mutagenesis of target gene in situ followed by recovery and analysis (i.e., sequencing, etc.)
Promotable oncogene (e.g. SV40 T antigen)	Determine mechanisms of oncogene activation in vitro and/or its role in cell transformation and population expansion (metastasia)
P448/450 genes with promotion region	Development of fibroblast cell lines with intrinsic metabolic enzymes capable of activating procarcinogens

ficulties associated with variable spontaneous backgrounds, sensitivity to specific media growth factor (e.g., serum), and poor laboratory-to-laboratory transferability have limited their use in routine testing. The problems cited above are compounded by difficulties with the use of S9 mix as a source of exogenous activation.

Several investigators have been working to solve many of the technical problems which have plagued these potentially promising methods. With cell transformation, for example, changes in media composition (53) and dose selection regimens (54) appear to have significantly improved their reproducibility and accuracy. Severe osmolality changes appear to modulate expansion of transformants in the Balb/c 3T3 cells and by setting the upper dose limit to 50 mOsm goods discrimination of carcinogens and noncarcinogenes has been obtained. Preliminary results with 66 chemicals (26 carcinogens and 40 noncarcinogens) showed the ability of the Balb/c 3T3 phenotype not only to match the results of rodent cancer tests (53), but it appears from this relatively small sample of chemicals, also tested in the Ames assay, that the Balb/c 3T3 test truly complements the Salmonella assay, meeting at least one of the essential criteria for a reliable in vitro test.

An additional feature of cell transformation tests is that they can respond to a wide range of rodent carcinogens believed to be nongenotoxic. This feature meets the second essential criteria for adequate in vitro tests.

CONCLUSIONS

Substantial time and resources have been devoted during the past 20 years to a search for reliable short-term tests able to identify animal and, presumed, human carcinogens. To date, the efforts have not produced a test or battery of tests which satisfy the necessary requirements. Reasons for this involve several areas:

1. Limited understanding of the full range of critical events involved in cancer initiation and tumor expression. Tests have been developed for some, but not all of the events.
2. Differences in the approaches to interpretation of animal cancer test results and data from short-term tests. Current methods almost assure a lack of concordance.
3. The lack of a validation standard for the rodent model so that an estimate of its false-positive and false-negative responses can be made.
4. Unavailability of in vitro tests which cover both genotoxic and nongenotoxic mechanisms and which truly complement each other across a range of chemical classes.

Research activities in the areas of in vitro cell transformation, in vitro cell line development using shuttle vectors and the development of transgenic animal models offer hope that short-term tests for carcinogens are not far from a reality.

REFERENCES

1. Peto, R. (1979). Detection of risk cancer to man. *Proc. R. Soc. Lond. B.* **205**: 111-120.
2. Mulvihill, J. J. (1977). Genetic repertory of human neoplasia. In *Genetics of Human Cancer.* J. J. Mulvihill, R. W. Miller, and J. F. Fraumeni, Jr. (Eds.). Raven Press, New York, pp. 137-143.
3. Xiaoping, Z., Dunn, J. M., Phillips, R. A., Goddard, A. D., Paton, K. E., Becker, A. and Gallie, B. L. (1989). Preferential germline mutation of the paternal allele in retinoblastoma. *Nature* **340**: 312-313.
4. Scott, D., and Heighway, J. (1986). Identification of individuals of risk: Cytogenetic and molecular methods. In *Genetic Toxicology of Environmental Chemicals,* Part B: *Genetic Effects and Applied Mutagenesis.* C. Ramel, B. Lambert, and J. Magnusson (Eds.). Liss, New York, pp. 205-212.
5. Ames, B. N. (1989). What are the major carcinogens in the etiology of human cancer? Environmental pollution, natural carcinogens, and the causes of human cancer: six errors. In *Important Advances in Oncology 1989.* V. T. DeVita, Jr., S. Hellman, and S. A. Rosenberg (Eds.). J. B. Lippincott, Philadelphia, pp. 237-247.
6. Falkow, P. J. (1977). Clonal origin and stem cell evaluation of human tumors. In *Genetics of Human Cancer.* J. J. Mulvihill, R. W. Miller, and J. F. Fraumeni, Jr. (Eds.). Raven Press, New York, pp. 439-453.
7. Barbacid, M. (1987). Mutagens, oncogenes and cancer. In *Oncogenes and Growth Factors.* R. A. Bradshaw and S. Prentis (Eds.). Elsevier, Amsterdam, pp. 90-99.
8. Shelby, M. D. (1988). The genetic toxicity of human carcinogens and its implications. *Mutat. Res.* **204**: 3-15.

9. Garrett, N. E., Stack, H. D., Gross, M. R., and Waters, M. D. (1984). An analysis of the spectra of genetic activity produced by known or suspected human carcinogens. *Mutat. Res.* **134**: 89-111.
10. Bern, H. A., Edery, M., Mills, K. T., Kohrman, A. F., Mori, T., and Larson, L. (1987). Long term alterations in histology and steroid receptor levels of the genital tract and mammary gland following neonatal exposure of female BALB/c Crgl mice to various doses of diethylstilbestrol. *Cancer Res.* **47**: 4167-4172.
11. Lechner, J. F., Tokiwa, T., LaVeck, M., Benedict, W. F., Banks-Schlegel, S., Yeager, Jr., H., Banerjee, A., and Harris, C. (1985). Asbestos-associated chromosomal changes in human mesothelial cells. *Proc. Natl. Acad. Sci., U.S.A.,* **82**: 3884-3888.
12. Kunkel, T. A., and Loeb, L. A. (1979). On the fidelity of DNA replication: Effect of divalent metal ion activators and deoxyribonucleotide triphosphate pools on in vitro mutagenesis. *J. Biol. Chem.* **254**: 5718-5720.
13. Sirover, M. A., and Loeb, L. A. (1976). Infidelity of DNA synthesis in vitro: Screening for potential metal mutagens or carcinogens, *Science* **194**: 1434-1436.
14. Lave, L. B., Ennever, F. K., Rosenkranz, H. S., and Omen, G. S. (1988). Information value of the rodent bioassay. *Nature* **336**: 631-633.
15. Purchase, I. F. H., and Paddle, G. M. (1989). Does formaldehyde cause nasopharyngeal cancer in man? *Cancer Lett.* **46**: 79-85.
16. Ames, B. N., Durston, W. E. Yamasaki, E., and Lee, F. D. (1973). Carcinogens are mutagens: A simple test system combining liver homogenates for activation and bacteria for detection. *Proc. Natl. Acad. Sci. U.S.A.* **70**: 2281-2285.
17. Ames, B. N., Sims, P., and Grover, P. L. (1972). Epoxides of polycyclic hydrocarbons are frameshift mutagens. *Science* **176**: 47-49.
18. Mukai, F. and Troll, W. (1969). The mutagenicity and initiating activity of some aromatic animal metabolites. *Ann. N.Y. Acad. Sci.* **163**: 828-834.
19. Brusick, D. J. (1983). Mutagenicity and carcinogenicity correlations between bacteria and rodents. In *Cellular Systems for Toxicity Testing.* G. M. Williams, V. C. Dunkel, and V. A. Ray (Eds.). New York Academy of Sciences, New York, pp. 164-176.
20. Tennant, R. W., Margolin, B. H., Shelby, M. D., Zeiger, E., Haseman, J., Spalding, W., Caspary, W., Resnick, M., Stasiewicz, S., Anderson, B., and Minor, R. (1987). Prediction of chemical carcinogenicity in rodents from in vitro genetic toxicity assays. *Science* **236**: 933-941.
21. Shelby, M. D., and Stasiewicz, S. (1984). Chemicals showing no evidence of carcinogenicity in long-term, two-species rodent studies: The need for short-term data. *Environ. Mutagen.* **6**: 971-878.
22. Lijinsky, W. (1989). A view of the relation between carcinogenesis and mutagenesis. *Environ. Mol. Mutagen.* **14**: 78-84.
23. Trosko, J. E., Chang, C. C., and Netzloff, M. (1983). Mechanisms of tumor promotion: Potential role of intercellular communication. *Cancer Invest.* **1**: 511-526.
24. Butterworth, B. E. (1989). Nongenotoxic carcinogens in the regulatory environment. *Reg. Toxicol. Pharmacol.* **9**: 244-256.
25. Kunkel, T., Shearman, C., and Loeb, L. (1981). *Nature* **291**: 349-351.

26. Miller, J. A., and Miller, E. C. (1977). Ultimate chemical carcinogens as reactive mutagenic electrophiles. In *Origins of Human Cancer.* H. H. Hiatt, J. D. Watson, and J. A. Winsten (Eds.). Cold Spring Harbor Laboratory, Cold Spring Harbor, New York, pp. 605-628.
27. Ashby, J. (1985). Fundamental structural alerts to potential carcinogenicity or non-carcinogenicity. *Environ. Mutagen.* **7**: 919-921.
28. Mitchell, C. S., Klopman, G., and Rosenkranz, H. S. (1986). In *Polynuclear Aromatic Hydrocarbons: Chemistry, Characterization and Carcinogenesis.* Ninth International Symposium. M. Cooke and A. J. Dennis (Eds.). Batelle Press, Columbus, Ohio, pp. 611-624.
29. Enslein, K. (1984). Estimation of toxicological endpoints by structure activity relationships. *Pharmacol. Rev.* **36**: 131S-135S.
30. Brockman, H. E., and DeMarini, D. M. (1988). Utility of short-term tests for genetic toxicity in the aftermath of the NTP's analysis of 73 chemicals. *Environ. Mol. Mutagen.* **11**: 421-436.
31. McCann, J., Choi, E., Yamasaki, E., and Ames, B. N. (1975). Detection of carcinogens as mutagens in the *salmonella*/microsome test: Assay of 300 chemicals. *Proc. Natl. Acad. Sci. U.S.A.* **72**: 5135-5139.
32. Sugimura, T., Sato, S., Nagao, M., Yakagi, T., Matsushima, T., Seino, Y. H., Takeuchi, M., and Kawachi, T. (1976). Overlapping of carcinogens and mutagens. In *Fundamentals in Cancer Prevention.* P. N. Magee, S. Takayoma, T. Sugimura, and T. Matsushima (Eds.). University Park Press, Baltimore, pp. 191-215.
33. Purchase, I. F., Longstaff, E., Ashby, J., Styles, J. A., Anderson, D., LaFevre, P. A., and Westwood, F. R. (1978). On evaluation of 6 short-term tests for detecting organic chemical carcinogens. *Br. J. Cancer* **37**: 873-903.
34. Meselson, M., and Russell K. (1977). Comparisons of carcinogenic and mutagenic potency. In *Origins of Human Cancer.* H. Hiatt, J. Watson, and J. Winsten (Eds.). Cold Spring Harbor Laboratory, Cold Spring Harbor, New York, pp. 1473-1481.
35. Clive, D. (1977). A linear relationship between tumorigenic potency in vivo and mutagenic potency at the heterozygous thymidine kinase (TK +/−) locus of L51784 mouse lymphoma cells coupled with mammalian metabolism. In *Progress in Genetic Toxicology.* D. Scott, B. A. Bridges, and F. H. Sobels (Eds.). Elsevier, Amsterdam, pp. 241-247.
36. McCann, J., Gold, L. S., Horn, L., McGill, R. Graedel, T. E., and Kaldor, J. (1988). Statistical analysis of Salmonella test data and comparison to results of animal cancer tests. *Mutat. Res.* **205**: 193-195.
37. Metzger, B., Crouch, E., and Wilson, R. (1989). On the relationship between carcinogenicity and acute toxicity. *Risk Analysis* **9**: 169-177.
38. Ashby, J., and Ishidate, Jr., M. (1986). Clastogenicity in vitro of the Na, K, Ca and Mg salts of saccharin; and of magnesium chloride; consideration of significance. *Mutat. Res.* **163**: 63-73.
39. Brusick, D. J. (1987). Implications of treatment-condition-induced genotoxicity for chemical screening and data interpretation. *Mutat. Res.* **189**: 1-6.

40. Ashby, J. (1988). Comparison of techniques for monitoring human exposure to genotoxic chemicals. *Mutat. Res.* **204**: 543-551.
41. Perera, F. (1987). Molecular cancer epidemiology: A new tool in cancer prevention. *J. Natl. Cancer Inst.* **78**: 887-898.
42. Brusick, D., and Auletta, A. (1985). Developmental status of bioassays in genetic toxicology: A report of phase II of the U.S. Environmental Protection Agency Gene-Tox Program. *Mutat. Res.* **153**: 1-10.
43. Nesnow, S., and Bergman, H. (1988). An analysis of the GeneTox Carcinogen Data Base. *Mutat. Res.* **205**: 237-253.
44. Pet-Edwards, J., Chankong, V., Rosenkranz, H. S., and Haines, Y. Y. (1985). Applications of the carcinogenicity prediction and battery selection (CPBS) method to the GeneTox data base. *Mutat. Res.* **153**: 187-200.
45. Ennever, F. K., and Rosenkranz, A. S. (1986). Short-term test results for NTP carcinogens: An alternative, more predictive battery. *Environ. Mutagen.* **8**: 849-865.
46. Ashby, J., and Tennant, R. W. (1988). Chemical structure, Salmonella mutagenicity and extent of carcinogenicity as indicators of genotoxic carcinogenesis among 222 chemicals tested in rodents by the U.S. NCI/NTP. *Mutat. Res.* **204**: 17-115.
47. Ashby, J., Tennant, R. W., Zeiger, E., and Stasiewiez, S. (1989). Classification according to chemical structure of mutagenicity to Salmonella and level of carcinogenicity of a further 42 chemicals tested for carcinogenicity by the U.S. National Toxicology Program. *Mutat. Res.* **223**: 73-103.
48. Moslen, M. T., and Legator, M. S. (1988). Advantages of a combined testing protocol (CTP) with multiple endpoints: The reverse tier approach. *Mutat. Res.* **205**: 91-97.
49. U.S. Patent No. 4, 736, 866. Transgenic Non-human Mammals. P. Leder and T. A. Stewart. April 12, 1988.
50. Cordaro, J. C. (1989). Transgenic mice as future tools in risk assessment. *Risk Analysis* **9**: 157-168.
51. Cepko, C. L., Roberts, B. E., and Mulligan, R. C. (1984). Construction and application of a highly transmissible murine retrovirus shuttle vector. *Cell* **37**: 1053-1062.
52. McCormick, J. J., and Maher, V. M. (1989). Malignant transformation of mammalian cells in culture, including human cells. *Environ. Mol. Mutagen.* **16**: 105-113.
53. LeBoeuf, R. A., and Kerckaert, G. A. (1987). Enhanced morphological transformation of early passage Syrian hamster embryo cells cultured in medium with a reduced bicarbonate concentration and pH. *Carcinogenesis* **8**: 589-697.
54. Matthews, E. (1990). Chemical-induced transformation in Balb/c-3T3 cells: Relationship between in vitro transformation and cytotoxicity, carcinogenesis, and genotoxicity. In *Mutation and the Environment*, Part D, M. Mendelsohn and R. Albertini (Eds.). Wiley-Liss, Inc., New York, pp. 229-238.
55. Gold, L. S., Sawyer, C. B., Magan, R., Backman, G. M., deVeciana, M., Levinson, R., Hooper, N. K., Havender, W. R., Bernstein, L., Peto, R., Pike, M. C., and Ames, B. N. (1984). A carcinogenic potency database of the standized results of animal bioassays. *Environ. Health Perspect.* **58**: 9-319.

56. Myhr, B., and Brusick, D. (1991). A transgenic mouse model for genetic toxicology studies. *Lab. Animal* **20**: 31-35.
57. Anderson, M., Binderup, M. L., Kiel, P., and Larsen, H. (1979). Evaluation of the Ames test. *Ugeskr. Laeg.* **14**: 305-307.
58. Rinkus, S. J., and Legator, M. S. (1979). Chemical characterization of 465 known or suspected carcinogens and their correlation with mutagenic activity in the *Salmonella typhimurium* system. *Cancer Res.* **39**: 3289-3318.
59. Dunkel, V. C., Zeiger, E., Brusick, D., McCoy, E., McGregor, D., Mortelmans, K., Rosenkranz, H., and Simmon V. (1984). Preproducibility of microbial mutagenicity assays; I. Tests with *Salmonella typhimurium* and *Escherichia coli* using a standardized protocol. *Environ. Mutagen.* **6**: 1-25.
60. Kier, L. D., Brusick, D. J., Auletta, A. E., Von Halle, E. S., Brown, M. M., Simmon, V. F., Dunkel, V., McCann, J., Mortelmans, K., Prival, M., Rao, T. K., and Ray, V. (1986). The *Salmonella typhimurium*/mammalian microsomal assay: A report of the U. S. Environmental Protection Agency GeneTox Program. *Mutat. Res.* **168**: 69-240.
61. Waters, M. D., Bergman, H. B., and Nesnon, S. (1988). The genetic toxicity of GenTox non-carcinogens. *Mutat. Res.* **205**: 139-182.

11

Validation of In Vitro Toxicity Tests

John M. Frazier

The Johns Hopkins University School of Hygiene and Public Health
Baltimore, Maryland

INTRODUCTION

An in vitro toxicity test consists of three components: (1) biological component, (2) endpoint measurement, and (3) timing of activities. Variations in any one of these components will result in a new test. For example, switching from hepatocytes to renal tubular cells will reflect differences in target organ responses; replacing the MTT-tetrazolium dye reduction endpoint measurement (which evaluates mitochondrial function) with a protein synthesis inhibition measurement alters the cellular target which is being investigated; or, switching from a 1-h exposure to a 48-h exposure will relate to issues of acute toxicity versus more chronic responses. In any particular situation, each of these three components must be carefully considered and the most appropriate choice selected for the particular toxicological problem at hand. Given three components, each of which can take on a large number of possible choices, the number of potential tests which can be constructed is quite large and is increasing steadily with new developments in cell culture techniques and bioanalytical methods. Before any new method can be incorporated into a strategy for toxicological evaluation, the method must be validated.

Validation is the process by which the credibility of a new method is established for a particular purpose (1-3). This process consists of two distinct aspects: (1) reliability and (2) relevance. Reliability implies that results of a testing method can be reproduced in the same laboratory over time and between laboratories. Relevance means that the data generated by the test can be effectively utilized in a toxicological decision-making process. Neither aspect—reliability or relevance—alone is sufficient to validate a new method. On the contrary, successful performance in both aspects is necessary for a test to be considered for implementation in a toxicological testing program.

It is useful when discussing the evolution of new testing methods to distinguish between three fundamental activities involved in their introduction: (1) test development, (2) validation, and (3) acceptance. Test development is the process by which a creative idea is converted into a specific, experimental protocol. During this process, the investigator developing the new method will undertake preliminary evaluations to demonstrate the feasibility of the method for answering toxicological questions. By the time the method is put forward as a candidate for validation, performance of the test should be optimized.

On the other end of the process, acceptance of a method is determined by the user's needs. A screening test for selection of candidate drugs for product development may be effective and accepted by a pharmaceutical company and yet not adequate for regulatory decision making. On the other hand, a sophisticated testing method which may be acceptable to a regulatory agency for product registration may be too expensive for screening purposes and thus not accepted by a company which must perform many such tests.

Validation is the process which falls between test development and acceptance. The validation process takes a documented test procedure and generates the information necessary for the users to make a decision as to whether the test is acceptable for their particular purposes. It should be clearly recognized that validation of a method can only take place in the context of the purpose for which the test is intended. It is essential to carefully define the intended purposes of a test before the validation study is designed rather than conduct a more or less random evaluation and then try to decide for what purposes the test can be used post hoc.

THE VALIDATION PROCESS

Having developed a candidate test (or tests) for a particular purpose, the actual validation process can be carried out in four stages: (1) intralaboratory assessment, (2) interlaboratory assessment, (3) database development, and (4) evaluation (4). Each of these stages requires careful attention to quality control in both data generation and record keeping.

The first stage of the validation process is an intralaboratory assessment. This is usually conducted in the laboratory which originally developed the method (the primary laboratory), although this is not essential. The purpose of this stage is to document the feasibility of the method for its intended purpose and to establish basic performance criteria for the method. Using the standard protocol for the test, a small set of calibration chemicals (n = 10-20) should be evaluated for two purposes: (1) to act as benchmarks for interpreting test results, and (2) for quality control purposes. The identity of these chemicals should be known to the investigator involved in the study, thus they can be used repeatedly as internal standards. This same set of calibration chemicals will be used in later stages of the validation process (see Interlaboratory Assessment below). As a second phase of the Intralaboratory Assessment, an additional set of chemicals—the Intralaboratory Assessment Set—consisting of 20-40 chemicals should be tested by the primary laboratory in a blind study (to eliminate any investigator bias). The results of the blind study should be utilized to decide whether the method is reproducible and whether the method demonstrates feasibility for providing data relevant to the intended purpose.

Assuming the test (or tests) successfully passes the Intralaboratory Assessment, the second stage is the Interlaboratory Assessment. This assessment involves three phases. The first phase is to set up the test undergoing validation in several laboratories other than the laboratory which developed the test; these laboratories are referred to as secondary laboratories. The number of secondary laboratories participating in this project is not well defined, but three to five laboratories are sufficient to answer most questions from a statistical point of view. The criteria for deciding when the secondary laboratories have successfully set up the test in question can be based on a comparison of the test performance using the Calibration Chemical Set between the secondary laboratory and the quality control data provided by the primary laboratory in the Intralaboratory Assessment stage. Having confirmed that the participating laboratories can successfully perform the tests, the second phase would be a trial run using a blind study with several chemicals selected from the Intralaboratory Assessment Chemical Set. This trial run is to guarantee that data collection techniques and quality control standards are satisfactorily implemented. The final phase of the Interlaboratory Assessment is to evaluate a collection of test materials, the Interlaboratory Assessment Chemical Set (n = 10-20) in a blind study to evaluate the performance of the method.

Again, if all goes well, the method can proceed to the third stage, Database Development. In this stage a large number of chemicals must be evaluated in a blind study to fully define the capabilities and limitations of the test. The number of chemicals required to fully validate a method can be quite large; based on an analysis of chemical structures and structural fragments, it has been estimated that approximately 250 chemicals are needed to evaluate the majority of toxicologically active structural entities. At least this many chemicals must be tested if the method is being proposed to be applied to the universe of all chemical structures. If the test is to be used to evaluate only a select class of chemicals, then the chemical set for Database Development can be significantly reduced. In addition, if the mechanistic basis for a test is well established, then a rationale exists to extrapolate the domain of validity of the method from a smaller set of validation chemicals to the larger universe of all chemicals. Unfortunately, the scientific basis for selection of test chemicals for validation purposes has not been fully explored; consensus on this issue would improve the efficiency of validation activities.

Returning to the process of Database Development, the large number of chemicals to be evaluated need not be undertaken by one laboratory. Several laboratories could collaborate on Database Development and with adequate coordination and quality control procedures the task could be completed relatively rapidly. Once the database is in hand, the final stage of validation, the Evaluation Process, is conducted; this process takes into consideration all the data developed in the three previous stages to evaluate fully the performance of the candidate test in the context of the proposed purpose. Based on the collective performance characteristics of the test, various users can decide whether the test suits their purposes. If the test is adequate for a particular situation, then the users will accept the test and implement it in their safety/hazard evaluation strategy.

As has been widely recognized, the utilization of in vitro toxicity tests to answer complex toxicological questions will require test batteries rather than a single test. The implication of such an assumption is that it will be necessary to validate batteries of tests rather than individual test methods; to date, the scientific basis for evaluating batteries of tests has not been fully defined. This is an area of active research which must be resolved in order to allow for more rapid progress.

It should be realized that there are many ways to conduct validation studies, and the outline described above is not to be construed as the only, or even necessarily the best, procedure. However, the discussion above attempts to identify the major issues which must be addressed by any validation study. The order of conducting the process or the criteria for successful accomplishment of each stage may vary, but the basic questions of reliability and relevance must always be answered.

IMPLEMENTATION OF VALIDATION STUDIES

As should be evident from the discussion above, the basic process of test method validation has many common characteristics whether the test is intended for screening for ocular irritation or for determining relative potency of chemicals to elicit neurotoxicity. Because of the universal character of certain components of the validation process, it should be possible to establish institutional mechanisms to facilitate these processes. Three important components for validation are: (1) a Chemical Bank, (2) an In Vitro Toxicity Testing Data Bank, and (3) Reference Laboratories.

The first component of an infrastructure to support validation activities is a Chemical Bank. A major limitation to rapid evaluation of new methods is the lack of availability of quality controlled reference chemicals (5). In many cases, initial evaluations of new methods utilize whatever chemicals are available in the primary laboratory. Many research investigators do not have the time, knowledge or inclination to carefully select reference chemicals for validating new methods. To solve this problem, a Chemical Bank should be established (optimally at an international level) to provide sets of quality controlled reference chemicals. As discussed above, several sets of reference chemicals should be available. The Calibration Set for a particular category of testing (e.g., ocular irritation testing, neurotoxicity testing) should be available to all researchers. Making these chemicals available to researchers developing new methods will facilitate the Intralaboratory Assessment phase of the validation process and allow for a rapid preliminary evaluation of the performance of a new test compared to existing tests. In later stages of the validation process, the various sets of chemicals which must be provided for blind studies could be easily supplied by the Chemical Bank, thus relieving researchers of the burden of organizing blind studies. In the long run, by providing well-documented and uniform sets of test chemicals, the process of validating methods and then deciding which methods to accept for specific purposes will be greatly facilitated by a Chemical Bank.

A second component is an In Vitro Toxicity Testing Data Bank. Currently, available data on the performance of new testing methods is widely dispersed in the literature and research laboratories. The collection, compilation, and availability of in vitro test performance data will reduce ad hoc efforts to collect this information for each new validation project. The availability of a data bank which provides on-line search and retrieval capabilities will allow those interested in validating new methods the opportunity to clarify the current status of methods of interest, and thus efficiently design validation studies to provide complementary data for evaluation purposes. In addition to supporting validation efforts, a data bank would be of significant importance to commercial activities by providing in vitro testing data on raw materials used in formulations, as well as response data for chemicals structurally related to new chemical entities. In the latter case, the toxicity of newly designed and synthesized chemicals can be predicted on the basis of structure-activity relationships using the nearest chemical neighbors in the database. Confirmation of predictions by actually conducting in vitro testing would give significant credibility to predictions of expected toxicity and thus enhance confidence in the safety/hazard evaluation process.

The third component to support validation activities would be Reference Laboratories. Currently, when new validation studies are organized, it is necessary to recruit several laboratories to participate in the study, particularly for the Interlaboratory Assessment stage. Historically, validation studies have been set up in an ad hoc fashion, thus each project must be initiated de novo. If a small number of Reference Laboratories (three to five) were in place, this phase of the validation study could be significantly accelerated. Standards for quality control and safety would have been previously established for each reference laboratory thus assuring reliable performance. The availability of reference laboratories would also allow for the preliminary evaluation of promising methods which are not fully developed by the primary laboratory.

Taken together, these three components—a Chemical Bank, an In Vitro Toxicity Testing Data Bank, and Reference Laboratories—can significantly improve the efficiency and speed of the validation process. Performance data on Reference Chemical Sets provided by the Chemical Bank to primary laboratories as well as Reference Laboratories can be collected by the In Vitro Toxicity Data Bank and made available for validation activities as well as product development and safety/hazard evaluation purposes. Such an integrated infrastructure is needed to support the validation activities which must be expanded to accommodate the increasing number of new tests.

FUTURE RESEARCH NEEDS

The issue of validation is not new; this problem has been plaguing researchers involved in the implementation of new toxicity testing methods for a long time. At the moment, there is a keen interest in the problem from many different perspectives, including regulatory and commercial interests. Several recently published documents (3,4) have highlighted the issues of importance. In light of this heightened interest, the question arises as to the most pressing research needs to address these issues.

Three important areas of research can be highlighted. First, much of our conceptualization of how to define a good test is flavored by past experience with carcinogenicity testing where the objective was to categorize a chemical into a bimodal classification scheme (i.e., a chemical was either a carcinogen or a noncarcinogen). Within this context it is easy to define theoretically what is meant by false positives and false negatives, although from an experimental point of view problems arose owing to uncertainty in the definitive classification of reference chemicals. In spite of the difficulties encountered, test performance could be evaluated by computing the parameters referred to as sensitivity, specificity, and predictive value (1). When dealing with other categories of toxicity, this simplistic situation cannot be applied directly. In certain types of toxicity, such as ocular irritation, the biological response to test chemicals can be categorized into a set of classes: non-, slight, mild, moderate, severe irritants. It is possible to expand the analysis of the bimodal classification to the multimodal classification scheme; however, when the response takes on a continuous range of values, such as the LD_{50}, new approaches must be adapted. Rank correlations or more advanced approaches, such as the concordance/discordance analysis, are attempts to address the issue of evaluating tests which are designed to measure continuous responses. Even these evaluating methods have their limitations, particularly since they do not take into consideration the mechanistic basis of test performance. What is needed are new approaches to the problem of defining what constitutes a good test and how "goodness" can be experimentally evaluated.

A second major research question is how to select and validate a battery of tests to answer a particular toxicological testing problem. Most of the current attempts to validate methods consider each test separately. If multiple tests are considered, the approach to evaluation is statistical in nature with little regard for mechanistic implications (6). To a certain extent the empirical approach is a result of the lack of basic knowledge concerning the mechanisms of in vivo pathogenesis. However, research should be focused on new approaches which integrate statistical and mechanistic perspectives to select and validate batteries of tests.

Finally, a major problem is the integration of multiple in vitro data into the decision-making process. Can an algorithm be defined which takes specific results of several in vitro toxicity tests and weights them appropriately to reach a final estimation of the likelihood of adverse effects? If such an algorithm can be generated, then the contribution of in vitro toxicity testing to the safety/hazard evaluation process will be greatly enhanced.

These are some of the major research problems which must be resolved. As with any new technology, it takes a period of time for it to find its ultimate niche in the arena to which it is applied. In the case of interest here, in vitro toxicity testing, new methods are currently being investigated and implemented in tier testing strategies. Validation is a critical component of this process. The better we understand validation and develop the tools to carry out the process in an efficient manner, the more rapidly new tests can progress from laboratory curiosities to full fledged components of the safety/hazard evaluation process.

REFERENCES

1. Scala, R. A. 1987. Theoretical approaches to validation. In *In Vitro Toxicology-Approaches to Validation. Alternative Methods in Toxicology.* Vol. 5. A. M. Goldberg (Ed.), Mary Ann Liebert, New York, pp. 1-10.

2. Frazier, John M. (1990). Validation of *in vitro* models. *J. Am. Coll. Toxicol.* **9**: 355-359.
3. OECD. (1990). *Scientific Criteria for Validation of In Vitro Toxicity Tests.* Environmental Monographs No. 36. OECD Publishing Office, p. 62.
4. Balls, M., Blaauboer, B., Brusick, B., Frazier, J., Lamb, D., Pemperton, M., Reinhardt, C., Roberfroid, M., Rosenkranz, H., Schmid, B., Spielmann, H., Stammati, A.-L., and Walum, E. (1990). Report and recommendations of the CAAT/ERGATT workshop on the validation of toxicity test procedures. *ATLA* **18**: 313-368.
5. Purchase, I. F. H. (1990). An international reference chemical databank would accelerate the development, validation and regulatory acceptance of alternative toxicology tests. *ATLA* **18**: 345-348.
6. Hellberg, S., Eriksson, L., Jonsson, J., Lindgren, F., Sjöström, M., Wold, S., Ekwall, B., Gómez-Lechón, M. J., Clothier, R., Accomando, N. J., Grimes, A., Barile, F. A., Nordin, M., Tyson, C. A., Dierickx, P., Shrivastava, R. S., Tingsleff-Skaanild, M., Garza-Ocañas, and L., Fiskesjö, G. (1990). Analogy models for prediction of human toxicity. *ATLA* **18**: 103-116.

12

Industrial Applications for In Vitro Toxicity Evaluation: A Tier Testing Strategy for Product Safety Assessment

Shayne Cox Gad

Becton Dickson and Company
Research Triangle Park, North Carolina

INTRODUCTION

The test methods designed and used to evaluate the potential of a man-made material to cause harm to the people who make, transport, use or otherwise come in contact with it hold a unique and ambivalent place in our society. On one hand, our society is not only critically dependent on technological advances to improve and/or maintain standards of living, but is also intolerant of risks (real or potential) to life and health; e.g., diseases like AIDS and multiple sclerosis and illness or disability caused by household products, pesticides, or waste products. At the same time, the traditional tests (with both their misuse and misunderstanding of their use) have served as the rallying point for those concerned about the humane and proper use of animals. This has caused the field of testing for potential to cause irritation or damage to the eyes to become both the most active area for the development of alternatives and innovations and the most sensitive area of animal testing and use in research. But all testing using animals has come under question.

In recent years, tremendous progress has been made in our understanding of biology down to the molecular level. This has translated to multiple modifications and improvements to in vivo testing procedures which now give us tests which (1) are more reliable, reproducible, and predictive of potential hazards in humans; (2) use fewer animals; and (3) are considerably more humane than earlier test forms. At the same time, a multitude of in vitro test systems have been proposed, developed, and validated to at least some extent. Yet the perception persists that little has changed in how safety assessment is performed by or for industry. Why?

It is hoped that this volume will serve to make more people aware of the new techniques which are available. But more importantly, it is hoped that the whole process involved in testing can be modified so that only what needs to be done will be done, and that such tests will answer the desired questions in a manner which maximizes efficiency, effectiveness, and animal welfare.

The entire product safety assessment process, in the broadest sense, is a multistage process in which none of the individual steps is overwhelmingly complex, but the integration of the whole process involves fitting together a large complex pattern of pieces. This volume as a whole seeks to address the questions of the use of in vitro test methods. How the data generated by the various test systems and models described elsewhere in this volume can be used by government and private enterprise to provide for a safe product life cycle is the subject of this chapter. As will be seen, this calls for a modification of the approach to the general product safety assessment problem, and it will be addressed by starting with the current general case and progressing to plans and a means for changing the process in an iterative fashion. Along the way, the limitations of current models and approach and places where testing and research data could be made more practically useful will be pointed out. Particularly with an understanding of mechanisms becoming increasingly important in both product design and evaluating the relevance of findings, the integration of in vitro methodologies into the product safety assessment process has become essential.

The single most important part of a product safety evaluation program is, in fact, the initial overall process of defining and developing an adequate data package on the potential hazards associated with the product life cycle (1) (the manufacture, sale, use, and disposal of a product and associated process materials). To do this, one must ask a series of questions in a highly interactive process, with many of the questions designed to identify and/or modify their successors. The first question is: What information is needed?

This calls for understanding the way in which a product is to be made and used, and the potential health and safety risks related to exposure of humans who will be associated with these processes. This is the basis of a hazard and toxicity profile. Once such a profile is established (as illustrated in Fig. 1), then the available literature is searched to determine what is already known.

Taking into consideration this literature information and the previously defined exposure profile, a tier approach (Table 1) has traditionally been used to generate a list of tests or studies to be performed.* What goes into a

*There is also the special case of pharmaceutical and pesticide products, where there are regulatory mandated minimum test batteries.

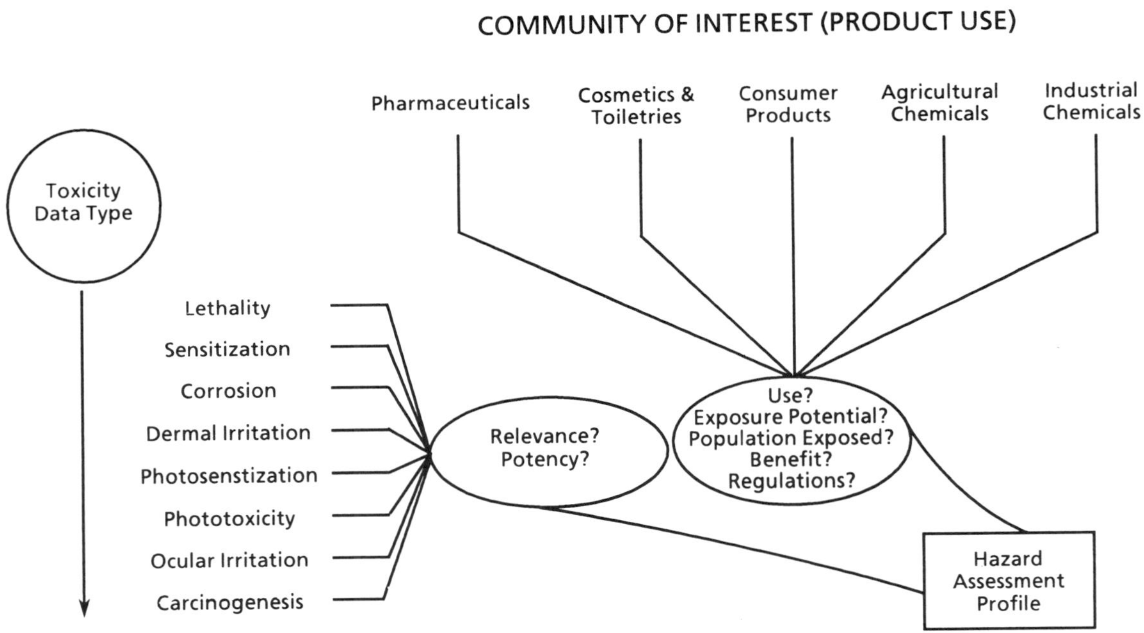

Figure 1 What hazards are associated with a new product is a multidimensional problem depending on the products intended use, its innate toxicity, its physiochemical properties, and the potential human and environmental exposure. This matrix diagramatically illustrates the key questions involved in developinng the final hazard assessment profile.

Table 1 Tier Testing

Testing Tier	Mammalian toxicology	Genetic toxicology	Remarks
0	Literature review	Literature review	Upon identification of a problem database of existing information and particulars of use of materials are established.
1	Cytotoxicity screens Dermal sensitization Acuted systemic toxicity Lethality screens	Ames test In vitro SCE In vitro cytogenetics Forward mutation/CHO	R&D materials and low volume chemicals with severely limited exposure
2	Subacute studies Metabolism Primary dermal irritation Eye irritation	In vivo SCE In vivo cytogenetics	Medium volume materials and/or those with a significant chance of human exposure
3	Subchronic studies Reproduction Teratology Chronic studies Mechanistic studies	—	Any material with a high volume or a potential for widespread or long-term human exposure or one which gives indications of specific long-term effects

The usual plan for characterizing the toxicity of a compound or product is to develop information in a tier approach. More information is required (a higher tier level is attained) as the volume of production and potential for exposure increases. A common scheme is shown.

tier system is determined by both regulatory requirements imposed by government agencies, the philosophy of the parent organization, economics, and available technology. How such tests are actually performed is determined on one of two bases. The first (and most common) is the menu approach: selecting a series of standard design tests as "modules" of data. The second, is an interactive/iterative approach, where strategies are developed and studies are designed based both on needs and what has been learned to date about the product.

DEFINING TESTING OBJECTIVES

The initial and most important aspect of a product safety evaluation program is the series of steps that leads to an actual statement of the problem or of the objectives of any testing and research program. This definition of objectives is essential and, as proposed here, consists of five steps: (1) defining product or material use, (2) estimating or quantitating exposure potential, (3) identifying potential hazards, (4) gathering baseline data, and (5) designing and defining the actual research program to answer outstanding questions. Later we will look at the specific application of this to dermal and ocular toxicity cases, where the concept of *communities of interest* (i.e., an understanding of the needs of the organization producing the material and the users) will become essential. This concept will be discussed in detail later.

Define Product/Material Use

Identifying how a material is to be used, what it is to be used for, and how it is to be made are the essential first three questions to be answered before a meaningful assessment program can be performed. These three factors determine, to a large extent, how many people are potentially exposed, to what extent and by what routes they are exposed, and what benefits they perceive or gain from product use. The answers to these questions are generally categorical or qualitative, and become quantitative (as will be reviewed in the next section) at a later step (frequently long after initial toxicity testing has been initiated).

Starting with an examination of how a material is to be made (or how it is already being made), it generally occurs that there are several process segments, each representing separate problems. Commonly, much of a manufacturing process is "closed" (i.e., it occurs in sealed airtight systems) thereby limiting exposures to (1) leaks with low-level (generally) inhalation and dermal exposures to significant portions of a plant work force, and (2) maintenance and repair workers (generally short-term, higher level inhalation and dermal exposures to small numbers of personnel, usually resulting from industrial accidents). Smaller segments of the process will almost invariably not be closed. These segments are most common either where some form of manual manipulation is required, or where the segment requires a large volume of space (such as when fibers or other objects are spun, formed, or individually coated with something), or where the product is packaged (such as powders being put into bags or polymers being removed from molds). The exact manner and quantity of each segment of the manufacturing process, in conjunction with the development of a categorization of exposures for each of these segments, will then serve to help quantitate the identified categories of exposure.

Likewise, consideration of what a product is to be used for and how it is to be used should be of help in identifying who, outside of the manufacturing process, may be exposed, by what routes, and to what extent.

The answers to these questions, again, will generate a categorical set of answers, but will also serve to identify which particular aspects of regulatory toxicity testing may be operative (such as those for the Department of Transportation or Consumer Product Safety Commission). If a product is to be worn (such as clothing or jewelry) or used on, or as, an environmental surface (such as household carpeting or wall covering), the potential for the exposure of a large number of people (albeit at low levels in the case of most materials) is large. If the product is to be used on exterior portions of buildings, the potential for exposure to a large number of individuals would be smaller. Likewise, the nature of the intended use (say, as a true consumer product versus an industrial product) determines the potential for extent and degree of exposure in overt and subtle manners. For example, a finish for carpets to be used in the home has a much greater potential for dermal and even oral (in the case of infants) exposure than such a product used only for carpeting in offices. Likewise, in general, true consumer products (such as household cleaners) have a greater potential for both accidental exposure and misuse.

Evaluate Exposure Potential

The next problem (or step) is quantitating the exposure of the human population, both in terms of how many people are exposed by what routes (or means) and to what quantities of an agent they are exposed.

This process of identifying and quantitating exposure groups within the human population is beyond the scope of this chapter, except for some key points. Classification is a collection of essential techniques which constitutes one aspect of "rule making" for data collection and analysis.

Data classification serves two purposes: data simplification (also called a descriptive function) and prediction. Simplification is necessary because there is a limit to both the volume and complexity of data that the human mind can comprehended and deal with conceptually. Classification allows us to attach a label (or name) to each group of data, to summarize the data (i.e., assign individual elements of data to groups and to characterize the population of the group), and to define the relationships between groups (i.e., develop a taxonomy).

Prediction is the use of summaries of data and knowledge of the relationships between groups to develop hypotheses as to what will happen when further data are collected (as when production or market segments are expanded) and as to the mechanisms which cause such relationships to develop. Indeed, classification is the prime device for the discovery of mechanisms in all of science. A classic example of this was Darwin's realization that there were reasons (the mechanisms of evolution) behind the differences and similarities in species which had helped Linaeus to earlier develop his classification scheme (or taxonomy) for animals.

To develop a classification, one first sets bounds wide enough to encompass the range of data to be considered, but not unnecessarily wide. This is typically done by selecting some global variables (variables all data have in common) and limiting the range of each so that it just encompasses all the cases on hand. One then selects a set of local variables (characteristics that only some of the cases have, such as certain skin types, enzyme activity levels, or dietary preferences). These local variables then serve to differentiate between groups. Data are then collected, and a system for measuring differences and similarities is developed.

Classification of biological data based on qualitative factors has been well discussed by Glass (2), and Gordon (3) does an excellent job of introducing the entire field and mathematical concepts. The specific problem of assessing exposure potential has also been addressed by Jayjock and Gad (4).

When these concepts are utilized for the problems of hazard assessment, the general case questions are as below:

1. Which groups are potentially exposed?
2. What are parts of groups? Consumers, production workers, neonatal patients, etc.
3. What are routes of potential exposure?
4. Which group does each route occur in?
5. Which sex is exposed?
6. Which age groups are potentially exposed?

An investigator must first understand the process involved in making, shipping, using, and disposing of a material. The Environmental Protection Agency (5) has proposed guidelines for such identification and exposure quantitation. The exposure groups may be very large or relatively small populations, each with a markedly different potential for exposure. Additional differences to be considered in assessing systemic exposure (such as the absorption by the lung for inhalation exposures) and special toxicity problems (such as delayed contact dermal sensitization) will also need to be incorporated. Though almost always ignored, there may also be populations with peculiar characteristics (such as extremes of age, preexisting diseases, or substandard nutritional states) which make them particularly susceptible.

All estimates of exposure in humans (and of the number of humans exposed) are subject to a large degree of uncertainty.

Identify Potential Hazard

Once the types of exposures have been identified and the quantities approximated, a toxicity matrix can be developed by identifying the potential hazards. Such an identification can proceed by one of three major approaches:

1. Analogy from data reported in the literature
2. Structure-activity relationships
3. Predictive testing

The first two of these approaches are beyond the scope of this chapter, and the interested reader should see Gad (1) and Gad and Chengelis (29) for discussions of these aspects.

For the third approach, the tests and their objectives (the questions they ask) can be categorized in two groups. The first catagory is single endpoint-type tests:

Primary dermal irritation (PDI): Evaluate potential of a single dermal exposure to cause skin irritation.
Primary eye irritation: Evaluate potential of a single ocular exposure to cause eye irritation.
Dermal corrosivity: Determine potential of a single 4-h dermal exposure to cause skin corrosion.
Dermal sensitization: Evaluate the potential of a material to cause delayed contact hypersensitivity.
Photosensitization: Evaluate the potential of a material to cause sunlight-activated delayed contact hypersensitivity.
Lethality screen: Determine the potential of a single dose of a material, at a predetermined level, for lethality.
Mutagenicity: Determine the potential of a material to cause undesirable genetic events.

The second category of predictive tests contains the "shotgun" (or multi-endpoint) tests. The name shotgun suggests itself for these studies because it is not known in advance what endpoints are being aimed at. Rather, the purpose of the study is to identify and quantitate all potential system effects resulting from a single exposure to a compound. Once known, specific target organ effects can then be studies in detail if so desired. Accordingly, the generalized design of these studies is to expose groups of animals to controlled amounts or concentrations of the material of interest, then to observe for and measure as many variables as practical over a period during or past the exposure. Further classification of tests within this category is defined either by the route by which test animals are exposed or dosed (generally oral, dermal, or inhalation are the options here) or by the length of dosing. Acute studies, for example, imply a single exposure interval (24 h or less) or dosing of test material. The longer term ("chronic") systemic toxicity, carcinogenicity, and developmental and reproductive toxicity tests also generally fit into this class:

Systemic toxicity: Determine the potential of a material to cause target organ toxicity at a site other than that of application.

Carcinogenicity: Determine the potential of a material to induce the occurrence of neoplasms.

Reproductive and developmental toxicity: Determine the potential of a material to adversely effect either the reproductive process or the normal structural and functional development of offspring.

Having completed these first three steps in defining testing objectives, one can proceed on to gathering from the literature or other sources, the available baseline data before actually designing and executing a testing program.

Collect Baseline Data

Before actually designing and executing any testing program, the toxicologist (or any biological scientist) should first (on both ethical and economic grounds) gather and evaluate the information already available to the scientific community. The classification scheme (as described in step 2) and information already gathered in the first three steps of this process should serve to refine the data gathering process. There are four major sources for such information.

1. Published information sources
2. On-line literature searches
3. Other sources: colleagues and in-house databases

Also to be considered is maintenance of a database once it is established (in many places this is called product surveillance).

However, before review of the literature is initiated, it is important to obtain as much of the following product composition and exposure information as practical:

1. Chemical composition and major impurities
2. Chemical production and use information; i.e., manufacturing process, exposure patterns, and other commercial uses.
3. Correct chemical identity including formula, Chemical Abstract Service Number, common synonyms, and trade names
4. Selected physical properties; i.e., physical state, vapor pressure, chemical reactivity, and pH
5. Other chemical substances exhibiting similar physical chemical characteristics, and if some toxicity data is available, similar toxicity and/or structure/activity relationships

This is, by the way, the cornerstone of the analogy approach to toxicity assessment.

Collection of the aforementioned information is not only important for the hazard assessment (high vapor pressure would indicate high inhalation potential just as high or low pH would indicate high irritation potential), but prior identificatino of all product uses and exposure patterns can identify alternative information sources; e.g., chemicals formerly used as anesthetics, food additives, or pesticides may have extensive toxicology data obtainable from government or private sources.

Published Information Sources

There are numerous published texts for use in literature reviewing. An alphabetic listing of 19 of the more commonly used texts is provided in Table 2. Obviously, this is not a complete listing and consists of only the general multipurpose texts that have a wider range of applicability for the toxicity of commercial products (current or potential). Texts dealing with specialized classes of chemicals, e.g., petroleum hydrocarbons, plastics, or those with specific target organ toxicities (neurotoxins and teratogens), are not considered to be within the scope of this section and the interested reader is referred to Wexler (6) or Parker (7) for further details.

On-Line Literature Searches

In the last 10 years, the use of on-line literature searches by many toxicologists has changed from an occasional, sporadic request to the semicontinuous need for computerized search capabilities. Usually nontoxicology-related

Table 2 Published Information Sources for Toxicology Data

Title	Ref.
Annual Report on Carcinogens	8
Burger's Medicinal Chemistry	9
Chemical Hazards of the Workplace	10
Clinical Toxicology of Commercial Products	11
Contact Dermatitis	12
Criteria Documents	13
Current Intelligence Bulletins (NIOSH)	14
Dangerous Properties of Industrial Materials	15
Documentation of the Threshold Limit Values (AIHA)	16
Handbook of Toxic and Hazardous Chenmicals	17
Hygienic Guide Series (AIHA)	18
Industrial Toxicology	19
International Agency for Research on Cancer (IARC)	20
Merck Index	21
Occupational Health Guidelines for Chemical Hazards (NIOSH/OSHA)	22
Patty's Industrial Hygiene and Toxicology	23
Physicians' Desk Reference	24
Registry of Toxic Effects of Chemical Substances (RETECS)	25
Toxicology of the Eye	26

search capabilities are already in place in many companies. Therefore, all that is needed is to expand the information source to include some of the databases that cover the types of toxicology information needed. A university or a private contract laboratory can often provide this service. Most of the databases of interest to toxicologists are parts of the National Library of Medicine (NLM) system.

The NLM information retrieval service (27) contains Medline, Toxline, and Cancerline databases. Databases commonly used by industrial toxicologists in the NLM service are briefly discussed below.

1. Toxline (Toxicology Information Online) is a bibliographic database covering the pharmacological, biochemical, physiological, environmental, and toxicological effects of drugs and other chemicals. It contains approximately 1.7 million citations, most of which are complete with abstract, index terms, and Chemical Abstracts Service (CAS) Registry Numbers. Toxline citations have publication dates of 1981 to the present. Older information is on Toxback 76 (1976-1980) and Toxback 65 (pre-1965 through 1975). Information on Toxline comes from 13 secondary subfiles.
2. Medline (Medical Information Online) is a database containing approximately 800,000 references to biomedical journal articles published since 1980. These articles, usually with an English abstract, are from over 3000 journals. Coverage of previous years (back to 1966) is provided by back files searchable online, which total some 3.5 million references.
3. Toxnet (Toxicology Data Network) is a computerized network of toxicologically oriented data banks. Toxnet offers a sophisticated search and retrieval package which accesses the following three subfiles:

   a. Hazardous Substances Data Bank (HSDB) is a scientifically reviewed and edited data bank containing toxicological information strengthened with additional data related to the environment, emergency situations, and regulatory issues. Data are derived from a variety of sources, including government documents and special reports. This database contains records for over 4100 chemical substances.
   b. Toxicology Data Bank (TDB) is a peer-reviewed data bank focusing on toxicological and pharmacological data, environmental and occupational information, manufacturing and use data, and chemical and physical properties. References have been extracted from a selective list of standard source documents.
   c. CCRIS (Chemical Carcinogenesis Research Information System) is a National Cancer Institute-sponsored database derived from both short- and long-term bioassays on 1200 chemical substances. Studies cover carcinogenicity, mutagenicity, promotion, and cocarcinogenicity.

4. Registry of Toxic Effect of Chemical Substances (RTECS) is the NLM online version of NIOSH's annual compilation of substances with toxic activity (25). The original collection of data was derived from the 1971 Toxic Substances Lists. The RTECS data contain threshold limit values, aquatic toxicity ratings, air standards, National Toxicology Program (NTP) carcinogenesis bioassay information, and toxicological/carcinogenic review information. The National Institute of Occupation, Safety and Health (NIOSH) is responsible for the file content in RTECS, and for providing quarterly updates to NLM. Currently, RTECS covers toxicity data on more then 61,000 substances. Greater detail on available data sources and their use in toxicology can be found in Wexler (6) or Parker (7).

5. Other: There are at least two other sources of information which are not generally publicly available. These are in-house databases (the results of past testing which has never been published) and information from colleagues in other organizations with access to similar databases.

Designing and Research Program

The next step, given that no data are found from any of these sources (and that it has been determined that data is needed) is to perform appropriate predictive tests. The bulk of this volume addresses specifics of performing such tests. Before considering how to design and conduct a testing program, we must first consider how the practice of safety assessment came to its current state in the employment of such tests.

To understand how product safety and toxicity data are used, and how the data generation process might be changed to better meet the product safety assessment needs of society, it is essential to understand that different commercial and regulatory organizations have different answers to these questions. The ultimate answer is a multidimensional matrix, with the three major dimensions of the matrix being (1) the toxicity data type (lethality, sensitization, corrosion, irritation, photosensitization, phototoxicity, etc.), (2) exposure characteristics (extent, population size, population characteristics, etc.), and (3) type of commercial organization (or organizations) regulated (which we will call the community of interest). This matrix was shown in Figure 1.

Communities of interest are defined by how the products are to be used, who regulates their use, and what benefits are expected for the consumer. There are a number of ways of classifying such communities, but for our purposes we will divide and define them as follows.

Pharmaceuticals

Materials of concern are agents intended as therapeutics (or medical devices) where the production worker or health care provider (doctor, nurse, or pharmacist) may have a significant chance of exposure, but the major concern is for those patients who receive or use the drug or device. The Food and Drug Administration (FDA) is the United States (US) regulator.

Cosmetics and Toiletries

The materials are cosmetics, fragrances, shampoos, hand and body soaps, hair dyes, and other materials intended to improve appearance and personal presentation. These are intended to be either applied to the skin or to be applied or used in a manner that makes dermal or ocular exposure (at least) unavoidable. The major US regulators are the Food and Drug Administration and Consumer Product Safety Commission (CPSC).

Consumer Products

Products intended to be used by the average person in and around their home can be divided into those that have a high potential for exposure (dish and laundry detergents, for example), those that have low potential for such exposure (drain cleaners, oven cleaners, etc.), or those that have a wide range in between (such as window and carpet cleaners). The primary regulators are CPSC and Department of Transportation (DOT), but the Environmental Protection Agency (EPA) also is important in terms of new chemical entities and disposal and waste management.

Agricultural Products

These products are pesticides, herbicides, fertilizers, and other intentional food additives (preservatives, sterilants, etc.). The extent of dermal, inhalation, oral, and other routes of exposure will vary widely in use. Note that these could be subdivided into those agents used in the field (i.e., actually used in agriculture), those for home or inside use, and those agents used in the storage and processing of foods. Regulatory oversight is vested primarily in the EPA (under the Federal Insecticide, Fungicide and Rodenticide Act—FIFRA), with secondary considerations by DOT and FDA. The third group (those used on foods) has FDA as the primary driving force, with EPA and DOT concerns secondary.

Industrial Chemicals

These are materials to which the major exposure is to workers involved in the manufacture and transportation of products. In a sense, all the materials (e.g., the above categories) fall into this group at some time, plus a number of other chemicals that never appear (as such) in those categories (such as hydroflouric acid and plasticizers). These are handled by a smaller population relative to most other products. Direct contact is never intended; in fact, active measures are taken to prevent it. The use of safety assessment data in these cases is to fulfill labeling requirements for shipping (DOT) and protecting workers (OSHA) and to provide hazard assessment information for accidental exposures and its treatment (DOT and OSHA). The results of such tests do not directly affect the economic future of a material.

Each of these communities have different needs and uses for each of the kinds of data produced and these must be considered independently.

What is called for is a careful consideration of what the optimum product safety assessment strategy would be. A framework for such an strategy is as shown in Figure 2. The components that constitute each of the data generation tool boxes shown (screens, confirmatory tests, higher tier tests, and mechanistic evaluations) are common to all safety assessment programs in some form. But what is actually used for each of these tasks—and how the judgment ovals (here labeled acceptance criterion and risk/benefit judgment) operate are not. The selection of these details are what constitutes the actual formulation of a strategy. Before formulating such a strategy and deciding what mix of tests should be used, it is first necessary to decide criteria for what would constitute an ideal (or acceptable) test system.

Testing Tier	Mammalian Toxicology	Genetic Toxicology	Remarks
0	Literature review	Literature review	Upon initial identification of a problem data base of existing information and particulars of use of materials are established
1	Cytotoxicity screens Dermal sensitization Acuted sytemic toxicity Lethality screens	Ames test In vitro SCE In vitro cytogenetics Forward mutation/CHO	R&D materials and low volume chemicals with severely limited exposure
2	Subacute studies Metabolism Primary dermal irritation Eye irritation	In vivo SCE In vivo cytogenetics	Medium volume materials and/or those with a significant chance of human exposure
3	Subchronic studies Reproduction Teratology Chronic studies Mechanistic studies	-	Any material with a high volume or a potential for widespread or long term human exposure or one which gives indications of specific long-term effects

Figure 2 Within a tiered product safety assessment approach, it is possible to ask each question to a different degree of detail. If an early evaluation provides sufficient information testing may be complete with relatively low expense. Conversely it may also be determined that either a more detailed (or specific) assay must be performed. Shown here is such an interactive approach which identifies points where in vitro systems could readily be utilized in place of in vivo systems.

TEST SYSTEMS: CHARACTERISTICS, DEVELOPMENT, AND SELECTION

Any useful test system must be sufficiently sensitive that the incidence of false negatives is low. Clearly a high incidence of false negatives is intolerable. In such a situation, large numbers of dangerous chemical agents would be carried through extensive additional testing only to find that they possess undesirable toxicological properties after the expenditure of significant time and money. On the other hand, a test system which is overly sensitive will give rise to a high incidence of false positives which will have the deleterious consequence of rejecting potentially beneficial chemicals. The "ideal" test will fall somewhere between these two extremes and thus provide adequate protection without unnecessarily stifling development.

The "ideal" test should have an endpoint measurement which provides data such that dose-response relationships can be obtained. Furthermore, any criterion of effect must be sufficiently accurate in the sense that it can be used to reliably resolve the relative toxicity of two test chemicals which produce distinct (in terms of hazard to humans) yet similar responses. In general, it may not be sufficient to classify test chemicals into generic toxicity categories, such as "intermediate" toxicity, since a test chemical which falls in a given category, yet is borderline to the next more severe toxicity category, should be treated with more concern than a second test chemical which falls at the less toxic extreme of the same category. Therefore, it is essential for a test system to be able to both place test chemicals in an established toxicity category and rank materials relative to others in the category.

The endpoint measurement of the "ideal" test system must be objective. This is important so that a given test chemical will give similar results when tested using the standard test protocol in different laboratories. If it is not possible to obtain reproducible results in a given laboratory over time or between various laboratories, then the historical database against which new test chemicals are evaluated will be time/laboratory dependent. If this condition is the case, then there will be significant limitations on the application of the test system, since it could potentially produce conflicting results. From a regulatory point of view this possibility would be highly undesirable. Along these lines, it is important for the test protocol to incorporate internal standards to serve as quality controls. Thus, test data could be represented utilizing a reference scale based on the test system response to the internal controls. Such normalization, if properly documented, could reduce interest variability.

Alternatives to current in vivo test systems basically should be designed to evaluate the toxic response of concern in a manner as closely predictive of the outcome of interest in man as possible.

From a practical point of view, there are several additional features of the "ideal" test which should be satisfied. The test should be fast enough that the turnaround time for a given test chemical is reasonable for the intended purpose (very rapid for a screen, timely for a definitive test). Obviously the speed of the test and the ability to conduct tests on several chemicals simultaneously will determine the overall productivity. The test should be inexpensive so that it is economically competitive with current testing practices. And finally, the technology should be easily transferred from one laboratory to another without excessive capital investment (relative to the value of the test performed) for test implementation. It should be kept in mind that though some of these practical considerations may appear to present formidable limitations for any given test system at the present time, the possibility of future developments in testing technology could overcome these obstacles. Additionally, in the real world environment, these practical considerations represent the grounds for consideration of multiple new candidate tests on competitive grounds. The most predictive test system in the universe of possibilities will never gain wide acceptance if it takes years to produce an answer or costs substantially more than other test systems which are only marginally less predictive.

The point is that these characteristics of the "ideal" test system provides a general framework for evaluation of alternative test systems in general. No test system is likely to be ideal. Therefore, it will be necessary to weigh the strengths and weaknesses of each proposed test system in order to reach a conclusion on how "good" a particular test is. The next section will present the basis for the specific test evaluation.

In both theory and practice in vivo and in vitro tests have potential advantages and disadvantages. Tables 3 and 4 summarize the advantages and disadvantages in vivo testing. How then might the proper tests be selected, especially in the case of the choice of staying with an existing test system or adopting a new one.

Considerations in Adopting New Test Systems

Conducting toxicological investigations in two or more species of laboratory animals is generally accepted as being a prudent and responsible practice in developing a new chemical entity, especially one that is expected to receive widespread use and to have exposure potential over human lifetimes. Adding a second or a third species to the testing regimen offers an extra measure of confidence to the toxicologist and the other professionals who will be responsible for evaluating the associated risks, benefits, and exposure limitations or protective measures. Although undoubtedly broadening and deepening a compound's profile of toxicity, the practice of enlarging on the num-

Table 3 Rationale for Using In Vivo Test Systems

1.	Provides evaluation of actions/effects on intact animal and organ/tissue interactions.
2.	Either pure chemicals or complete formulated products (complex mixtures) can be evaluated.
3.	Either concentrated or diluted products can be tested.
4.	Yields data on the recovery and healing processes.
5.	Required statutory tests for agencies under such laws as the Federal Hazardous Substances Act (unless data are already available), Toxic Substances Control Act, Federal Insecticides, Fungicides and Rodenticides Act (FIFRA), Organization for Economic Cooperation (OECD), and Food and Drug Administration Laws.
6.	Quantitative and qualitative tests with scoring system generally capable of ranking materials as to relative hazards.
7.	Amenable to modifications to meet the requirements of special situations (much as multiple dosing or exposure schedules).
8.	Extensive available database and cross-reference capability for evaluation of relevance to human situation.
9.	The ease of performance and relative low capital costs in many cases.
10.	Tests are generally both conservative and broad in scope, providing for maximum protection by erring on the side of overprediction of hazard to man.
11.	Tests can be either single end point (such as lethality, corrosion, etc.) or shot-gun (also called multiple endpoint, and include such test systems as a 13-week oral toxicity study).

Table 4 Limitations of In Vivo Testing Systems Which Serve as a Basis for Seeking In Vitro Alternatives for Toxicity Tests

1.	Complications (and potential confounding or masking findings) of animal and tissue/organ in vivo evaluation.
2.	In vivo systems may only assess short-term site of application or immediate structural alterations produced by agents. Note, however, that specific in vivo tests may only be intended to evaluate acute local effects (i.e., this may be a purposeful test system limitation).
3.	Technician training and monitoring are critical (particularly due to the subjective nature of evaluation).
4.	If our objective is either the total exclusion of a particular type of agent or the identification of truly severe acting agents on an absolute basis (that is, without false positives or negatives), in vivo tests in animals do not perfectly predict results in humans.
5.	Clearly, there are structural and biochemical differences between test animals and humans which make extrapolation from one to the other difficult.
6.	Lack of standardization of in vivo systems.
7.	Variable correlation with human results.

Table 4 Continued

8.	Large biological variability between experimental units (i.e., individual animals).
9.	Large, diverse, and fragmented databases which are not readily comparable.

ber of test species is, as has been demonstrated in multiple points in the literature (see Ref. 29, for example), an indiscriminate scientific generalization. Moreover, such a tactic is certain to generate the problem of species-specific toxicoses; that is, a toxic response or an inordinately low biological threshold for toxicity is evident in one species or strain, whereas all other species examined are either unresponsive or strikingly less sensitive. The investigator confronting such findings must be prepared to address the all-important question, Are humans likely to react positively or negatively to the test agent under similar circumstances?

Assuming that numerical odds prevail and humans automatically fit into the predominant category, whether on the side of being safe or at risk, would be scientifically irresponsible. Far from being an irreconcilable nuisance, however, such a confounded situation can be an opportunity to advance more quickly into the heart of the search for predictive information. A species-specific toxicosis can frequently contribute toward better understanding of the general case if the underlying biological mechanism either causing or enhancing toxicity is defined, and especially if it is discovered to uniquely reside in the sensitive species.

A mention of species-specific toxicoses usually implies that either different metabolic pathways for converting or excreting xenobiotics or anatomical differences are involved. The design of our current tests appear to serve society reasonably well (i.e., significantly more times than not) in identifying hazards that would be unacceptable. However, the process can just as clearly be improved from the standpoints of both improving our protection of society and doing necessary testing in a manner that uses fewer animals and uses these fewer animals in a more humane manner.

In Vitro Models

In vitro models, at least as screening tests, have been with us in toxicology for some 20 years now. The last 5-10 years has brought a great upsurge in interest in such models. This increased interest is due to economic and animal welfare pressures and technological improvements.

Criteria against which an in vitro model should be evaluated for its suitability in replacing (partially or entirely) an accepted in vivo model are incorporated in the process detailed in Table 5, which presents the steps in one

Table 5 Multistage Scheme for the Development, Validation, and Transfer of In Vitro Test System Technology in Toxicology

Stage I: Statement of Test Objective
A. Identify existing test system and its strengths and weaknesses.
B. Clearly state objectives for alternative test system.
C. Identify potential alternative test system.

Stage II: Define Developmental Test Design
A. Identify relevant variables.
B. Evaluate effects of variables on test system.
C. Optimize test performance.
D. Understand what the test does in a functional sense;
  1. Is it a simulation of an in vivo event?
  2. Is this simply a response to the presence of the agent?
  3. Is the measured response a functional step or link in the in vivo event of interest?
  4. Is this response an event or a property mechanistically linked to the in vivo event of interest or some intermediate stage?
  5. Is this an effect on some structure or function analogous to the in vivo structure or function?

Stage III: Evaluate Performance of Optimum Test
A. Develop library of known positive and negative response materials of diverse structure and a range of response potencies (i.e., if the endpoint is irritation, then materials should range from nonirritating to severity irritating).
B. Use optimum test design to evaluate the library of "knowns" under "blind" conditions.
C. Compare correlation of test results to those of other test systems and to real case of interest—results in humans.

Stage IV: Technology Transfer
A. Present and publish results though professional media (at society meetings, in peer reviewed journals).
B. Provide hands-on training to personnel from other facilities and facilitate their performing internal evaluations of test methods.

Stage V: Validation
A. Arrange for test of coded samples in multiple labs (i.e., interlaboratory evaluation).
B. Compare, present, and publish results.

Stage VI: Continue to Refine and Evaluate Test System Performance and Utilization
A. Continually strive for an understanding of why the test "works" and its relevance to effects in man.
B. Remain skeptical. Why should any one of us be the one to make the big breakthrough? Clearly there is some basic flaw in the design or conduct of the study

Table 5 Continued

which has given rise to these promising results. Doubt, check, and question, then let your most severe critic review the data; then go to a national meeting and give a presentation; then go back home and doubt, check and question some more!

proposed process for taking a new in vitro testing technology from being a research construct to a validated and accepted test system.

It should be noted that, in addition to potential advantage, in vitro systems per se also have a number of limitations which can contribute to their not being acceptable models. Findings from an in vitro system which either limit their use in predicting in vivo events or make them totally unsuitable for the task include there being wide differences in the doses needed to produce effects or differences in the effects elicited. Some reasons for such findings are detailed in Table 6.

At the same time there are substantial potential advantages in using in vitro system. These advantages of using cell or tissue culture in toxicological testing are isolation of test cells or organ fragments from homeostatic and hormonal control, accurate dosing, and quantitation of results. It is important to devise a suitable model system which is related to the mode of toxicity of the compound. Tissue and cell culture has the immediate potential to be used in two very different ways by industry. First, it has been used to examine a particular aspect of the toxicity of a compound in relation to its toxicity in vivo (i.e., mechanistic or explanatory studies). Second, it has been used as a form of rapid screening to compare the toxicity of a group of compounds for a particular response. Indeed, the pharmaceutical industry has used in vitro test systems in these two ways for years in the search for new potential drug entities.

The theory and use of screens in toxicology have previously been reviewed (28). Mechanistic and explanatory studies are generally called for when a traditional test system gives a result that is either unclear or for which the relevance to the real life human exposure is doubted. In vitro systems are particularly attractive for such cases because they can focus on very defined single aspects of a problem or pathogenic response, free of the confounding influence of the multiple responses of an intact higher level organism. Note, however, that first one must know the nature (indeed the existence of) the questions to be addressed.

NEAR-TERM ADVANCES: THE MIXED BATTERY

From the review and discussion presented in this chapter, four key points stand out.

Table 6 Possible Interpretations When In Vitro Data Do Not Predict Results of In Vivo Studies

1. Chemical is not absorbed at all or is poorly absorbed in in vivo studies.
2. Chemical is well absorbed but is subject to "first-pass effect" in the liver.
3. Chemical is distributed so that less (or more) reaches the target tissue than would be predicted on the basis of its absorption.
4. Chemical is rapidly metabolized to an active or inactive metabolite that has a different profile of activity and/or different duration of action than the parent drug.
5. Chemical is rapidly eliminated (e.g., through secretory mechanisms).
6. Species of the two test systems used are different.
7. Experimental conditions of the in vitro and in vivo experiments differed and may have led to different effects than expected. These conditions include factors such as temperature or age, sex, and strain of animal.
8. Effects elicited in vitro and in vivo by the particular test substance in question differ in their characteristics.
9. Tests used to measure responses may differ greatly for in vitro and in vivo studies, and the types of data obtained may not be comparable.
10. The in vitro study did not use adequate controls (e.g., pH, vehicle used, volume of test agent given, samples taken from sham-operated animals), resulting in "artifacts" of methods rather than results.
11. In vitro data cannot predict the volume of distribution in central or in peripheral compartments.
12. In vitro data cannot predict the rate constants for chemical movement between compartment.
13. In vitro data cannot predict the rate constants of chemical elimination.
14. In vitro data cannot predict whether linear or nonlinear kinetics will occur with specific dose of a chemical in vivo.
15. Pharmacokinetic parameters (e.g., bioavailability, peak plasma concentration, half-life) cannot be predicted based solely on in vitro studies.
16. In vivo effects of chemical are due to an alteration in the higher order integration of an intact animal system, which cannot be reflected in a less complex system.

1. As a result of advancements in toxicology as a science, product safety assessment should not continue to be performed as it traditionally has been.
2. There are no generally accepted in vitro test systems immediately available to completely replace all (or, indeed, any) of the in vivo testing requirements.
3. There are some steps which can be taken to move development and acceptance of in vitro systems along.
4. There are some modifications to current in vivo testing methods which both can and should be adopted.

Before developing these points, however, one must consider the needs of the communities of interest responsible for testing and understand the basic concept of a screen (as opposed to a definitive test).

Screens are simple tests which try to answer single questions. Many of the currently proposed in vitro systems show immediate promise as screens. As such, they would be employed to rapidly and efficiently identify those materials which were clearly strong irritants or corrosives, for example, which would therefore not need further evaluation.

Until in vitro tests are further developed and accepted, the appropriate strategy (or mix of tests) for industrial safety assessment should be a mixed tier approach (such as Fig. 3) utilizing in vitro tests as screens. The tier approach presented in Figure 4 is one form which can be (and is being) utilized currently for ocular irritation, but this can be improved on. For the near term, a better system could be used which employs a mixed series of screening steps. Such a system would have the following stages (using the particular case of evaluation of potential eye irritants as an example).

In Vitro Screen

1. Extremely active compounds in a cytotoxicity assay should be considered strong irritants (or worse) and classified/handled as such. Note that this

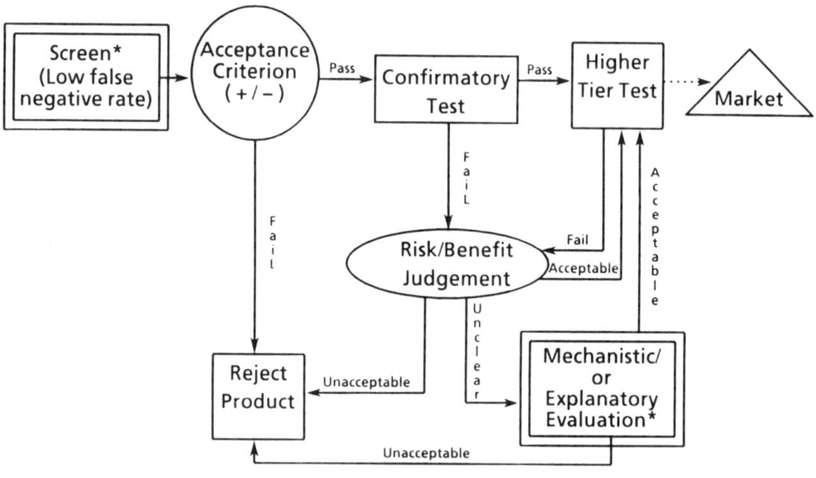

Figure 3 Shown here is a now widely adopted example of an iterative/tier approach to toxicity testing which utilizes range of test systems (physics—chemical, in vitro and in vivo) to minimize both cost and animal usage and distress.

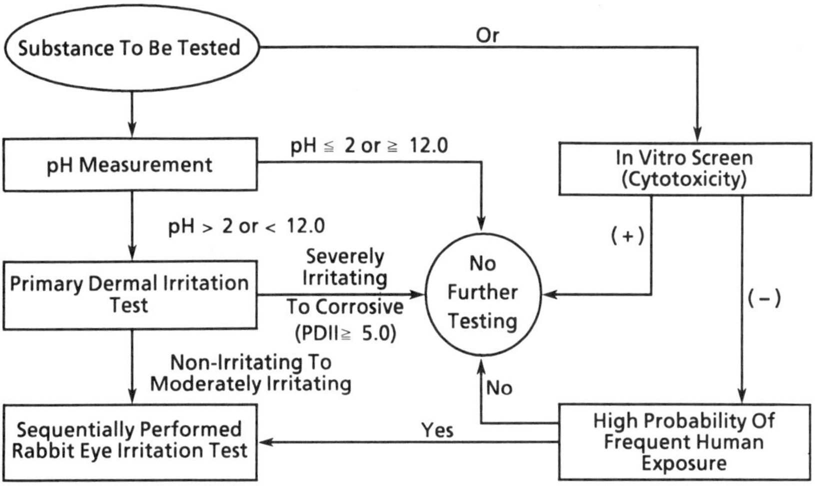

Figure 4 Tiered procedure for test articles prior to conduct of acute ocular irritation procedures. This approach serves to identify corrosive and almost all strong irritants before they are tested in the rabbit eye.

should also serve to identify (among others) the same compounds as the current pH screen, and therefore that step may not be required.

2. Less active or inactive compounds would pass on, unless the testing need was only to identify (item 1) type compounds (in which case testing is complete).

Primary Dermal Irritation

1. Severely irritating to corrosive compounds should be treated as item 1 under in vivo screen above.
2. Mild to nonirritants should be treated as item 1.

Staggered Eye Irritation Test

Using a low volume form test, materials should be evaluated using a single animal. If no irritation was seen at 24 h, a second (and 24 h later, a third) rabbit would be added to the test. Clear positive findings would stop the test.

FAR HORIZONS AND HOW TO GET THERE

Clearly great progress has been made both in improving practices as to the conduct of safety assessment tests in intact animals and in developing an array of promising in vitro candidates for replacement of the in vivo test.

Where we would like to be is to have in place (i.e., accepted and used by industry and regulation agencies) one or a battery of in vitro systems which would reduce the need for intact animal testing in vivo to only necessary cases, and to have duplicate or unnecessary testing in vivo of materials reduced to a minimum. These goals are dictated as much by economic reasons and the need to do better science as they are by ethical and humane concerns. The efficient and effective safety assessment/toxicology laboratory of the very near term future will have as its "front door" in vitro screening shops which will "draw" validated specific target organ screens from a library, as needed, to perform the initial go/no go evaluations on new compounds (or at least provide guidance as to where further evaluation is required). This same shop would also provide (again, from its established collection) in vitro system models to elucidate mechanistic questions later in the assessment process. Some would say that this is the current state-of-the-art. Clearly much of the necessary library could be assembled now.

Though substantial progress has been made in improving the design and conduct of in vivo tests, it does not appear that we are currently closer to achieving the optimum case than we were in 1980 (though we clearly understand it better), and minimal progress toward the specific objectives of improved strategy is immediately apparent. How does the science and practice of toxicology go about getting to this point?

There are two critical steps that must be taken for the eventual fulfillment of these objectives. The first of these is the need for acceptance of a scientific approach to the problem of safety assessment. The second is to develop an operative validation and acceptance process for new test procedures.

A scientific approach to safety assessment, such as the one presented in this chapter, does have proponents and adherents. Such an approach requires those involved in both the management and conduct of the safety assessment process to continually question (and test) both the efficiency and the validity of their evaluation systems and processes. More to the point, it requires recognition of the fact that "we have always done it this way" is not a reason for continuing to do so. Ask first what is the objective behind the testing, and then how well is our current testing meeting this objective. Such questions are exemplified by efforts such as those questioning if the information given by using six rabbits in an eye irritation test is more predictive than that obtained by using two or three (and determining that it is not [32,33]).

The second necessary step which is currently totally absent, is that there needs to be a collaborative process involving industrial, academic, and regulatory agencies in place for the validation and "acceptance" of new test systems. The general model of peer recognition leading to acceptance by the scientific community (34) is not working in this case, as should have been expected from a situation where politics, social policy, and litigation have as much influence as science itself.

One approach to this integrated approach is the use of a properly developed battery of tiered in vitro and in vivo tests, as is now sured in much of the pharmaceutical industry (35).

CONCLUSIONS

The first principle in hazard assessment is to have your actual data as similar to the real life situation of concern as possible. That is, the nearer the model to man, the better the quality of the prediction of any potential hazards (37).

The second principle should now also be clear—to be able to translate toxicity to hazard, and to be able to manage such hazards, it is essential to know how the agent is to be used and the marketplace of which it is to be a part. It is hoped that this chapter makes these relationships clear.

Finally, alternatives of both in vitro and in vivo types are in the process of development for almost all the different endpoints of concern in safety assessment (29,36). Many of these have great promise, and could be used as screens for many of the purposes presented here or as mechanistic tools. But complete replacement is clearly not near at hand, particularly for the most complicated endpoints. How these then can (and should) be integrated into strategies for product safety assessment is the key scientific and managerial challenge for the next decade. For not only are there strong reasons making it difficult to continue as in the past, but there are also the potentials for tremendous competitive advantage to those who successfully manage to integrate in vitro tools as both efficient screens and effective means of detecting and understanding the mechanistic underpinning for toxic and pathogenic processes.

REFERENCES

1. Gad, S. C. (1988). Defining product safety information and testing requirements. In *Handbook of Product Safety Evaluation*. S. C. Gad (Ed.). Marcel Dekker, New York, pp. 1-22.
2. Glass, L. (1975). Classification of biological networks by their qualitative dynamics. *J. Theoret. Biol.* **54**: 85-107.
3. Gordon, A. D. (1981). *Classification*. Chapman and Hall, New York.
4. Jayjock, M. A., and Gad, S. C. (1988). Hazard and risk assessment. In *Handbook of Product Safety Evaluation*. S. C. Gad (Ed.). Marcel Dekker, New York, pp. 558-628.
5. EPA (1986). Guidelines for carcinogen risk assessment. *Fed. Reg.* **51**(185): 33992-34054.

6. Wexler, P. (1988). *Information Resources in Toxicology*. Elsevier, New York.
7. Parker, C. M. (1987). Available toxicology information source and their use. In *Handbooks for Product Safety Evaluation*. S. C. Gad (Ed.). Marcel Dekker, New York, pp. 23-41.
8. National Toxicology Program (1985). Fourth Annual Report on Carcinogens, Washington, D. C., Department of Health and Human Services, PB 85-134633.
9. Wolff, M. E. (Part II, 1979; Part III, 1981). *Burger's Medicinal Chemistry*. J Wiley, New York.
10. Proctor, N. H., and Hughes, J. P. (1978). *Chemical Hazards of the Workplace*. Philadelphia, Lippincott.
11. Gosselin, R. E., Smith, R. P., and Hodge, H. C. (1984). *Clinical Toxicology of Commercial Products*. 5th Ed. Williams & Wilkens, Baltimore.
12. Cronin E. (1980). *Contact Dermatitis*. Churchill Livingstone, Edinburgh.
13. National Institute for Occupational Safety and Health, *NIOSH Criteria for a Recommended Standard for Occupational Exposure to . . .* Ohio, Cincinnati, Department of Health, Education and Welfare.
14. National Institute for Occupational Safety and Health. *NIOSH Current Intelligence Bulletins*. Cincinnati, Ohio, Department of Health, Education and Welfare.
15. Sax, N. I. (1985). *Dangerous Properties of Industrial Materials*. 6th Ed. Van Nostrand Reinhold, New York.
16. American Conference of Governmental Industrial Hygienists (ACGIH) (1986). *Documentation of the Threshold Limit Values*. 5th Ed. Cincinnati, Ohio.
17. Sittig, M. (1981). *Handbook of Toxic and Hazardous Chemicals*. Noyes, Park Ridge, New Jersey.
18. American Industrial Hygiene Association (1980). *Hygienic Guide Series*. Vols. I, II. AIHA, Akron, Ohio.
19. Finkel, A. J. (1983). *Hamilton and Hardy's Industrial Toxicology*. 4th Ed. John Wright PSG, Boston.
20. International Agency for Research on Cancer (1982). *Evaluation of the Carcinogenic Risks of Chemicals to Human,* Monograph Suppl. 4, Volumes 1-29, Lyon, France.
21. Budavari (1989). *The Merck Index,* Eleventh Ed. Merck and Company, Rahway, New Jersey.
22. Mackison, F. (1981). National Institute for Occupational Health and Safety/ Occupational Safety and Health Administration (1981). *Occupational Health Guidelines for Chemical Hazards*. Department of Health and Human Services (NIOSH)/Department of Labor (OSHA) DHHS No. 81-123, Washington, D.C., Government Printing Office.
23. Clayton, D. G., and Clayton, F. E. (1981). *Patty's Industrial Hygiene and Toxicology,* 3rd Rev. Ed., Vols. 2A, 2B, and 2C. J Wiley, New York.
24. Barnhart, E. R. (1991). *Physicians' Desk Reference,* Medical Economics, Oradell, New Jersey.
25. National Institute of Occupational Safety and Health (1984). *Registry of Toxic Effects of Chemical Substances,* 11th Ed. Vols. 1-3. Washington, DC, Depart-

ment of Health and Human Services DHHS No. 83-107, 1983 and RTECS Supplement DHHS 84-101.
26. Grant, W. M. (1974). *Toxicology of the Eye.* 2nd Ed., Vols. I and II. Thomas, Springfield, Illinois.
27. National Library of Medicine, Office of Inquiries and Publications Management, 8600 Rockville Pike, Bethesda, MD, 20209.
28. Gad, S. C. (1988). An approach to the Design and Analysis of Screening Data in Toxicology. *J. Am. Coll. Toxicol.* **7**(2): 127-138.
29. Gad, S. C., and Chengelis, C. P. (1989) *Acute Toxicology.* Telford Press, Caldwell, New Jersey.
30. Jackson, J., and Rutty, R. A. (1985). Ocular Tolerance Assessment Integrated Tier Policy. *Food Chem. Toxicol.* **23**: 309-310.
31. Jackson, E. M. (1983). Industrial practices in safety testing. In *Product Safety Evaluation.* A. M. Goldberg Ann Liebert, New York, 51-65.
32. De Sousa, D. J., Rouse, A. A., and Smolon, W. J. (1984). Statistical consequences of reducing the number of rabbits utilized in eye irritation testing. Data on 67 petrochemicals. *Toxicol. Appl. Pharmacol.* **76**: 234-242.
33. Talsma, D. M. Leach, C. L., Hatoum, N. S., Gibbons, R. D., Roger, J. C., and Garvin, P. J. (1988). Reducing the number of rabbits in the Draize eye irritancy test: A statistical analysis of 155 studies conducted over 6 years. *Fund. Appl. Toxicol.* **10**: 146-153.
34. Greim, H., Andrae, U., Forster, U., and Schwarz, L. (1986) Application, limitation and research requirements of in vitro test systems in toxicology. *Arch. Toxicol.* **9**: (Suppl.): 225-236.
35. Gad, S. C. (1989). A tier testing strategy incorporating in vitro testing methods for pharmaceutical safety assessment. *Humane Innovations Alternatives in Animal Exp.* **3**: 75-79.
36. Enslein, K. (1984). Estimation of toxicology endpoints by structure activity relationships. *Pharmacol. Rev.* **36**: 131-134.
37. Calabrese, E. J. (1984). *Principles of Animal Extrapolation.* J Wiley, New York, pp. 391-402.

13

Regulatory Law and the Use of In Vitro Methods for the Assessment of Various Toxicities

Sidney Green and June A. Bradlaw

Food and Drug Administration
Washington, D.C.

INTRODUCTION

For the democratic process to foster the needs of an industrial, high-tech, and space-age society, good tools and people of integrity and ability to use them are required. Legal authority provides the mechanism to impose a measure of control to correct abuses, and technology and information serve to implement this authority. The challenge for scientists and regulators is how to merge a rapidly growing and evolving in vitro technology with often inflexible tradition that mandates testing with whole animals for safety and risk assessments.

In vitro toxicity testing is often accomplished by alternative techniques such as cell and tissue culture or physicochemical tests (1). Studies with isolated cells, tissues, and organs cultured in vitro have directed the scientific community toward developing, evaluating, and validating alternative test systems (2). As sophisticated in vitro technology advances, the multidisciplinary science of toxicology also continues to advance and broaden. These alternative approaches provide additional data to support the enforcement of several laws and amendments passed by the Congress since 1950, such as (1) the Food Additives Amendment of 1958 to the Federal Food, Drug, and Cosmetic (FD&C) Act of 1938, (2) the Federal Insecticide, Fungicide and Rodenticide Act (FIFRA) of 1947 and its amended version of 1972, (3) the Toxic Substance Control Act (TSCA) of 1976, and (4) the Occupation Safety and Health Act of 1971. Each law or amendment is the product of a long developmental process that required much thought and great debate. Each Act provides new and expanded authority over potential health risks posed by chemicals and other environmental agencies. Although the laws finally passed by Congress are not ideal, they do serve as a springboard for the future, to be updated and improved as new scientific information becomes available. In vitro toxicological methods are being used more frequently to screen substances that may pose a threat to human safety, to set priorities for further testing, and to study toxic mechanisms. In this chapter we review current amendments and laws concerning in vitro toxicity testing methods, laws that are implemented by federal agencies such as the Food and Drug Administratin (FDA), the Environmental Protection Agency (EPA), the Occupational Safety and Health Administration (OSHA), and the Consumer Product Safety Commission (CPSC).

HISTORICAL PERSPECTIVE

Societies have demanded protection from adulterated food and drink since the beginning of recorded history. The early work "A Treatise on Adulteration of Foods and Culinary Poisons" included a discussion on water purity (3). This treatise was reviewed in the *London Literary Gazette* and other publications with criticism and skepticism, not unlike reactions today by persons opposed to current laws and amendments directed toward regulating chemicals and other environmental agents. These early comments included statements referring to the impossible task of identifying the myriad of substances that could be harmful and the possible panic of an over-concerned public (4), concerns that are applicable to modern times. Nevertheless, momentum was created for enactment of laws prohibiting adulteration of foods.

In the United States, regulation of foods originated during colonial times and federal controls over drugs were enacted in 1848. Before 1950, many legislative mandates had been enacted to regulate foods, drinks, drugs, and biological materials. Most prominent of these were (1) the original Food and Drugs Act of 1906, which prohibited interstate commerce in misbranded and adulterated foods, drinks, and drugs and (2) the FD&C Act of 1938, which extended coverage to cosmetics, required clearance for the safety of new drugs, and provided for tolerances for unavoidable poisonous subtances.

After 1950, revolutionary changes took place as the result of new advances in the food and pharmaceutical sciences. Numerous new materials, products, and methods of production and packaging created the problem of how to protect the consumer and enforce laws without impeding progress. The FDA, concerned about the increased use of new substances, became involved in identifying problems and seeking solutions. Hearings in 1951 before the House Select Committee to Investigate the Use of Chemicals in Foods and Cosmetics, otherwise known as the Delaney Committee, led to three major laws: (1) the Pesticide Chemicals Act of 1954, (2) the Food Additives Amendment of 1958, which contained a provision prohibiting the use of an additive if it was found to cause cancer in man or experimental animals, and (3) the Color Additive Amendments of 1960, which contained a similar provision regarding carcinogenesis. All three laws required the manufacturer to submit scientific data pertaining to the safety of a chemical before distribution. Previously, the FDA could initiate court proceedings against a chemical only after it had produced evidence that a chemical was harmful.

In the area of drug legislation, the Kefauver-Harrise Drug Amendments of 1962 required that pharmaceutical manufacturers back their claims with scientific data about effectiveness as a function of safety. Another broad-reaching legislative mandate, the TSCA, was enacted in 1976 and the EPA was charged with its enforcement. The TSCA is both controversial and complicated, and Walsh predicted that its scientific uncertainty could lead to questions about the enforceability of the law (5). Nevertheless, these laws provide the legal authority that may encourage the future use of in vitro methods in the safety evaluation and regulatory processes.

DIRECTION OF METHODOLOGY

Scientific technology has increased the scope and complexity of scientific problems and activities in regulatory agencies. Historically, emphasis was placed on the chemistry, pharmacology, and animal toxicology of the many substances that were new to the human environment. Often the results from chronic toxicologic tests, which require several years for completion, led only to vague conclusions about the safety of a test substance. No possible expansion of scientific effort in a federal agency can cope with the backlog and projected list of untested substances. Thus, alternative testing methods with less resources invested, both in material requirements and time, are being considered. In the future, increased reliance will be placed on a composite approach in which information from in vitro procedures will be combined with additional information obtained from intact animal models. The in vitro component may be particularly useful for identifying the comparative metabolism of certain agents in a variety of tissues from several animal species, as well as the intrinsic toxic effects of the agent on a biological system (e.g., tissue explants or cells in culture). In vitro methods will probably serve as a bioassay designed for rapid screening of certain groups of structurally related substances before chemical identification or as a means of alerting the agency to substances that require further testing. A need exists for the development and validation of these new methods for use in toxicology testing and safety evaluation. In the future, safety decisions may be based on toxicological testing performed with in vitro methods.

FEDERAL AGENCIES AND REGULATIONS

Food and Drug Administration (FDA)

The FD&C Act of 1938, with its subsequent amendments and provisions, gives FDA authority to ensure the safety of foods, cosmetics, medical devices, veterinary medicines, and biological materials, certain types of radiation exposure, and the safety and efficacy of drugs. In several of these areas, animal toxicologic tests are necessary at some point either during product development or when additional information is needed to assess the safety of a product already being marketed.

The FDA has not yet adopted a program for the full use of in vitro methods for general toxicologic testing; however, it has encouraged the development of in vitro methods and recognizes the contribution that could be made by use of such methods. In the Center for Food Safety and Applied Nutrition (CFSAN), for example, plans are under way to develop in vitro testing for certain areas of toxicity to augment results from animal studies. In some instances in vitro testing would allow a more definitive evaluation of safety (e.g., studies of mechanisms) than is presently achieved by animal tests alone. Other centers of the FDA are using in vitro methods for a variety of purposes. For example, the Center for Devices and Radiological Health and the Center for Biologic Evaluation and Research use in vitro methods in their research programs, and these data are used in making regulatory decisions.

In the 1960s, FDA became the first federal agency to include a mutagenicity testing program as a component of toxicology. This unit, as originally conceived, performed in vitro techniques exclusively. In January of 1977, at the request of the Associate Commissioner for Sciences, a group of scientists within the FDA was organized as a panel to determine how short-term tests for neoplasia could serve the regulatory functions of the FDA. Because many of these methods were mutagenicity methods, the panel recognized that they also had to consider the utility of these tests for mutagenicity purposes.

The panel included many whole animal methods in their definition of short-term tests. In vitro methods with mammalian cells in culture and bacteria were described for use in investigations of potential mutagenicity and carcinogenicity of chemicals. Flamm (6) and Green (7) have discussed the rationale for the use of in vitro methods in general and by their use in FDA in particular. These methods were used in a tier-type fashion and as part of a battery of mutagenicity test procedures. Each method was selected on the basis of its relationship to a chromosomal or gene mutational endpoint.

Mutagenicity data may be considered in two ways; as a means of detecting genetic damage and as a signal of potential carcinogenicity of a substance. Although there is no general agency policy on the latter, certain programs treat positive in vitro mutagenicity results as indicators of potential carcinogenicity. This philosophy is embodied in a compendium of toxicologic principles used for the safety assessment of food additives published by CFSAN (8) and in the Threshold Assessment Genetic Toxicology Guidelines of the Center for Veterinary Medicine (CVM) (9). The CFSAN compendium, also known as the Redbook, recommends three tests: the *Salmonella typhimurium* microsome test (10), the L5178-Y (TK-locus) mouse lymphoma test (11), and unscheduled DNA synthesis in primary rat hepatocyte (12). These tests are used as preliminary screens and positive results are not interpreted as conclusive evidence of carcinogenicity. A minimum of three genetic toxicity test systems is recommended in the CVM guidelines. These tests have been validated and shown to exhibit a high degree of correlation with in vivo chronic bioassay results. The generally recommended tests are the Ames *Salmonella typhimurium* microsome assay (9,13), a gene mutational assay in mammalian cells (14,15), and an assay for detection of DNA repair in mammalian cells (16,17). The guidelines emphasize that when a given test or battery of tests is considered inappropriate, alternative assay systems may be used.

The Center for Food Safety and Applied Nutrition is currently revising the Redbook (8). The revised document will include an expanded guideline recommending a battery of short-term tests for genotoxicity of food and color additives. Genotoxicity test results can not yet be used for making estimates of heritable genetic risk in humans. However, the tests are used for (1) considering genotoxic activity with respect to potential carcinogenic effects, (2) evaluating ambiguous animal bioassay data, (3) assessing the need for additional toxicity tests, and (4) considering mechanistic explanations of toxicological activity. In addition, FDA may recommend that substances of low concern that produce strong positive results undergo carcinogenicity bioassay testing.

With the increased emphasis on using fewer animals in toxicity testing, agencies are investigating in vitro methods for teratogenicity and general systemic toxicity studies. Cell cultures or whole embryo cultures are the primary methods used as screens for teratogenicity. Neonatal rat myocardial cells, kidney cells from adults rats, and hepatocytes from the mini-pig represent other in vitro methods in general systemic toxicity and safety assessment. A number of in vitro assays that are currently being investigated may reduce or eliminate the use of rabbits for ocular toxicity testing. These efforts have only recently become a part of the FDA's in vitro program. Consequently, it is too early to evaluate these assays as screens or to provide information on mechanisms of test substances.

Environmental Protection Agency (EPA)

Toxic Substances Control Act

The EPA is authorized by the 1976 TSCA to require that potentially harmful chemical substances and mixtures already on the market be tested for effects on health and the environment. The EPA also requires testing of new chemicals and existing chemical substances for which there is a substantial new use.

Before President Ford signed the TSCA into law, a great debate ensued for several years between lawmakers and scientists about whether the United States had the resources to conduct a large-scale toxicologic testing of numerous substances. Many scientists testified that large-scale toxicologic testing was possible, provided that short-term in vitro toxicologic procedures (such as the *Salmonella* microsome test and mammalian cell neoplastic transformation tests) had the potential to provide relevant information on large numbers of substances. This information is necessary for predicting long-term effects such as cancer and gene mutation. The scientific community, however, has not yet decided whether these methods can be used to predict long-term effects. The TSCA consists of 31 sections, most of which are not relevant to the subject of this chapter; thus, only sections 4 and 5 will be addressed here.

Under section 4 of TSCA, EPA has the authority to require manufacturers or processors of chemicals distributed in commerce to test their chemicals for health and environmental effects. Testing is required when there is evidence of potential risk, insufficient evidence on which to make a judgment of risk, or no information about the chemical. Data may be requested for carcinogenesis, mutagenesis, teratogenesis, and behavioral disorders, and other effects that may present an unreasonable risk to human health (18).

The EPA has published guidelines for 19 in vitro and in vivo assays for genotoxicity. Whenever testing is required by the agency, the appropriate guideline is specified. EPA is presently revising the guidelines for some of these tests, however, most of the data accumulated thus far do not address the question of heritable genetic effects in mammals.

The EPA uses mutagenicity data to evaluate potential genetic damage and to predict carcinogenicity. Two testing schemes are used by the agency, and both use a tier approach (18).

With respect to section 5 of TSCA, a manufacturer must notify EPA 90 days before manufacturing, processing, or importing a new chemical substance. The following information is required for the new chemical: chemical identity, production volume, proposed users, estimates of exposure and release, and any health or environmental test data that are available to the submitter. There is no explicit authority to require manufacturers to conduct testing of a new chemical before its entry into the market, and therefore little actual testing data are provided to the agency. Thus, to evaluate the potential toxicity of a new chemical, EPA uses a Structure Activity Team (SAT), composed of chemists, toxicologists, and environmental scientists, who use professional judgment to express concern for potential environmental or health effects that may be caused by the use of the chemical (18).

If the SAT determines there is insufficient information to evaluate the chemical and that use of the chemical may present an unreasonable risk, the agency may issue a proposed order to prohibit or limit production of the substance. The company may also be required to submit data after testing the substance for certain specific effects.

In vitro data are used primarily for mutagenesis studies. Mutagenicity data, in turn, are used for three purposes: (1) to require manufacturers to test compounds produced at certain high volumes, (2) to assess the potential of the new chemical to induce heritable genetic effects, and (3) to provide part of the weight of evidence that a chemical may or may not be a potential oncogen (18). The principal use of mutagenicity data under section 5 has been a part of the weight-of-evidence approach for oncogenicity. However, if there is no information on an analog of the new chemical with respect to oncogenicity testing, in vitro mutagenicity data alone are not enough to support a concern for potential oncogenicity. In vitro methods have not reached the state of development to be incorporated into testing guidelines for teratogenicity, neurobehavioral studies, or several other areas.

Federal Insecticide, Fungicide, and Rodenticide Act (FIFRA)

The FIFRA requires that all pesticides sold or distributed in commerce be registered. The agency must have data to evaluate the risk and benefits that serve as the basis for the registration. The types of data and information that must be submitted to the agency are detailed in the Code of Federal Regulations (CFR) Part 158 (19).

In general, the standard toxicologic tests that are required by EPA range from acute to carcinogenicity tests. All of these tests, with the exception of mutagenicity, specify animals as the means of providing the data. Efforts are under way to study the recent advances in ocular toxicology which include the development of in vitro and in vivo assays to reduce or eliminate the use of rabbits for ocular toxicity testing.

Mutagenicity data are required if a pesticide meets the following criteria.

1. The use of the pesticide requires (a) a tolerance, (b) exemption from the requirement to obtain a tolerance, or (c) issuance of a food additive regulation.
2. The pesticide is likely to result in significant human exposure.
3. The active ingredient or any metabolite is structurally related to a mutagen or oncogen, or belongs to any chemical class of compounds containing a significant number of mutagens or oncogens.

See specifically the CFR, Title 40, Parts 158.50 and 258.135 to determine whether mutagenicity data must be submitted. Section II-A of this subdivision contains an additional discussion of the formulator's exemption and who must submit the required data as a general rule.

A battery of mutagenicity tests is required, and the substance should be tested with and without metabolic activation. The EPA stipulates certain standards for metabolic activation and negative and positive controls. For a discussion of these, see the "Pesticide Assessment Guidelines, Subdivision F, Hazard Evaluation, Human and Domestic Animals" (20). The battery must include tests for gene mutations, structural chromosomal aberrations, and other effects appropriate for the test substance. For gene mutation tests, prokaryotic and eukaryotic organisms are recommended, with forward and reverse mutations measured in eukaryotes. Mammalian cells in culture for forward and reverse mutations are also included. For structural chromosomal aberrations, eukaryotic microorganisms and mammlian cells in culture may be used. Tests for other genotoxic effects include the use of bacteria, yeast, and mammlian cells in culture for DNA damage and repair. With respect to numerical chromosomal damage, eukaryotic microorganisms and cells in culture may be used. For a more complete discussion of the in vitro and other tests recommended by the EPA, see the Pesticide Assessment Guidelines (20).

The Consumer Product Safety Commission (CPSC)

The CPSC, established in 1973 as part of the FDA Bureau of Product Safety, has the responsibility to maintain a clearing house for information about the hazards associated with consumer products, to conduct investigations of the hazards, and to perform research on the safety of consumer products.

In the *Federal Register* of June 13, 1978, the CPSC issued an interim statement of policy and procedure in regard to classifying, evaluating, and regulating carcinogens in consumer products. The CPSC concluded that because positive results in these in vitro tests suggest the need for carcinogenicity testing in whole animals, the CPSC would consider performing, requiring, or encouraging further use of in vitro testing. Thus, in vitro methods will probably be used as preliminary screens for carcinogenicity.

The CPSC is in the process of publishing guidelines on classifying, evaluating, and regulating carcinogens and teratogens in consumer products; the possible use of in vitro tests is also discussed.

The Occupational Safety and Health Administration (OSHA)

Since its creation in 1971, OSHA has issued rules for regulating carcinogens in the workplace. These regulations stipulate that a chemical may be identified and classified as a potential occupational carcinogen on the basis of human epidemiological studies and/or experimental carcinogenesis bioassay in mammals. Positive results in short-term tests will also be used as concordant evidence. Short-term tests are defined as tests for neoplastic cell transformation, tests in *Drosophila melanogaster,* and tests involving in vitro mutagenesis methods which include those methods in which mammalian germinal and somatic cells are used (21). The regulations are somewhat ambiguous as to what is meant by tests in mammalian germinal and somatic cells. Tests could include whole animal methods as well as in vitro procedures. Regardless of the intent, the short-term tests would serve only to provide concordant information and by themselves would not provide the basis for a regulatory decision. The regulations disregard the use of mutagenicity tests for making decisions related to mutagenicity per se. Thus, OSHA has a policy similar to that of the FDA; that is, results from short-term tests are used as evidence to demonstrate potential carcinogenicity or as concordant evidence of the carcinogenicity of a substance after it has been tested in animals.

SUMMARY AND FUTURE PROJECTIONS

Numerous and diverse in vitro test systems that represent a wide range of methodological developments and applications have been described in the literature. Many of these tests will be improved and changed with the introduction of new information and advances in in vitro toxicology and related fields, such as molecular biology and biotechnology. In the future, several different in vitro tests performed in concert may be necessasry to provide useful information for the regulatory process.

We have learned much about in vitro test systems in developing genetic toxicology methods. In spite of the progress made in short-term tests for carcinogenicity, these methods have come under severe criticism. The evolution of their use has been previously reviewed (22).

The impact that mutagenicity and carcinogenicity in vitro tests make on the regulatory process is very likely to affect the future use of in vitro methods in other areas of toxicology. How these methods are used, how they are interpreted, and how they are phased into a regulatory program will affect the acceptance of in vitro procedures for teratogenicity and general toxicology.

We conclude that in vitro methodology and its application to toxicology will continue to grow in importance and that the contribution of these methods to the regulatory process will be substantial. In vitro methods in toxicologic testing may one day be included as part of the evaluation of chemicals and environmental agents, just as in vitro clinical diagnostic methods are used today in the evaluation of biological materials.

The applications of such methods are not without problems and several questions can be asked about the usefulness of in vitro methods. Are the methods adequate for estimates of risk? Can they serve as models for estimating the potency of a toxicant to humans? Are these methods sufficiently accepted by the scientific community to support current legislation?

If these methods can be used, how can they be related to the problem of individual genetic variability of humans and the myriad of environmental and dietary factors? Would the use of in vitro tests be more cumbersome when one is forced to make regulatory decisions? None of these questions has simple answers, but we should seek answers to resolve scientific and policy considerations raised by this new technology.

In vitro systems may be important in determining the intrinsic toxicologic properties of substances, such as the mechanisms of action of a toxic agent. Knowledge of the basic biochemical, physiological, and genetic events in the cell or tissue may allow a relevant extrapolation to be made from animal species to humans and even to a specific human tissue. This extrapolation would require consideration of metabolic differences within the animal species and humans. In vitro systems may also be used to extrapolate the data from high dosage concentrations to low concentrations. In the past, several statistical models have been proposed for carcinogenicity tests but the rationale for selecting one statistical model over another is often unclear. In vitro approaches and applications to risk estimation are becoming more important for carcinogenicity and mutagenicity. In vitro methods may also have applications for teratogenesis and general toxicology responses, because the intrinsic potency of a substance and the molecular basis for toxic action may be determined. Although this approach may also involve problems of validation and reliability, it may bring some order to the staggering problem of regulating thousands of substances.

In an attempt to coordinate and focus the activities of several agencies, a National Toxicology Program was established by Joseph A. Califano, Jr., the Secretary of the Department of Health, Education, and Welfare (HEW), in November 1978. The purpose was to strengthen the Department's activities in testing chemicals of public health concern and in developing and validating new and better integrated test methods to provide needed scientific information to the regulatory and research agencies. In vitro methodology as applied to toxicology is included in the overall plan.

Throughout the world, scientists are attempting to develop, evaluate, and validate in vitro toxicologic methods. The Organization for Economic Co-operation Development's monograph on Scientific Criteria for Validation of In Vitro Toxicity Tests identifies several initiatives, including The Center for Alternatives to Animal Testing at The Johns Hopkins University, the Fund for the Replacement of Animals in Medical Experiments, and the Tufts Center for Animals and Public Policy (23). In addition, special groups within scientific societies (e.g., the Tissue Culture Association) and several agencies (e.g., EPA, FDA and CPSC) are presently attempting to assess the usefulness of various in vitro procedures for general toxicity testing.

The problems concerning the enforcement of legislative mandates with regard to human safety of environmental and consumable substances and products are obvious. It is not necessary to reiterate here the content of several reports and articles dealing with difficulties associated with the toxic substances legislation, risk assessment based on chemical carcinogenicity and mutagenicity data, and implementation of the laws (24-26). Given the magnitude of the problems involved, the development, validation, and evaluation of in vitro test methods, alternatives to animal tests will be achieved slowly and by degrees. While the search for relevant and suitable alternative tests continues, efforts will be made to improve toxicity testing for the benefit of public safety and for more informed and conservative use of experimental animals. Only the test of time and specific case examples can demonstrate the effectiveness of current and future scientific technology in the regulation of toxic materials.

ACKNOWLEDGMENTS

The authors gratefully acknowledge the helpful discussions and assistance of Dr. H. Blumenthal, previous director, Division of Toxicology, and Dr. W. Gary Flamm, previous director, Office of Toxicological Sciences, FDA; Dr. Michael Waters, Office of Health and Ecological Effects, and Office of Research and Development, EPA; Dr. Angela Auletta, Office of Toxic Substances, EPA; Dr. I. Mauer, Office of Pesticide Products, EPA; Drs. R. Osterberg and L. Schechtman, Centers for Drug Evaluation and Research and for Veterinary Medicine, respectively. We also acknowledge the helpful assistance of Dr. K. Gupta of the CPSC, Dr. L. Schuman of the OSHA, and Ms. Shonda Enlow of the FDA in the preparation of this manuscript.

REFERENCES

1. Goldberg, A. M., and Frazier, J. M. (1989). Alternatives to animals in toxicity testing. *Sci. Am.* **261**: 24-30.

2. McKeehan, W. L., Barnes, D., Reid, L., Stanbridge, D., Murakami, H., and Sato, G. (1990). Frontiers in mammalian cell culture. *In Vitro Cell. Dev. Biol.* **26**: 9-23.
3. Accum, F. (1820). *A Treatise on Adulterations of Foods and Culinary Poisons.* Abraham Small Publishers Philadelphia, Pennsylvania.
4. Schuette, H. A. (1943). *Wisconsin academy of science, arts and letters transactions.* **35**: 285-303.
5. Walsh, J. (1978). *EPA and toxic substances law: Dealing with uncertainty science.* **202**: 598-602.
6. Flamm, W. G. (1974). A tier system approach to mutagen testing. *Mutat. Res.* **26**: 329-333.
7. Green, S. (1977). Present and future uses of mutagenicity tests for assessment of the safety of food additives. *J. Environ. Pathol. Toxicol.* **1**: 49-54.
8. U.S. Food and Drug Administration (1982). *Toxicological Principles for the Safety Assessment of Direct Food Additives and Color Additives Used in Food.* National Technical Information Service Pub. No. PB-83-170696. Department of Health and Human Services. Washington, DC.
9. *Fed. Regist.* (1985). *Sponsored Compounds in Food-Producing Animals: Criteria and Procedures for Evaluating the Safety of Carcinogenic Residues.* Vol. 50, No. 211; *Code of Federal Regulations* (CFR) Title 21, Parts 500, 514, and 571.
10. Maron, D. M., and Ames, B. N. (1983). Revised methods for the *Salmonella* mutagenicity test. *Mutat. Res.* **113**: 173-215.
11. Clive, D., McCuen, R., Spector, J. F. S., Piper, C., and Mavouria, K. H. (1983). A report of the U. S. Environmental Protection Agency Gene-Tox Program. *Mutat. Res.* **115**: 225-251.
12. Williams, G. M. (1980). The detection of chemical mutagens/carcinogens by DNA repair and mutagenesis in liver cultures. In *Chemical Mutagens.* Vol. VI. F. J. Deserres and A. Hollander (Eds) Plenum Press, New York; pp. 66-79.
13. Ames, B. N., McCann, J., and Yamasaki, E. (1975). Methods for detecting carcinogens and mutagens with the *Salmonella*/mammalian microsome mutagenicity test. *Mutat. Res.* **31**(6): 347-364.
14. Hsie, A. W., Casciano, D. A., Couch, D. B., Krahn, D. F., and Oneill, J. P. (1981). The use of Chinese hamster ovary cells to quantify specific locus mutations and to determine mutagenicity of chemicals. A report of the Gene-Tox Program. *Mutat. Res.* **86**: 193-214.
15. Clive, D., Johnson, K. O., Spector, J. F. S., Batson, A. G., and Brown, M. M. (1979). Validation and characterization of the L5178Y/TK t1-mouse lymphoma mutagen assay system. *Mutat. Res.* **59**: 61-108.
16. Williams, G. M. (1977). Detection of chemical carcinogens by unscheduled DNA synthesis in rat liver primary cell cultures. *Cancer Res.* **37**: 1845-1851.
17. Butterworth, B. E., Ashby, J., Bermudez, E., Cascinno, D., Mirsalis, J., Probst, G., and William, G. (1987). A protocol and guide for the *in vitro* rat hepatocyte DNA-repair assay. *Mutat. Res.* **189**: 113-121.
18. Aulette, A. (1991). *Regulatory Perspectives: TSCA in Genetic Toxicology. A Treatise.* A. P. Li and R. H. Heflich (Eds) (In press).

19. *Code of Federal Regulations* (CFR), Title 40, Part 158 (1984). *Data Requirements for Pesticide Registration—Final Rule.*
20. U. S. Environmental Protection Agency (1984). *Pesticide Assessment Guidelines, Subdivision F.* Hazard evaluation of human and domestic animals. Washington, DC, EPA, pp. 149-151.
21. *Fed. Regist.* (January 1980) *Part 1990—Identification, Classification and Regulation of Potential Occupational Carcinogens.* **45**(15): 5282-5285.
22. Prival, M. J., and Dellarco, V. L. (1989). Evolution of social concerns and environmental policies for chemical mutagens. *Environ. Mol. Mutagen.* **14**, (16): 46-50.
23. Frazier, J. M. (1990). *Scientific Criteria for Validation of In Vitro Toxicity Test. Organization for Economic Cooperation and Development.* Environment Monograph. No. 36.
24. Culliton, B. J. (1978). Toxic substance legislature: How well are laws being implemented? *Science* **201**: 1198-1199.
25. Maugh, T. H. (1978). Chemical carcinogens: The scientific basis for regulation. *Science* **201**: 1200-1205.
26. Maugh, T. H. (1978). Chemical carcinogens: How dangerous are low dosages? *Science* **202**: 37-41.

Index